Transdermal and Topical Drug Delivery

Transdermal and Topical Drug Delivery
Principles and Practice

Edited by

Heather A.E. Benson
School of Pharmacy, CHIRI, Curtin University, Perth, Australia

Adam C. Watkinson
Storith Consulting Limited, Kent, UK

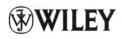

A John Wiley & Sons, Inc., Publication

Published by John Wiley & Sons, Inc., Hoboken, New Jersey.
Published simultaneously in Canada.

For general information on our other products and services or for technical support, please contact our
Customer Care Department within the United States at (800) 762-2974, outside the United States at
(317) 572-3993 or fax (317) 572-4002.

Wiley also publishes its books in a variety of electronic formats. Some content that appears in print
may not be available in electronic formats. For more information about Wiley products, visit our web
site at www.wiley.com.

Library of Congress Cataloging-in-Publication Data

Topical and transdermal drug delivery : principles and practice / edited by Heather A. E. Benson,
Adam C. Watkinson.
    p. ; cm.
  Includes bibliographical references and index.
    ISBN 978-0-470-45029-1 (hardback)
  1. Transdermal medication. 2. Drug delivery systems. 3. Skin absorption. I. Benson, Heather
A. E. II. Watkinson, Adam C.
  [DNLM: 1. Administration, Cutaneous. 2. Administration, Topical. 3. Drug Delivery
Systems–methods. 4. Skin Absorption. WB 340]
  RM151.T656 2011
  615'.19–dc23

                                    2011019937

Printed in Singapore.

10 9 8 7 6 5 4 3 2 1

For my husband Tony for his patience and support, and Tom, Sam, and Victoria for their inspiration.

Heather

For my wife Becky, my mum and dad, and my brother Tom.

Adam

Contents

Preface

The premise for this book was to provide a single volume covering the principles of transdermal and topical drug delivery and how these are put into practice during the development of new products. We have divided the book into two sections to deal with each of these perspectives and hope that their contents will appeal equally to readers based in academia and industry. We also hope that it will help each of these readers better understand the perspective of the other and therefore aid communication between them.

The first section of the book describes the major principles and techniques involved in the conduct of the many experimental approaches used in the field. We appreciate that these have been covered in previous texts but feel that this section provides a fresh and up-to-date look at these important areas to provide a fundamental understanding of the underlying science in the field. The authors have aimed to provide both the science and practical application based on their extensive experience. The second section of the book provides an insight into product development with an emphasis on practical knowledge from people who work in and with the industry. Designing a new product is about taking different development challenges and decisions into account and always understanding how they may impact the process as a whole. An understanding of the complete process is therefore a prerequisite to maximizing the quality of the product it produces.

As with any such book, we are heavily indebted to our contributors who have all worked hard to produce a text that we believe will be of interest to a cross-section of professionals involved in topical and transdermal product development.

HEATHER A.E. BENSON
ADAM C. WATKINSON

About the Editors

HEATHER A.E. BENSON has extensive experience in drug delivery with particular focus in transdermal and topical delivery. She is an Associate Professor at Curtin University, Perth, Australia, where she leads the Drug Delivery Research Group. In addition she is a director in Algometron Ltd., a Perth-based company involved in the development of a novel pain diagnostic technology, which she co-invented. This technology received the Western Australian Inventor of the Year (Early Stage Category) award in 2008. She is also a scientific advisor to OBJ Ltd., a Perth-based company involved in the development of magnetically enhanced transdermal delivery technologies. Prior to Perth Dr. Benson was at the University of Manitoba, Canada, where she won Canadian Foundation for Innovation funds to establish the Transdermal Research Facility. Before this 2-year period in Canada, she was a senior lecturer at the University of Queensland, Australia, where she worked closely with Professor Michael Roberts to establish a highly successful topical and transdermal research group at the university. Heather has a PhD from Queen's University in Belfast in the area of transdermal delivery and a BSc (Hons) in Pharmacy from Queen's University. She has published extensively on her research and holds a number of patents related to transdermal delivery. She has supervised numerous Masters and PhD students in drug delivery research areas, many of whom now have successful careers in R&D in industry. She is on the editorial board *of Current Drug Delivery* and acts as a reviewer for many journals. She is a member of the CRS Australian Chapter Executive Committee and the Australian Peptide Society Conference Organising Committee.

ADAM C. WATKINSON has a wealth of experience in the area of drug delivery in general, and transdermal and topical delivery in particular. Until May 2011 he was Chief Scientific Officer at Acrux Ltd. in Melbourne, Australia, where his responsibilities included the strategic leadership of product development, provision of technical support to commercial partnering activities, and regulatory affairs. During his 6 years with Acrux he was a key member of the senior management team and played a pivotal role in the development and approval of Axiron™, a novel transdermal testosterone product that was subsequently licensed to and launched by Eli Lilly in the United States. Prior to Acrux he worked at ProStrakan in Scotland as a Project Manager and Drug Delivery Research Manager. While at ProStrakan he initiated and managed the early development of Sancuso™, the first transdermal granisetron patch that was launched by ProStrakan in the United States in 2008. Before his 5-year stint at ProStrakan, Adam played key roles at An-eX in Wales, a company that provides R&D development services in the area of percutaneous absorption to the pharmaceutical, cosmetic, and agrochemical industries. Adam has an MBA from Cardiff University, a PhD from the Welsh School of Pharmacy in the area of trans-dermal delivery, and a BSc in Chemistry from the University of Bath. He has published extensively on his research, is the author of several patents, and holds an Honorary Chair at the School of Pharmacy at the University of London. He is also an Associate Lecturer at Monash University in Melbourne, Australia, and has long been a member of the Scientific Advisory Board for the international PPP (Perspectives on Percutaneous Penetration) conference. Despite his lengthy allegiance to industry he has co-supervised several PhD students and is an advocate of encouraging students to interact with industry as early and as much as possible. Having recently returned from Australia he has set up a U.K.-based consultancy firm (Storith Consulting Limited in Kent) offering advice in the areas of drug development and topical and transdermal drug delivery.

Contributors

HUGH ALSOP, Acrux Ltd., West Melbourne, Australia

EVA BENFELDT, Department of Environmental Medicine, Copenhagen University, Copenhagen, Denmark

HEATHER A.E. BENSON, School of Pharmacy, CHIRI, Curtin University, Perth, Australia

MARC B. BROWN, MedPharm Ltd., Guildford, Surrey, UK, and School of Pharmacy, University of Hertfordshire, College Lane Campus, Hatfield, Hertfordshire, UK

MICHAEL J. CORK, Academic Unit of Dermatology Research, Department of Infection and Immunity, Faculty of Medicine, Dentistry and Health, The University of Sheffield Medical School, Sheffield, UK, and The Paediatric Dermatology Clinic, Sheffield Children's Hospital, Sheffield, UK

SIMON G. DANBY, Academic Unit of Dermatology Research, Department of Infection and Immunity, Faculty of Medicine, Dentistry and Health, The University of Sheffield Medical School, Sheffield, UK

SACHIN DUBEY, School of Pharmaceutical Sciences, University of Geneva, Geneva, Switzerland

GORDON W. DUFF, Academic Unit of Dermatology Research, Department of Infection and Immunity, Faculty of Medicine, Dentistry and Health, The University of Sheffield Medical School, Sheffield, UK

BARRIE FINNIN, Monash Institute of Pharmaceutical Sciences, Faculty of Pharmacy and Pharmaceutical Sciences, Monash University, Parkville, Australia

THOMAS J. FRANZ, Cetero Research, Fargo, ND, USA

JEFFREY E. GRICE, School of Medicine, The University of Queensland, Princess Alexandra Hospital, Woolloongabba, Australia

JONATHAN HADGRAFT, Department of Pharmaceutics, The School of Pharmacy, University of London, London, UK

JON R. HEYLINGS, Dermal Technology Laboratory, Med IC4, Keele University Science and Business Park, Keele University, Keele, Staffordshire, UK

RIKKE HOLMGAARD, Department of Dermato-Allergology, Copenhagen University, Gentofte Hospital, Copenhagen, Denmark, and Department of Environmental Medicine, University of Southern Denmark, Odense, Denmark

DHAVAL R. KALARIA, School of Pharmaceutical Sciences, University of Geneva, Geneva, Switzerland

YOGESHVAR N. KALIA, School of Pharmaceutical Sciences, University of Geneva, Geneva, Switzerland

MARK A.F. KENDALL, Australian Institute for Bioengineering & Nanotechnology, The University of Queensland, St. Lucia, Australia

MAJELLA E. LANE, Department of Pharmaceutics, The School of Pharmacy, University of London, London, UK

PAUL A. LEHMAN, Cetero Research, Fargo, ND, USA

SIAN T. LIM, MedPharm Ltd., MedPharm Research and Development Centre, Guildford, Surrey, UK

HOWARD I. MAIBACH, Department of Dermatology, School of Medicine, University of California, San Francisco, CA, USA

ANDREW MAKIN, LAB Research, Lille Skensved, Denmark

KENNETH J. MILLER, Mylan, Morgantown, WV, USA

JENS THING MORTENSEN, LAB Research, Lille Skensved, Denmark

SARA NICOLI, Department of Pharmacy, University of Parma, Parma, Italy

JESPER B. NIELSEN, Department of Environmental Medicine, University of Southern Denmark, Odense, Denmark

TARL W. PROW, School of Medicine, The University of Queensland, Princess Alexandra Hospital, Woolloongabba, Australia

SAM G. RANEY, Cetero Research, Fargo, ND, USA

Belum Viswanath Reddy, Skin and VD Center, Hyderabad, India

Michael S. Roberts, School of Medicine, The University of Queensland, Woolloongabba, Australia

Paulo Santos, Department of Pharmaceutics, University of London, London, UK

Geetanjali Sethi, Skin and VD Center, Hyderabad, India

William K. Sietsema, INC Research, Cincinnati, OH, USA, and University of Cincinnati, Cincinnati, OH, USA

Robert Turner, MedPharm Ltd., MedPharm Research and Development Centre, Guildford, Surrey, UK

Kenneth A. Walters, An-eX Analytical Services Ltd., Cardiff, UK

Adam C. Watkinson, Storith Consulting Ltd., Kent, UK

Sandra Wiedersberg, Research & Development, LTS Lohmann Therapie-Systeme AG, Andernach, Germany

Part One

Current Science, Skin Permeation, and Enhancement Approaches

Chapter 1

Skin Structure, Function, and Permeation

Heather A.E. Benson

INTRODUCTION

The skin is the largest organ of the body, covering about 1.7 m^2 and comprising approximately 10% of the total body mass of an average person. The primary function of the skin is to provide a barrier between the body and the external environment. This barrier protects against the permeation of ultraviolet (UV) radiation, chemicals, allergens and microorganisms, and the loss of moisture and body nutrients. In addition, the skin has a role in homeostasis, regulating body temperature and blood pressure. The skin also functions as an important sensory organ in touch with the environment, sensing stimulation in the form of temperature, pressure, and pain.

While the skin provides an ideal site for administration of therapeutic compounds for local and systemic effects, it presents a formidable barrier to the permeation of most compounds. The mechanisms by which compounds permeate the skin are discussed later in this chapter, and methods to enhance permeation are described in Chapters 2–4. An understanding of the structure and function of human skin is fundamental to the design of optimal topical and transdermal dosage forms. The structure and function of healthy human skin is the main focus of this chapter. Physiological factors that can compromise the skin barrier function, including age-related changes and skin disease, are also reviewed. Chapter 19 describes the current and future trends in the treatment of these and other skin diseases.

HEALTHY HUMAN SKIN: STRUCTURE AND FUNCTION

Human skin is composed of four main regions: the stratum corneum, the viable epidermis, dermis, and subcutaneous tissues (Fig. 1.1). A number of appendages are

Transdermal and Topical Drug Delivery: Principles and Practice, First Edition. Edited by Heather A.E. Benson, Adam C. Watkinson.

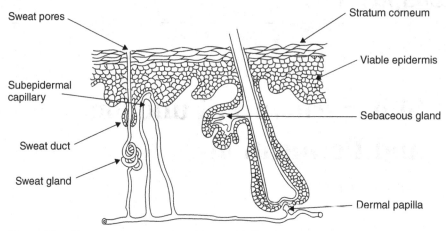

Figure 1.1   Diagrammatic cross-section of human skin.[96]

associated with the skin: hair follicles and eccrine and apocrine sweat glands. From a skin permeation viewpoint, the stratum corneum provides the main barrier and therefore the structure of this layer will be discussed in most detail. The other layers and appendages contribute important functions and are important target sites for drug delivery.

Epidermis

The epidermis is a multilayered region that varies in thickness from about 0.06 mm on the eyelids to about 0.8 mm on the palms of the hands and soles of the feet. There are no blood vessels in the epidermis, therefore epidermal cells must source nutrients and remove waste by diffusion across the epidermal–dermal layer to the cutaneous circulation in the dermis. Consequently, cells loose viability with increasing distance from the basal layer of the epidermis. The term "viable epidermis" is often used for the epidermal layers below the stratum corneum, but this terminology is question-able, particularly for cells in the outer layers. The epidermis is in a constant state of renewal, with the formation of a new cell layer of keratinocytes at the stratum basale, and the loss of their nucleus and other organelles to form desiccated, proteinaceous corneocytes on their journey toward desquamation, which in normal skin occurs from the skin surface at the same rate as formation. Thus the structure of the epi-dermal cells changes from the stratum basale, through the stratum spinosum, stratum granulosum, and stratum lucidum to the outermost stratum corneum (Fig. 1.2). The skin possesses many enzymes capable of metabolizing topically applied compounds. These are involved in the keratinocyte maturation and desquamation process,[1] for-mation of natural moisturizing factor (NMF) and general homeostasis.[2]

While the stratum corneum provides an efficient physical barrier, when damaged, environmental contaminants can access the epidermis to initiate an immunological response. This includes (1) epithelial defense as characterized by antimicrobial

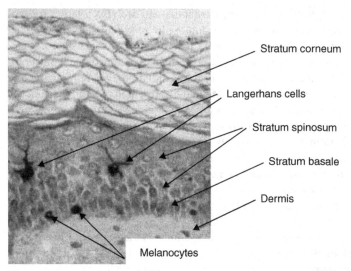

Stratum corneum

Langerhans cells

Stratum spinosum

Stratum basale

Dermis

Melanocytes

Figure 1.2   Human epidermis.[97]

peptides (AMP) produced by keratinocytes—both constitutively expressed (e.g., human beta defensin 1 [hBD1], RNAse 7, and psoriasin) and inducible (e.g., hBD 2-4 and LL-37); (2) innate-inflammatory immunity, involving expression of pro-inflammatory cytokines and interferons; and (3) adaptive immunity based on antigen presenting cells, such as epidermal Langerhans and dendritic cells, mediating a T cell response.[3] An understanding of these systems is important as they can be involved in skin disease and may also be therapeutic targets for the management of skin disease. The importance of these systems as therapeutic targets is highlighted in Chapter 19.

Stratum Basale

The stratum basale is also referred to as the stratum germinativum or basal layer. This layer contains Langerhans cells, melanocytes, Merkel cells, and the only cells within the epidermis that undergo cell division, namely keratinocytes. The keratinocytes of the basal lamina are attached to the basement membrane by hemi-desmosomes, which are proteinaceous anchors.[4,5] The absence of this effective adhesion results in rare chronic blistering diseases such as pemphigus and epidermolysis bullosa. Within the epidermis, desmosomes act as molecular rivets, interconnecting the keratin of adjacent cells, thereby ensuring the structural integrity of the skin.

Langerhans cells are dendritic cells and the major antigen presenting cells in the skin. They are generated in the bone marrow, and migrate to and localize in the stratum basale region of the epidermis. When activated by the binding of antigen to the cell surface, they migrate from the epidermis to the dermis and on to the regional lymph nodes, where they sensitize T cells to generate an immune response.

Langerhans cells are implicated in allergic dermatitis and are also a target for the mediation of enhanced immune responses in skin-applied vaccine delivery.

Melanocytes produce melanins, high molecular weight polymers that provide the pigmentation of the skin, hair, and eyes. The main function of melanin is to protect the skin by absorbing potentially harmful UV radiation, thus minimizing the liberation of free-radicals in the basal layer. Melanin is present in two forms: eumelanins are brown-black, whereas pheomelanins are yellow-red. Melanin is synthesized from tyrosine in the melanosomes, which are membrane-bound organelles that are associated with the keratinocytes and widely distributed to ensure an even distribution of pigmentation. Regulation of melanogenesis involves over 80 genes, many of which have now been characterized and cloned.[6] Mutations in these genes can result in conditions such as albinism and vitiligo, production of melanin with reduced photoprotective effects, and they may offer immune targets for the management of malignant melanoma.

Merkel cells are associated with the nerve endings and are concentrated in the touch-sensitive sites of the body such as the fingertips and lips.[7,8] Their location suggests that their primary function is in cutaneous sensation.

Stratum Spinosum

The stratum spinosum or prickle cell layer consists of the two to six rows of keratinocytes immediately above the basal layer (Fig. 1.3). Their morphology changes from columnar to polygonal, and they have an enlarged cytoplasm containing many organelles and filaments. The cells contain keratin tonofilaments and are interconnected by desmosomes.

Stratum Granulosum

Keratinocytes in the stratum granulosum or granular layer continue to differentiate. Present are intracellular keratohyalin granules and membrane-coating granules containing lamellar subunits arranged in parallel stacks, which are believed to be the precursors of the intercellular lipid lamellae of the stratum corneum.[9] The lamellar granules also contain hydrolytic enzymes including stratum corneum chymotryptic enzyme (SCCE), a serine protease that has been associated with the desquamation process.[10,11] Overexpression of SCCE has been implicated in psoriasis[12] and dermatitis.[13] As the cells approach the upper layers of the stratum granulosum, the lamellar granules are extruded into the intercellular spaces.

Stratum Lucidum

Within the stratum lucidum the cell nuclei and other organelles disintegrate, keratinization increases, and the cells are flattened and compacted. This layer takes on the typical structure common also to the stratum corneum of intracellular protein matrix and intercellular lipid lamellae, which is fundamentally important to the permeability barrier characteristics of the skin.

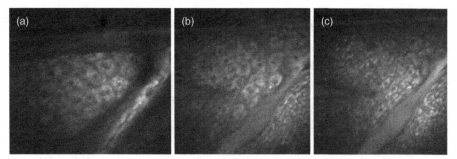

Figure 1.3   Multiphoton microscopy and fluorescence lifetime imaging (MPM-FLIM) images of human epidermis. (A) Stratum granulosum; (B) stratum spinosum; (C) stratum basale.[98]

Stratum Corneum

The outermost layer, the stratum corneum (or horny layer), consists of 10–20 μm of high density (1.4 g/cm^3 in the dry state) and low hydration (10%–20% compared with about 70% in other body tissues) cell layers. Although this layer is only 10–15 cells in depth, it serves as the primary barrier of the skin, regulating water loss from the body and preventing permeation of potentially harmful substances and microorganisms from the skin surface. The stratum corneum has been described as a brick wall-like structure of corneocytes as "bricks" in a matrix (or "mortar") of intercellular lipids, with desmosomes acting as molecular rivets between the corneocytes.[14,15] While this is a useful analogy, it is important to recognize that the corneocytes are elongated and flattened, often up to 50 μm in length while only 1.5 μm thick and is more like a brick wall built by an amateur. The corneocytes lack a nucleus and are composed of about 70%–80% keratin and 20% lipid within a cornified cell envelope (~10 nm thick). The cornified cell envelope is a protein/lipid polymer structure formed just below the cytoplasmic membrane that subsequently resides on the exterior of the corneocytes.[16] It consists of two parts: a protein envelope and a lipid envelope. The protein envelope is thought to contribute to the biomechanical properties of the cornified envelope due to cross-linking of specialized structural proteins by both disulfide bonds and N-(γ-glutamyl) lysine isopeptide bonds formed by transglutaminases. Some of the structural proteins involved include involucrin, loricrin, small proline-rich proteins, keratin intermediate filaments, elafin, cystatin A, and desmosomal proteins. It has been proposed that the corneocyte envelope plays an important role in the assembly of the intercellular lipid lamellae of the stratum corneum. The lipid envelope comprised of N-ω-hydroxyceramides, which is covalently bound to the protein matrix of the cornified envelope,[17] has been shown to be essential for the formation of normal stratum corneum intercellular lipid lamellae, and in its absence, the barrier function of the skin is disrupted.[18] Thus, the anchoring of the intercellular lipids to the corneocyte protein envelope is important in providing the structure and barrier function of the stratum corneum.

The unique composition of the stratum corneum intercellular lipids and their structural arrangement in multiple lamellar layers within a continuous lipid domain

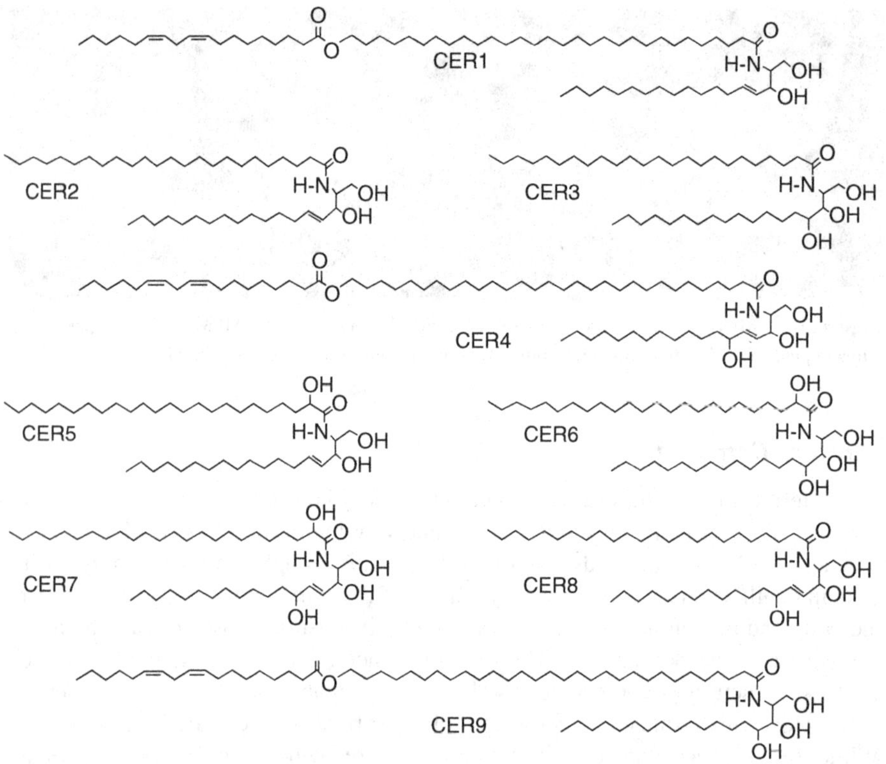

Figure 1.4   Molecular structure of ceramides (CER) in human stratum corneum. CER1, CER4 and CER9 have an ω-hydroxy acyl chain to which a linoleic acid is chemically linked.[26]

is critical to the barrier function of the stratum corneum. In recent years, our knowledge of the structure and organization of the stratum cornuem lipids has been greatly enhanced by a range of sophisticated visualization techniques.[19] The major components of the lipid domains are ceramides, cholesterol, free fatty acids, cholesterol esters, and cholesterol sulfate, with the notable absence of phospholipids. The lipid content varies between individuals and with anatomical site.[20] Ceramide structures are based on sphingolipids (Fig. 1.4) and have been classified based on their polarity, with ceramide 1 being the least polar. New ceramide species continue to be identified using increasingly sophisticated analytical techniques.[21–23] The free fatty acids in the stratum corneum consist of a number of saturated long-chain acids, the most abundant being lignoceric acid (C24) and hexacosanoic acid (C26), with trace amounts of very long-chain (C32-C36) saturated and monounsaturated free fatty acids.[24] The presence of cholesterol and cholesterol esters is likely to reduce the fluidity of the intercellular lipid lamellae in the same way as incorporation of cholesterol into other lipid membranes, such as liposomes, provides a stabilizing effect.

   An increasing understanding of the biophysics of the stratum corneum intercellular lipid lamellae has been developed in recent years. It is clear that the intercellular

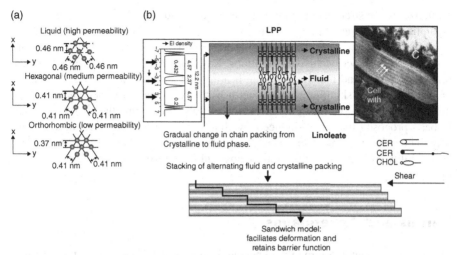

Figure 1.5   Lateral packing (a) and molecular arrangement (b) of stratum corneum lipids domains in the long periodicity phase (LPP) as determined from X-ray diffraction patterns. The presence of a broad–narrow–broad sequence in the repeating unit of the LPP (arrows) (left panel) is in agreement with the broad–narrow–broad pattern found in RuO_4-fixed stratum corneum (right panel). CER1 plays an important role in dictating the broad–narrow–broad sequence: fluid phase in the central narrow band and crystallinity gradually increasing from the central layer. Bouwstra-proposed "sandwich model": permits deformation as a consequence of shear stresses (skin elasticity) while barrier function is retained.[25]

lipid lamellae that are oriented parallel to the corneocytes cell wall are highly structured yet exhibit heterogeneous phase behavior with multiple states of lipid organization. Using X-ray diffraction, Bouwstra et al. identified two lamellar phases with periodicities of 6.4 (short periodicity phase, SPP) and 13.4 nm (long periodicity phase, LPP), together with a fluid phase.[25] They proposed a "sandwich model" consisting of three lipid layers: one narrow central lipid layer with fluid domains on both sides of a broad layer with a crystalline structure as most representative of the lamellar phase (Fig. 1.5).[25] The lattice spacing within these layers has been measured and lipid packing identified as orthorhombic (crystalline), hexagonal (gel-like), and liquid (Fig. 1.5).[26] These packing lattices correspond with low, medium, and high permeability, respectively. Within human stratum corneum, the orthorhombic lattice predominates, thus providing the main contribution to the permeability barrier function, while a transition to the less tightly packed hexagonal lattice structure increases toward the skin surface and is thought to be induced by sebum lipids.[27,28] An in-depth review of the structural organization of the stratum corneum in healthy and diseased skin has been provided by Bouwstra and Ponec.[26]

The stratum corneum contains about 15%–20% water that is primarily associated with the keratin in the corneocytes. Only small amounts of water are present in the intercellular polar head group regions.[29] The presence of water is essential to maintain the suppleness and integrity of the skin. NMF acts as a humectant and plasticizer in the stratum corneum, binding water to aid swelling of the corneocytes. Hydration within the stratum corneum is controlled by the conversion of filaggrin to NMF: conversion occurs only at high water activity, with low NMF levels present in corneocytes under occlusive conditions. Rawlings and Matts have reviewed the role of hydration and moisturization in healthy and diseased skin states.[30] Water is known to enhance skin permeability yet it has only a small presence and does not directly alter the organization of the intercellular lipid lamellae.[29] Walters and Roberts proposed that water-induced swelling of the corneocytes acts in a similar way to how the swelling of bricks in a wall could loosen the mortar, thus increasing permeability by loosening the lipid chains without exerting a direct effect on the lipid ordering.[31]

Dermis and Appendages

The dermis is about 2–5 mm in thickness and consists of collagen fibrils that provide support, and elastic connective tissue that provides elasticity and flexibility, embedded within a mucopolysaccharide matrix. Within this matrix is a sparse cell population, including fibroblasts that produce the components of the connective tissue (collagen, laminin, fibronectin, vitronectin), mast cells involved in immune and inflammatory response, and melanocytes responsible for pigment production. Due to this structure, the dermis provides little barrier to the permeation of most drugs, but may reduce the permeation to deeper tissues of very lipophilic drugs. A number of structures and appendages are contained or originate within the dermis, including blood and lymph vessels, nerve endings, hair follicles, sebaceous glands, and sweat glands.

Contained within the dermis is an extensive vascular network that acts to regulate body temperature, provides oxygen and nutrients to and removes toxins and waste products from tissues, and facilitates immune response and wound repair. In addition to fine capillaries, arteriovenous anastomoses are present throughout the skin. They permit direct shunting of up to 60% of the skin blood flow between the arteries and veins, thus permitting the rapid blood flow required in heat regulation.[32] This extensive blood supply ensures that most permeating molecules are removed from the dermo–epidermal junction to the systemic blood supply, thus establishing a concentration gradient between the applied chemical on the skin surface and the dermis.

Lymph vessels within the dermis play important roles in regulating interstitial pressure, mobilizing immune response and waste removal. As they also extend to the dermo–epidermal junction, they can also remove permeated molecules from the skin. While small molecule permeants such as water are primarily removed via the blood flow, it has been shown that clearance by the lymph vessels is important for large molecules such as interferon.[33]

There are three appendages that originate in the dermis: the hair follicles and associated sebaceous glands, eccrine, and apocrine sweat glands. Hair follicles are present at a fractional area of about 1/1000 of the skin surface, except on the lips, palms of the hands, and soles of the feet. The sebaceous gland associated with each hair follicle secretes sebum, which is composed of free fatty acids, triglycerides, and waxes. Sebum protects and lubricates the skin, and maintains the skin surface at pH of about 5. The erector pilorum muscle attaches the follicle to the dermis and allows the hair to respond to cold and fear. Eccrine glands, present at a fractional area of about 1 in 10,000 of the skin surface, secrete sweat (dilute salt solution of pH about 5) in response to exercise, high environmental temperature, and emotional stress. Apocrine glands are present in the axillae, nipples, and anogenital areas, and are about 10 times the size of eccrine glands. Their secretion consists of "milk" protein, lipoproteins, and lipids.

Subcutaneous Tissue

The subcutaneous tissue or hypodermis consists of a layer of fat cells arranged as lobules with interconnecting collagen and elastin fibers. Its primary functions are heat insulation and protection against physical shock, while also providing energy storage that can be made available when required. Blood vessels and nerves connect to the skin via the hypodermis.

PHYSIOLOGICAL FACTORS AFFECTING THE SKIN BARRIER

There are a number of physiological factors that affect the skin barrier and hence skin permeability.

Age

It is clear from visual inspection that the skin structure changes as the skin ages. It is important to recognize that while there are intrinsic aging processes, environmental factors such as exposure to solar radiation and chemicals, including cosmetics and soaps, will also influence skin structure and function over time.[34] Intrinsic aging causes the epidermis to become thinner and the corneocytes less adherent to one another. There is flattening of the dermoepidermal interface and a decrease in the number of melanocytes and Langerhans cells. The dermis becomes atrophic and relatively acellular and avascular, with alternations in collagen, elastin, and glycosaminoglycans. The subcutaneous tissue is diminished in some areas, especially the face, shins, hands, and feet, but increased in other areas, particularly the abdomen in men and the thighs in women.[35] As the stratum corneum constitutes the skin barrier function, it is important to understand age-related changes to this structure. While epidermal thickness alters with age, stratum corneum thickness has been shown not to significantly change.[36] However, the lipid composition did alter with age and also with seasons, as demonstrated from stratum corneum tape strips taken from three body sites (face, hand, leg) of female Caucasians of different age groups in winter, spring, and summer.[37] There were significantly decreased levels of all major lipid species (ceramides, ceramide 1 subtypes, cholesterol, and fatty acids), in particular ceramides, with increasing age. In addition, stratum corneum lipid levels were substantially depleted in winter compared with spring and summer.

Do these age-related changes alter skin barrier function? Studies of barrier function with age cohorts have generally involved biophysical measures such as transepidermal water loss (TEWL) and skin conductance (as a measure of stratum corneum hydration) *in vivo* or direct measurement of permeation *in vitro*. A number of studies have shown a decrease in TEWL with age.[38–41] However, aging has not been shown to significantly effect the skin permeation of compounds such as estradiol, caffeine, aspirin, nicotinates, or water.[35,42,43] These studies have been conducted in adults ranging from young adult (twenties) to aged (seventies to eighties). In contrast, skin barrier function in young children may be significantly reduced, particularly in newborn and neonatal (preterm) children.[44–47] This needs to be taken into account in topical therapy.

Anatomical Site

Skin permeability at different body sites has been widely studied over age range from neonates to adults. Feldman and Maibach[48] first described regional variation of ^{14}C-labeled hydrocortisone skin permeation and subsequent elimination in human volunteers over 40 years ago. Highest absorption was seen for the scrotal areas (42 times greater than the ventral forearm) and lowest absorption was observed on the heel. Rougier et al.[49] conducted a similar experiment with ^{14}C-labeled benzoic acid application, measuring elimination and amount in stratum corneum tape strip at 30 minutes, at six body sites on male volunteers. They reported that the 30-minute tape strip samples correlated well with skin absorption, and a similar regional variation with head and neck showing three times the permeability as back skin. Based on a number of studies, the regional variation in skin barrier function is in the following order:

Genitals > head and neck > trunk > arm and leg.

Transdermal patches are generally applied to the trunk where there is intermediate skin permeability, though there are examples of patches applied to areas where permeability is higher, such as the scopolamine patch to the postauricular region (behind the ear) and a testosterone patch to the scrotal region.

There is also variability within body regions as demonstrated by Marrakchi and Maibach for the face.[41,50] Basal TEWL measurements taken to map the skin barrier function on the face of 20 volunteers showed a twofold difference between nasolabial and forehead areas, with the following rank order:

Nasolabial > perioral > chin > nose > cheek > forehead > neck > forearm.

Ethnicity

Ethnic differences in skin barrier function have been extensively investigated in recent years, with the majority of studies reporting no significant difference across ethnic groups.[51,52] Some differences have been reported but these are inconsistent, suggesting that ethnic differences are much less profound than inter-individual differences within the ethnic groups.[53] Differences in skin lipid composition across ethnic groups have been reported and it is suggested that these may influence the prevalence of skin disease and sensitivity.[54] A comprehensive review of the literature on skin barrier function and ethnicity is provided by Hillebrand and Wickett.[55]

Gender

There is little if any difference in skin barrier function as determined by basal TEWL between male and female skin.[56,57] Differences in corneocytes size between pre- and postmenopausal women have been reported, but this did not correlate with any change in basal TEWL in this study.[57] Other groups have investigated skin barrier function during the menstrual cycle, reporting that skin barrier function is reduced in the days before the onset of menses.[58,59]

Skin Disorders

The clinical symptoms and pathophysiology of skin disorders has been extensively reviewed in dermatological textbooks. The focus here is on the effect of skin disorders on barrier function, and thus on topical and transdermal drug delivery. A number of common skin disorders compromise barrier function, including eczema (dermatitis), ichthyosis, psoriasis, and acne vulgaris. Skin infections that cause eruptions at the skin surface such as impetigo, Herpes simplex infections ("cold sores"), and fungal infections (such as "athlete's foot") reduce the barrier, but the effect is self-limiting and resolves as the infection is treated.

Atopic dermatitis is common in children and often associated with other atopic disorders such as asthma and hay fever. It is characterized by papules (solid, raised spot), itching, and thickened and hyperkeratotic (thickened, scaly stratum corneum) skin with reduced barrier function as demonstrated by elevated TEWL and hydrocortisone penetration compared to uninvolved skin on atopic patients, which is also higher than normal skin.[60–63] Contact or allergic dermatitis is characterized by erythema (skin reddening), papules, vesicles, and hyperkeratosis, which occurs in response to skin contact with allergenic substances. Sodium lauryl sulfate (SLS) has been used to experimentally generate contact dermatitis and the barrier reduction caused is dose dependent. Benfeldt et al.[64] reported a 46-fold and 146-fold increase in salicylic acid skin permeation in mild dermatitis (1% SLS) and severe dermatitis (2% SLS), respectively, relative to normal skin, as measured by microdialysis of skin tissue levels. This correlated with other measures of barrier perturbation (TEWL and erythema) in each individual.

Psoriasis is a chronic autoimmune disease characterized by red lesions and plaques (epidermal hyperproliferation), particularly at the knee, elbow, and scalp. Elevated TEWL and permeation of a range of compounds including electrolytes,[65] steroids,[66] and macromolecules[67,68] in psoriatic skin relative to normal skin has been reported.

SKIN PERMEATION

Compounds have been applied to the skin for thousands of years to enhance beauty and treat local conditions. More recently, transdermal delivery devices, primarily patches, have been successfully developed for a range of disorders. These include scopolamine for travel sickness, nitroglycerin for cardiovascular disorders, estradiol and testosterone for hormone replacement, fentanyl for pain management, nicotine for smoking cessation, rivastigmine for Alzheimer's disease, and methylphenidate for attention deficit hyperactivity disorder (ADHD). Transdermal delivery offers significant advantages over oral administration due to minimal first-pass metabolism, avoidance of the adverse gastrointestinal environment, and the ability to provide controlled and prolonged drug release. Despite these obvious advantages, the range of compounds that can be delivered transdermally is limited because permeability sufficient to provide effective therapeutic levels often cannot be achieved.

The outermost layer of the skin, the stratum corneum, is generally considered to be the main barrier to permeation of externally applied chemicals and loss of moisture (TEWL). Removal of the stratum corneum by tape stripping and reduced stratum corneum barrier integrity in psoriatic skin[66] have been shown to provide significantly increased permeability. This region therefore provides the primary protection of the body from external contaminants and limits the potential therapeutic effectiveness of topically applied compounds.

The therapeutic target sites within the skin must be considered. While for most applications this will involve permeation to the deeper skin tissues (e.g., antihistamines, anesthetics, anti-inflammatories, antimitotics) or systemic uptake, other applications may necessitate targeting the skin surface (e.g., sunscreens, cosmetics, barrier products) or appendages (e.g., antiperspirants, hair growth promoters, antiacne products). Thus the following consideration of skin permeation pathways must be viewed within the context of the therapeutic target site.

SKIN PERMEATION PATHWAYS

A penetrant applied to the skin surface has three potential pathways across the epidermis: through sweat ducts, via hair follicles and associated sebaceous glands, or across the continuous stratum corneum (Fig. 1.1). These pathways are not mutually exclusive, with most compounds possibly permeating the skin by a combination of pathways and the relative contribution of each being related to the physicochemical properties of the permeating molecule.

Permeation via Appendages

While it is generally accepted that the predominant permeation route is across the continuous stratum corneum, Scheuplein[69] suggested that the appendageal route dominates during the lag phase of the diffusional process. While the appendages have been considered as low resistance shunts, this is an overly simplistic view, as the sweat glands are filled with aqueous sweat and the follicular glands with lipoidal sebum. In addition, the appendages represent only 0.1%–1% of the total skin surface area, varying from the forearm to the forehead.[70] In recent years, there has been renewed interest in targeting the skin appendages, in particular targeted follicular delivery. This can be achieved by either manipulating the formulation or modifying the target molecule to target delivery, as recently reviewed by Lu et al.[71] Formulation approaches have included particle-/vesicle-based dosage forms and the use of sebum-miscible excipients, while molecular modification involves optimizing physicochemical properties such as size, lipophilicity, solubility parameter, and charge.

Permeation via the Stratum Corneum: Transcellular Route

The transcellular route (Fig. 1.6) has been regarded by some as a polar route through the stratum corneum.[72] While the corneocytes contain an intracellular keratin matrix that is relatively hydrated and thus polar in nature, permeation requires repeated partitioning between this polar environment and the lipophilic domains surrounding

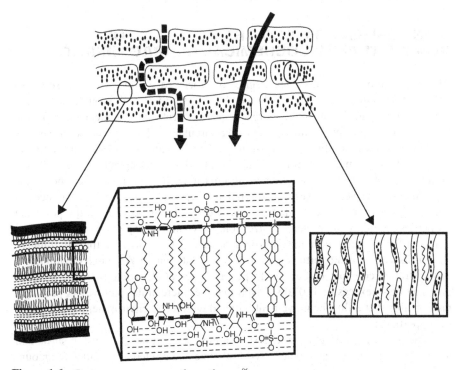

Figure 1.6   Stratum corneum permeation pathways.[96]

the corneocytes. Based on the large body of permeation data, the view of most skin scientists is that transport through the stratum corneum is predominantly by the intercellular route.

Permeation via the Stratum Corneum: Intercellular Route

While the intercellular lipid bilayers occupy only a small area of the stratum corneum,[73] they provide the only continuous route through the stratum corneum (Fig. 1.6). Evidence of the importance of the intercellular route has been generated over many years. This includes studies investigating the effects of solvents capable of delipidizing the stratum corneum bilayers[74] and microscopic studies providing direct evidence of the histological localization of topically applied compounds.[75]

The structure of the stratum corneum lipids contributes to the barrier properties of the skin. Within the intercellular lipid domains, transport can take place via both lipid (diffusion via the lipid core) and polar (diffusion via the polar head groups) pathways. The diffusional rate-limiting region of very polar permeants is the polar pathway of the stratum corneum, which is fairly independent of their partition coefficient, while less polar permeants probably diffuse via the lipid pathway, and their permeation increases with increase in lipophilicity.[73,76,77]

Clearly the relative contribution of these three pathways to skin permeation will depend on the physicochemical characteristics of the permeant.

SKIN PERMEATION AND THE INFLUENCE OF PERMEANT PHYSICOCHEMICAL CHARACTERISTICS

The permeation process involves a series of processes starting with release of the permeant from the dosage form, followed by diffusion into and through the stratum corneum, then partitioning to the more aqueous epidermal environment and diffusion to deeper tissues or uptake into the cutaneous circulation. These processes are highly dependent on the solubility and diffusivity of the permeant within each environment. Release of the permeant from the dosage form vehicle and uptake into the stratum corneum is dependent on the relative solubility in each environment, and hence the stratum corneum–vehicle partition coefficient. The diffusion coefficient or speed at which the permeant moves within each environment is dependent on the permeant properties including the molecular size, solubility and melting point, ionization and potential for binding within the environment, and factors related to the environment such as its viscosity and tortuosity or diffusional path length. Although the thickness of the stratum corneum is only 10–15 μm, the intercellular route is highly tortuous and may be in excess of 150 μm. Given that the intercellular pathway is predominant, factors that influence movement into and within this environment are of greatest importance.

The permeation of an infinite dose of a molecule applied to the skin surface in an *in vitro* experiment can be measured over time and plotted as cumulative amount permeating (Q) versus time. Steady-state permeation or flux (J) can be viewed fairly simplistically based on Fick's laws of diffusion:

$$J = \frac{dQ}{dt} = \frac{DPC_v}{h},\qquad(1.1)$$

where Q is the amount permeating a unit area of skin, D is the diffusion coefficient of the permeant in the skin, P is the partition coefficient between the stratum corneum and the vehicle, C_v is the applied concentration of permeant, and h is the diffusional path length. As the stratum corneum is the main barrier for most permeants, diffusion coefficient within and the path length of the intercellular route through the stratum corneum are most relevant.

A number of groups have developed more complex mathematical approaches to describe and/or predict skin permeation under a range of conditions and readers are referred to some of the more recent reviews of this area.[78–81] These models take into account key parameters such as partition coefficient, molecular size and aqueous solubility, and other factors such as ionization and permeant binding[82,83] within the stratum corneum.

Partition Coefficient

The first step in the skin transport process is partitioning of the permeant from the applied vehicle to the intercellular lipid domains of the stratum corneum, followed by diffusion within this relatively lipophilic environment. Many studies have demonstrated that increasing lipophilicity increases skin permeation,[84–87] with log P(o/w) of 2–3 being optimal. It is likely that these molecules with intermediate lipophilicity can permeate via both the lipid and polar microenvironments within the intercellular route. Very lipophilic molecules will have high solubility in the intercellular lipids but will not readily partition from the stratum corneum to the more aqueous viable epidermis, thus limiting their skin permeation rate.

Molecular Size

The size and shape of the permeant will influence the diffusivity within the stratum corneum. It has been shown that there is an inverse relationship between permeant size and skin permeation.[82,83,88–91] As a general rule, permeants selected for topical and transdermal delivery tend to be less than 500 Da, as larger molecules permeate poorly. Consequently, although molecular size is important and is incorporated as a parameter in many mathematical models, when considering the physicochemical factors influencing permeation of the molecules that tend to be applied to the skin (generally in the sub 500 Da range), other factors such as partition coefficient and ionization are more influential. It is important to note that large molecules such as proteins and peptides are not good candidates for topical and transdermal delivery unless their transport can be facilitated (usually by physical disruption of the barrier), as discussed in later chapters.

Solubility

The solubility of the permeant in the intercellular pathway will influence the diffusion coefficient within the stratum corneum. Lipophilic compounds have increased solubility in the intercellular domains and thus increased flux. However, the skin permeation rate is also dependent on the concentration of soluble permeant in the applied vehicle. Thus if a lipophilic compound has limited solubility in a topical vehicle, the compound may readily partition into the stratum corneum, resulting in depletion in the vehicle and thus reducing permeant flux. Therefore, the ideal permeant requires lipid solubility (high diffusion coefficient) but also reasonable aqueous solubility (high donor concentration) to maximize flux. In mathematical models, melting point is frequently used as a predictor of aqueous solubility.

Hydration

Increasing stratum corneum hydration increases skin permeability. Indeed, water is considered to be a natural skin penetration enhancer in topical formulation. This has been applied in the use of transdermal patches, occlusive dressings (e.g., Tegaderm dressing with EMLA™ cream; Tegaderm, 3M, Maplewood, MN; EMLA, AstraZeneca, Wilmington, DE), and occlusive or hydrating topical formulations. The formulation of topical and transdermal products, and their influence on skin hydration and permeability, is considered later in this book. In addition, the reader is referred to reviews on skin hydration and moisturization available in the literature.[92-95]

CONCLUSION

The successful development of products for topical and transdermal drug delivery relies on understanding skin permeation and designing a solute and/or formulation appropriately. Methods to assess and enhance skin permeation are discussed in the following chapters in Part One of this text.

ACKNOWLEDGMENTS

Thanks to Dr. Tarl Prow and Yousuf Mohammed for the MPM images of human epidermal layers (Fig. 1.4).

REFERENCES

1. ZEEUWEN PL. Epidermal differentiation: The role of proteases and their inhibitors. *Eur J Cell Biol* 2004; 83: 761–773.
2. HACHEM J-P, MAN M-Q, CRUMRINE D, et al. Sustained serine proteases activity by prolonged increase in pH leads to degradation of lipid processing enzymes and profound alterations of barrier function and stratum corneum integrity. *J Invest Dermatol* 2005; 125: 510–520.
3. MEYER T, STOCKFLETH E, CHRSTOPHERS E. Immune response profiles in human skin. *Br J Dermatol* 2007; 157: 1–7.

4. DOWLING J, YU QC, FUCHS E. Beta4 integrin is required for hemidesmosome formation, cell adhesion and cell survival. *J Cell Biol* 1996; 134: 559–572.

5. BURGESON RE, CHRISTIANO AM. The dermal-epidermal junction. *Curr Opin Cell Biol* 1997; 9: 651–658.

6. HEARING VJ. Biochemical control of melanogenesis and melanosomal organization. *J Investig Dermatol Symp Proc* 1999; 4: 24–28.

7. TACHIBANA T, NAWA T. Recent progress in studies on Merkel cell biology. *Anat Sci Int* 2002; 77: 26–33.

8. TACHIBANA T. The Merkel cell: Recent findings and unresolved problems. *Arch Histol Cytol* 1995; 58: 379–396.

9. LANDMANN L. The epidermal permeability barrier. *Anat Embryol (Berl)* 1988; 178: 1–13.

10. LUNDSTROM A, EGELRUD T. Stratum corneum chymotryptic enzyme: A proteinase which may be generally present in the stratum corneum and with a possible involvement in desquamation. *Acta Derm Venereol* 1991; 71: 471–474.

11. EGELRUD T. Purification and preliminary characterization of stratum corneum chymotryptic enzyme: A proteinase that may be involved in desquamation. *J Invest Dermatol* 1993; 101: 200–204.

12. EKHOLM E, EGELRUD T. Stratum corneum chymotryptic enzyme in psoriasis. *Arch Dermatol Res* 1999; 291: 195–200.

13. VASILOPOULOS Y, CORK MJ, MURPHY R, et al. Genetic association between an AACC insertion in the 3'UTR of the stratum corneum chymotryptic enzyme gene and atopic dermatitis. *J Invest Dermatol* 2004; 123: 62–66.

14. ELIAS PM. Epidermal lipids, membranes, and keratinization. *Int J Dermatol* 1981; 20: 1–19.

15. MICHAELS AS, CHANDRASEKARAN SK, SHAW JE. Drug permeation through human skin: Theory and in vitro experimental measurement. *AIChE J* 1975; 21: 985–996.

16. NEMES Z, STEINERT PM. Bricks and mortar of the epidermal barrier. *Exp Mol Med* 1999; 31: 5–19.

17. LAZO ND, MEINE JG, DOWNING DT. Lipids are covalently attached to rigid corneocyte protein envelopes existing predominantly as beta-sheets: A solid-state nuclear magnetic resonance study. *J Invest Dermatol* 1995; 105: 296–300.

18. BEHNE M, UCHIDA Y, SEKI T, et al. Omega-hydroxyceramides are required for corneocyte lipid envelope (CLE) formation and normal epidermal permeability barrier function. *J Invest Dermatol* 2000; 114: 185–192.

19. WARTEWIG S, NEUBERT RH. Properties of ceramides and their impact on the stratum corneum structure: A review. Part 1: Ceramides. *Skin Pharmacol Physiol* 2007; 20: 220–229.

20. LAMPE MA, BURLINGAME AL, WHITNEY J, et al. Human stratum corneum lipids: Characterization and regional variations. *J Lipid Res* 1983; 24: 120–130.

21. MASUKAWA Y, NARITA H, SATO H, et al. Comprehensive quantification of ceramide species in human stratum corneum. *J Lipid Res* 2009; 50: 1708–1719.

22. MASUKAWA Y, NARITA H, SHIMIZU E, et al. Characterization of overall ceramide species in human stratum corneum. *J Lipid Res* 2008; 49: 1466–1476.

23. MASUKAWA Y, TSUJIMURA H, NARITA H. Liquid chromatography-mass spectrometry for comprehensive profiling of ceramide molecules in human hair. *J Lipid Res* 2006; 47: 1559–1571.

24. NORLEN L, NICANDER I, LUNDSJO A, et al. A new HPLC-based method for the quantitative analysis of inner stratum corneum lipids with special reference to the free fatty acid fraction. *Arch Dermatol Res* 1998; 290: 508–516.

25. BOUWSTRA J, PILGRAM G, GOORIS G, et al. New aspects of the skin barrier organization. *Skin Pharmacol Appl Skin Physiol* 2001; 14(Suppl 1): 52–62.

26. BOUWSTRA J, PONEC M. The skin in healthy and diseased state. *Biochim Biophys Acta* 2006; 1758: 2080–2095.

27. PILGRAM GS, ENGELSMA-VAN PELT AM, BOUWSTRA JA, et al. Electron diffraction provides new information on human stratum corneum lipid organization studied in relation to depth and temperature. *J Invest Dermatol* 1999; 113: 403–409.

28. PILGRAM GS, van der MEULEN J, GOORIS GS, et al. The influence of two azones and sebaceous lipids on the lateral organization of lipids isolated from human stratum corneum. *Biochim Biophys Acta* 2001; 1511: 244–254.

29. SUHONEN TM, BOUWSTA JA, URTTI A. Chemical enhancement of percutaneous absorption in relation to stratum corneum structural alterations. *J Control Rel* 1999; 59: 149–161.

30. RAWLINGS AV, MATTS PJ. Stratum corneum moisturization at the molecular level: An update in relation to the dry skin cycle. *J Invest Dermatol* 2005; 124: 1099–1110.

31. WALTERS KA, ROBERTS MS. The structure and function of skin. In: Walters KA, ed. *Dermatological and Transdermal Formulations*. Marcel Dekker, New York, 2002.

32. HALE AR, BURCH GE. The arteriovenous anastomoses and blood vessels of the human finger. Morphological and functional aspects. *Medicine (Baltimore)* 1960; 39: 191–240.

33. CROSS SE, ROBERTS MS. Subcutaneous absorption kinetics and local tissue distribution of interferon and other solutes. *J Pharm Pharmacol* 1993; 45: 606–609.

34. LOBER CW, FENSKE NA. Photoaging and the skin: Differentiation and clinical response. *Geriatrics* 1990; 45: 36–40.

35. FENSKE NA, LOBER CW. Structural and functional changes of normal aging skin. *J Am Acad Dermatol* 1986; 15: 571–585.

36. BATISSE D, BAZIN R, BALDEWECK T, et al. Influence of age on the wrinkling capacities of skin. *Skin Res Technol* 2002; 8: 148–154.

37. ROGERS J, HARDING C, MAYO A, et al. Stratum corneum lipids: The effect of ageing and the seasons. *Arch Dermatol Res* 1996; 288: 765–770.

38. TAKAHASHI M, WATANABE H, KUMAGAI H, et al. Physiological and morphological changes in facial skin with aging (II). *J Soc Cosmet Chem Japan* 1989; 23: 22–30.

39. SHRINER DL, MAIBACH HI. Regional variation of nonimmunologic contact urticaria. Functional map of the human face. *Skin Pharmacol* 1996; 9: 312–321.

40. WILHELM KP, CUA AB, MAIBACH HI. Skin aging. Effect on transepidermal water loss, stratum corneum hydration, skin surface pH, and casual sebum content. *Arch Dermatol* 1991; 127: 1806–1809.

41. MARRAKCHI S, MAIBACH HI. Sodium lauryl sulfate-induced irritation in the human face: Regional and age-related differences. *Skin Pharmacol Physiol* 2006; 19: 177–180.

42. ROSKOS KV, BIRCHER AJ, MAIBACH HI, et al. Pharmacodynamic measurements of methyl nicotinate percutaneous absorption: The effect of aging on microcirculation. *Br J Dermatol* 1990; 122: 165–171.

43. ROSKOS KV, GUY RH. Assessment of skin barrier function using transepidermal water loss: Effect of age. *Pharm Res* 1989; 6: 949–953.

44. KALIA YN, NONATO LB, LUND CH, et al. Development of skin barrier function in premature infants. *J Invest Dermatol* 1998; 111: 320–326.

45. GIUSTI F, MARTELLA A, BERTONI L, et al. Skin barrier, hydration, and pH of the skin of infants under 2 years of age. *Pediatr Dermatol* 2001; 18: 93–96.

46. WILLIAMS ML, FEINGOLD KR. Barrier function of neonatal skin. *J Pediatr* 1998; 133: 467–468.

47. YOSIPOVITCH G, MAAYAN-METZGER A, MERLOB P, et al. Skin barrier properties in different body areas in neonates. *Pediatrics* 2000; 106: 105–108.

48. FELDMAN R, MAIBACH HI. Absorption of some organic compounds through the skin in man. *J Invest Dermatol* 1970; 54: 399–404.

49. ROUGIER A, DUPUIS D, LOTTE C, et al. Regional variation in percutaneous absorption in man: Measurement by the stripping method. *Arch Dermatol Res* 1986; 278: 465–469.

50. MARRAKCHI S, MAIBACH HI. Biophysical parameters of skin: Map of human face, regional, and age-related differences. *Contact Dermatitis* 2007; 57: 28–34.

51. BERARDESCA E, MAIBACH HI. Racial differences in sodium lauryl sulphate induced cutaneous irritation: Black and white. *Contact Dermatitis* 1988; 18: 65–70.

52. KOMPAORE F, MARTY JP, DUPONT C. In vivo evaluation of the stratum corneum barrier function in blacks, Caucasians and Asians with two noninvasive methods. *Skin Pharmacol* 1993; 6: 200–207.

53. WARRIER AG, KLIGMAN AM, HARPER RA, et al. A comparison of black and white skin using non-invasive methods. *J Soc Cosmet Chem* 1996; 47: 229–240.

54. MUIZZUDDIN N, HELLEMANS L, VAN OVERLOOP L, et al. Structural and functional differences in barrier properties of African American, Caucasian and East Asian skin. *J Dermatol Sci* 2010; 59: 123–128.

55. HILLEBRAND GG, WICKETT RR. Epidemiology of skin barrier function: Host and environmental factors. In: Walters KA, Roberts MS, eds. *Dermatologic, Cosmeceutic and Cosmetic Development.* Informa Healthcare, New York, 2008; 129–156.

56. CUA AB, WILHELM KP, MAIBACH HI. Frictional properties of human skin: Relation to age, sex and anatomical region, stratum corneum hydration and transepidermal water loss. *Br J Dermatol* 1990; 123: 473–479.

57. FLUHR JW, PELOSI A, LAZZERINI S, et al. Differences in corneocyte surface area in pre- and post-menopausal women. Assessment with the noninvasive videomicroscopic imaging of corneocytes method (VIC) under basal conditions. *Skin Pharmacol Appl Skin Physiol* 2001; 14(Suppl 1): 10–16.

58. HARVELL J, HUSSONA-SAEED I, MAIBACH HI. Changes in transepidermal water loss and cutaneous blood flow during the menstrual cycle. *Contact Dermatitis* 1992; 27: 294–301.

59. MUIZZUDDIN N, MARENUS KD, SCHNITTGER SF, et al. Effect of systemic hormonal cyclicity on skin. *J Cosmet Sci* 2005; 56: 311–321.

60. AALTO-KORTE K, TURPEINEN M. Transepidermal water loss and absorption of hydrocortisone in widespread dermatitis. *Br J Dermatol* 1993; 128: 633–635.

61. AALTO-KORTE K, TURPEINEN M. Quantifying systemic absorption of topical hydrocortisone in erythroderma. *Br J Dermatol* 1995; 133: 403–408.

62. AALTO-KORTE K, TURPEINEN M. Pharmacokinetics of topical hydrocortisone at plasma level after applications once or twice daily in patients with widespread dermatitis. *Br J Dermatol* 1995; 133: 259–263.

63. AALTO-KORTE K, TURPEINEN M. Transepidermal water loss predicts systemic absorption of topical hydrocortisone in atopic dermatitis [letter]. *Br J Dermatol* 1996; 135: 497–498.

64. BENFELDT E, SERUP J, MENNE T. Effect of barrier perturbation on cutaneous salicylic acid penetration in human skin: In vivo pharmacokinetics using microdialysis and non-invasive quantification of barrier function. *Br J Dermatol* 1999; 140: 739–748.

65. SHANI J, BARAK S, LEVI D, et al. Skin penetration of minerals in psoriatics and guinea-pigs bathing in hypertonic salt solutions. *Pharmacol Res Commun* 1985; 17: 501–512.

66. SCHAEFER H, ZESCH A, STUTTGEN G. Penetration, permeation, and absorption of triamcinolone acetonide in normal and psoriatic skin. *Arch Dermatol Res* 1977; 258: 241–249.

67. WHITE PJ, GRAY AC, FOGARTY RD, et al. C-5 propyne-modified oligonucleotides penetrate the epidermis in psoriatic and not normal human skin after topical application. *J Invest Dermatol* 2002; 118: 1003–1007.

68. GOULD AR, SHARP PJ, SMITH DR, et al. Increased permeability of psoriatic skin to the protein, plasminogen activator inhibitor 2. *Arch Dermatol Res* 2003; 295: 249–254.

69. SCHEUPLEIN RJ. Properties of the skin as a membrane. *Adv Biol Skin* 1972; 12: 125–152.

70. OTBERG N, RICHTER H, SCHAEFER H, et al. Variations of hair follicle size and distribution in different body sites. *J Invest Dermatol* 2004; 122: 14–19.

71. LU GW, CIOTTI SN, VALIVETI S, et al. Targeting the pilosebaceous gland. In: Walters KA, Roberts MS, eds. *Dermatologic, Cosmeceutic and Cosmetic Development.* Informa Healthcare, New York, 2008; 169–188.

72. SCHEUPLEIN RJ. Mechanism of percutaneous adsorption. I. Routes of penetration and the influence of solubility. *J Invest Dermatol* 1965; 45: 334–346.

73. SCHEUPLEIN RJ, BLANK IH. Permeability of the skin. *Physiol Rev* 1971; 51: 702–747.

74. HARADA K, MURAKAMI T, YATA N, et al. Role of intercellular lipids in stratum corneum in the percutaneous permeation of drugs. *J Invest Dermatol* 1992; 99: 278–282.

75. BODDE HE, van den BRINK I, KOERTEN H, et al. Visualization of in vitro percutaneous penetration of mercurin chloride: Transport through intercellular space versus cellular uptake through desmosomes. *J Control Release* 1991; 15: 227–236.

76. KIM YH, GHANEM AH, HIGUCHI WI. Model studies of epidermal permeability. *Semin Dermatol* 1992; 11: 145–156.

77. COOPER ER, KASTING GB. Transport across epithelial membranes. *J Control Rel* 1987; 6: 23–35.

78. WATKINSON AC, BRAIN KR. Mathematical principles in skin permeation. In: Walters KA, ed. *Dermatological and Transdermal Formulations.* Marcel Dekker, New York, 2002; 61–88.

79. ROBERTS MS, CROSS SE, PELLETT MA. Skin transport. In: Walters KA, ed. *Dermatological and Transdermal Formulations.* Marcel Dekker, New York, 2002; 89–196.
80. LIAN G, CHEN L, HAN L. An evaluation of mathematical models for predicting skin permeability. *J Pharm Sci* 2008; 97: 584–598.
81. HADGRAFT J. Skin deep. *Eur J Pharm Biopharm* 2004; 58: 291–299.
82. PUGH WJ, DEGIM IT, HADGRAFT J. Epidermal permeability-penetrant structure relationships: 4, QSAR of permeant diffusion across human stratum corneum in terms of molecular weight, H-bonding and electronic charge. *Int J Pharm* 2000; 197: 203–211.
83. PUGH WJ, ROBERTS MS, HADGRAFT J. Epidermal permeability—Penetrant structure relationships: 3. The effect of hydrogen bonding interactions and molecular size on diffusion across the stratum corneum. *Int J Pharm* 1996; 138: 149–165.
84. FLYNN GL, YALKOWSKY SH. Correlation and prediction of mass transport across membranes. I. Influence of alkyl chain length on flux-determining properties of barrier and diffusant. *J Pharm Sci* 1972; 61: 838–852.
85. BRONAUGH RL, CONGDON ER. Percutaneous absorption of hair dyes: Correlation with partition coefficients. *J Invest Dermatol* 1984; 83: 124–127.
86. BARRY BW, HARRISON SM, DUGARD PH. Vapour and liquid diffusion of model penetrants through human skin; correlation with thermodynamic activity. *J Pharm Pharmacol* 1985; 37: 226–236.
87. ANDERSON BD, HIGUCHI WI, RAYKAR PV. Heterogeneity effects on permeability-partition coefficient relationships in human stratum corneum. *Pharm Res* 1988; 5: 566–573.
88. IDSON B. Percutaneous absorption. *J Pharm Sci* 1975; 64: 901–924.
89. SCHEUPLEIN RJ, BLANK IH, BRAUNER GJ, et al. Percutaneous absorption of steroids. *J Invest Dermatol* 1969; 52: 63–70.
90. KASTING GB, SMITH RL, COOPER ER. Effect of lipid solubility and molecular size on percutaneous absorption. *Pharmacol Skin* 1987; 1: 138–153.
91. FLYNN GL. Mechanism of percutaneous absorption from physicochemical evidence. In: Bronaugh RL, Maibach HI, eds. *Percutaneous Absorption.* Marcel Dekker Inc, New York, 1985; 17–52.
92. RAWLINGS AV, MATTS PJ. Dry skin and moisturizers. In: Walters KA, Roberts MS, eds. *Dermatologic, Cosmeceutic and Cosmetic Development.* Informa Healthcare, New York, 2008; 339–371.
93. RAWLINGS AV, HARDING CR. Moisturization and skin barrier function. *Dermatol Ther* 2004; 17(Suppl 1): 43–48.
94. VERDIER-SEVRAIN S, BONTE F. Skin hydration: A review on its molecular mechanisms. *J Cosmet Dermatol* 2007; 6: 75–82.
95. ROBERTS MS, BOUWSTA JA, PIROT F, et al. Skin hydration-a key determinant in topical absorption. In: Walters KA, Roberts MS, eds. *Dermatologic, Cosmeceutic and Cosmetic Development.* Informa Healthcare, New York, 2008; 115–128.
96. BENSON HAE. Transdermal drug delivery: Penetration enhancement techniques. *Curr Drug Deliv* 2005; 2: 23–33.
97. WICKETT R, VISSCHER M. Structure and function of the epidermal barrier. *Am J Infect Control* 2006; 34: S98–S110.
98. MOHAMMED Y, PROW T. unpublished data.

Chapter 2

Passive Skin Permeation Enhancement

Majella E. Lane, Paulo Santos, Adam C. Watkinson, and Jonathan Hadgraft

SKIN AND PERCUTANEOUS ABSORPTION

The skin is the largest organ of the body and represents 10% of the total body mass in adults, with an average total surface area of 2 m^2.[1] It is a complex organ with a diverse cellular population and a range of physiological activities. The main function of the skin is the protection of internal organs from the external environment by preventing the egress of water and the ingress of toxins. Despite this barrier role, the skin is also an organ that is exploited for drug administration, both local and, to a lesser degree, transdermal.

Delivery of active compounds to the skin has three different goals: epidermal, topical, or transdermal absorption.[2] Cosmetics, insect repellents, and disinfectants are examples of common formulations designed to maintain the active compound on the surface of the skin. Topical formulations allow the active to penetrate into deeper regions of the skin. Finally, transdermal formulations aim to deliver the active into the systemic circulation.

The passive absorption of drugs through the skin occurs via diffusion[3] through intact epidermis (*transepidermal route*) and/or skin appendages (*transappendageal route*).[2] Two pathways through the bulk of the stratum corneum (SC) may exist: the intercellular lipid route between the corneocytes (A—*intercellular*) and the transcellular route through the corneocytes and interleaving lipids (B—*transcellular*).[4,5] Transcellular drug diffusion is often regarded as a polar route through the membrane as the predominantly highly hydrated keratin provides an aqueous environment for the diffusion of hydrophilic drugs. The intercellular route involves drug permeation only via drug partitioning and diffusing into the intercellular lipid matrix. Most drugs that are currently delivered transdermally are hydrophobic, and thus should

Transdermal and Topical Drug Delivery: Principles and Practice, First Edition. Edited by Heather A.E. Benson, Adam C. Watkinson.

preferentially be transported via the lipid channels, suggesting that the intercellular route is the main route of absorption for these drugs.[6–8]

Processes for Percutaneous Absorption

Drug absorption from a transdermal drug delivery system into the systemic circulation may be regarded as passage through consecutive skin layers (or barriers) and involves the following steps:

1. Release from the formulation;
2. Penetration into the SC and permeation/diffusion through it;
3. Partitioning from the SC into the viable epidermis (VE) before reaching the capillaries located in the dermis.

Drug partitioning into the SC is the first limiting factor as the drug diffuses rapidly in the vehicle for most formulations. At the formulation/skin interface, drug partitioning into the membrane is highly dependent on the relative solubility of the drug in the components of the delivery system and in the SC.[9] However, in some situations, drug delivery may also be controlled by the formulation, as is the case for patches with a rate-controlling barrier. After partitioning into the SC, the drug diffuses through the SC at a rate determined by the diffusivity within it.[3] In the deepest layers of the SC, the drug undergoes a second partitioning step at the SC/VE interface.[10,11] As a result, for highly hydrophobic drugs, the VE can constitute a major barrier for drug absorption, as the drug has to partition into this more hydrophilic region.[12] The dermis is also hydrophilic in nature. Once the drug reaches the deepest layers of the VE, the high vasculature of the dermis allows rapid distribution of the drug into the systemic circulation.[13,14]

Factors Affecting Drug Permeation: Properties of the Permeant

The capacity of a molecule to enter the skin depends on its ability to penetrate, consecutively, the hydrophobic and hydrophilic barrier layers of the skin. Permeation through the SC depends on the following physicochemical parameters presented in the succeeding sections.

Partition

Topically applied drugs must partition into the lipophilic domain of the SC (lipid bilayers), then into the more hydrophilic milieu of the VE before reaching the systemic circulation. Therefore, drugs must possess balanced lipid and water solubility in order to be systemically absorbed. Drugs that are too hydrophilic are unlikely to partition from the vehicle into the SC, whereas drugs that are too lipophilic will have a high affinity for the SC and are unlikely to partition (or readily partition) into the VE.

Molecular Size

The molecular weight (MW) of a chemical is a good indicator of its molecular size, which, in turn, is related to the diffusion coefficient according to the Stokes–Einstein equation.[15] As drug diffusion through the skin is a passive mechanism, small molecules traverse the human skin more rapidly than larger molecules.[16] Candidates for transdermal delivery generally have a MW ≤ 500 Da.

Solubility/Melting Point

Another important factor affecting drug permeation is drug solubility in the skin lipids.[8] The solubility of a solute in the intercellular SC lipid domain is determined by the melting point (MP) of the drug. Nitroglycerin (MP 13.5°C) and nicotine (−79°C) are examples of very good skin permeants as they have relatively low MPs and log $K_{oct/water}$ values between 1 and 3.[17]

Ionization

Permeation will also depend on the degree of ionization and how ionization influences the drug solubility in the formulation and drug partitioning into the skin.[8] The ionized species of a drug has a lower permeability coefficient than its respective unionized species, as the log $K_{oct/water}$ of ionized species is also lower.[18] Thus the free acid or free base should be preferentially used in order to improve permeation. However, as noted by Hadgraft and Valenta, the total flux (J_{total}) of a permeant through the skin is the sum of the transport of both the ionized and unionized species, according to Equation 2.1.[19]

$$ J_{total} = k_p^{union} \cdot C_{union} + k_p^{ion} \cdot C_{ion}. \tag{2.1} $$

Ionized species have a low k_p^{ion} and a high aqueous solubility, whereas unionized species will have a low aqueous solubility but a high k_p^{union}. Considering the relative solubilities of each species, it is possible that the lower permeability of the ionized species is compensated for by increased solubility, thus resulting in comparable flux from each species. As a result, the free acid or free base may not be the optimum form for maximizing drug permeation and therefore the influence of changing pH should be explored during formulation development .[19]

Passive Permeation Enhancement

The impermeable nature of the skin is critical for prevention of water loss from the body and to support life on dry land. This protective function also prevents the uptake of drugs and the systemic absorption of therapeutically relevant doses of compounds. Therefore, many strategies have been developed to facilitate drug permeation through the skin.[20] Physical enhancement strategies are not the focus of this chapter as they enhance drug delivery by active methods or by disrupting the skin.[21] Passive penetration enhancement can be achieved by:

1. Increasing the thermodynamic activity of the drug in formulations;
2. Use of chemicals or chemical penetration enhancers (CPE) that interact with skin constituents to promote drug flux.[22]

STRATEGIES TO INFLUENCE THERMODYNAMIC ACTIVITY

The use of supersaturated solutions in transdermal drug delivery was first considered by Higuchi.[23] Supersaturation is a state where the drug is at higher concentration or chemical potential than the solubility limit. As flux through a membrane is driven by the chemical potential gradient, the flux from supersaturated systems increases proportionally. Supersaturated formulations offer several advantages for topical and transdermal drug administration, namely:

1. Increased driving force, which enables molecules to better permeate across the SC;
2. Penetration enhancement without using CPE or physical methods;
3. Concentration reduction, as equivalent flux or enhancement may be achieved at lower doses. This is particularly important for very potent or expensive drugs (e.g., fentanyl).

However, since the activity of supersaturated formulations is higher than that of saturated systems, they are inherently unstable, which prevents their production and storage for long periods of time. Alternative strategies have been explored to produce supersaturated states *in situ* or immediately prior to application in order to avoid these stability issues.[24] Generally, a solution is defined as a molecular dispersion of a solute in a solvent. The activity of a solid in a solution saturated with that solid is equal to that of pure solid and maximal.[25] Supersaturated solutions are usually prepared by changing the drug solubility abruptly.[26] The dependence of the solubility with pH, temperature, and solvent composition is normally manipulated to produce transient metastable and supersaturated phases. The various approaches to produce such systems are described in more detail in the following sections.

Production of Supersaturated Systems

Mixed Cosolvent Systems

Solvents such as ethanol, propylene glycol (PG), and polyethylene glycol (PEG) are often used to increase drug solubility in water or aqueous vehicles. The solubilization effect is primarily dependent on the polarity (or solubility) of the drug with respect to the solvent (S) and cosolvent (CoS).[27] The molar solubility of drug (S_w) in water is defined by:

$$\log S_w = \frac{-\Delta S_f (MP - 25)}{1364} - \log \gamma_w. \tag{2.2}$$

Similarly, the molar solubility of drug in cosolvent (S_{Cos}) is:

$$\log S_{Cos} = \frac{\Delta S_f (MP - 25)}{1364} - \log \gamma_{Cos}, \qquad (2.3)$$

where ΔS_f is the enthalpy of fusion of the solute, MP is the melting point, and γ_w and γ_{Cos} are the activity coefficient of the drug in water and CoS, respectively. Assuming that the solubilization by a cosolvent mixture (S_{mix}) composed of a fraction f_{Cos} of cosolvent and $(1 - f_{Cos})$ of water is a direct contribution of the solubilization of the drug by each solvent, then:

$$\log S_{mix} = f_{Cos} \log S_{Cos} + (1 - f_{Cos}) \log S_w. \qquad (2.4)$$

Replacing the molar solubility defined by Equations 2.2 and 2.3 and simplifying, the following equation can be obtained:

$$\log S_{mix} = \log S_w + (\log \gamma_{Cos} - \log \gamma_w) f_{Cos}. \qquad (2.5)$$

According to Equation 2.5, the solubilization of a nonpolar compound in a mixture of water and CoS would be expected to increase exponentially with the fraction of CoS (Fig. 2.1; black curve). As a result, depending on the initial drug concentration in the solvent with higher solubility, it is possible to prepare saturated or supersaturated solutions, simply by adding the solvent with lower drug solubility. For example, by preparing a saturated solution in solvent b, and diluting with pure solvent a, supersaturated solutions can be obtained along the line $\overline{AB}$. The degree of saturation (DS) is calculated by dividing the theoretical drug concentration in solution by the solubility of the same cosolvent system in equilibrium (black curve).

Hadgraft and coworkers have shown the utility of supersaturated systems prepared by the mixed cosolvent technique for transdermal drug delivery.[28–35] As shown in Table 2.1, mixtures of PG and water have been predominantly used to create

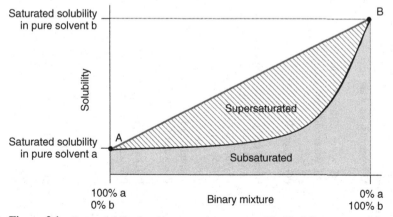

Figure 2.1   Drug solubility in a binary cosolvent system. The black line represents the saturated solubility of a drug in the binary mixture of solvent a and solvent b. By mixing a saturated solution in system b with pure system a, supersaturated ($\overline{AB}$) solutions can be obtained. Adapted from Davis et al.[28]

Table 2.1 Supersaturation Studies for Transdermal Drug Delivery (a Literature Review)

References	Formulation	Membrane	Study/dose	Drug	Polymers
Cosolvent systems					
39	Microemulsions water-free	Rabbit	*In vitro* and *in vivo*/infinite	Bupranolol	–
28	PG : water (different ratios)	Silicone	*In vitro*/0.5 g/cm^2	Hydrocortisone acetate	–
54	PG : water (different ratios)	Silicone and human skin	*In vitro*/~1 mL/cm^2	Oestradiol	HPC, PVA, PVP, PEG 4000, and PEG 8000
32,55	PG : water (40:60 v/v)	Silicone and human skin	*In vitro*/~1.5 mL/cm^2	Piroxicam	HPMC
101	Binary composition of System A (ethanol : PG 50:50 v/v) with System B (water : glycerol 50:50 v/v)	Silicone and human skin (occluded)	*In vivo*/human: 6 μL/cm^2 *In vitro*/silicone: 0.6 mL/cm^2	Fluocinonide	PVP K25
35,53	0.5% carbopol gel and solutions containing PG : water (20:80 v/v)	Silicone	*In vitro*/none	Hydrocortisone acetate	MC, HPMC
30,31	PG : water (40:60 v/v)	Silicone and human skin	*In vitro*/~0.8 mL/cm^2	Ibuprofen	HPMC, hydroxypropyl-β-CD
29	PG : buffer pH 3.0 (50:50 v/v)	Silicone	*In vitro*/0.5 mL/cm^2	Diclofenac	HPMC, hydroxypropyl-β-CD
102	PG : water (70:30 v/v)	Pig ear and silicone	*In vitro*	Lipophilic lavendustin derivative	–
103,104	PG : water (30:70 v/v) PEG400 : water (30:70 v/v) IPM : silicone (30:70 v/v)	Pig ear	*In vitro*/2 mL/cm^2	Lipophilic lavendustin derivative	–
37	pH 8.0 : pH 2.0 (80:20 v/v)	Silicone and human skin	*In vitro*/1 mL/cm^2	Salicylic acid	HPMC

Solvent evaporation

Ref.	Vehicle	Membrane	Dose	Drug	Polymer
40	PG or IPM (nonvolatile solvents) in isopropanol (volatile) at different concentrations	Human skin	In vitro/80 μL/cm²	Fluocinolide and fluocinolone acetonide	–
105	o/w cream or gels with ethanol as volatile solvent	Silicone	In vitro/16 mg/cm²	Hydrocortisone butyrate propionate	–
47	PG : water : ethanol (20:63:17 v/v)	Human skin	In vitro/~40 μL/cm²	Minoxidil	–
106	EtOH : pH 4.2 buffer (25:75 v/v)	Rat	In vitro/780 μL/cm²	Sodium nonivamide acetate	MC, HPC, HPMC, PVP and Eudragit®
104	EtOH : PG 50:50	Pig ear	In vitro/150 μL/cm²	Lipophilic lavendustin derivative	–
50–52	Binary and ternary mixtures with acetone (volatile solvent), PG (hydrophilic nonvolatile), and/or IPM (lipophilic nonvolatile)	Rat and silicone	in vivo/rat: 200 μL/cm²; in vitro/silicone: 1 mL/cm², rat: 125 μl/cm²	Nifedipine	Eudragit RS100L, PVP, PVP K30, EC, and HPMCP
107,108	PG : water : ethanol (1:1:4)	Rat	In vitro/5 μL/cm²	Testosterone	Vinylpyrrolidone/vinyl acetate copolymers and RAMEB

Heating and cooling

Ref.	Vehicle	Membrane	Dose	Drug	Polymer
43	Liquid paraffin and (1%–15%) hydrogenated soybean phospholipids	Cellulose	In vitro/0.1 g/cm²	Indomethacin, ketoprofen, flubiprofen, and ibuprofen	–
104	Cream	Pig ear	In vitro/150 mg/cm²	Lipophilic lavendustin derivative	–

The table shows transdermal and topical drug delivery studies conducted with supersaturated formulations prepared by solvent evaporation, cosolvent mixing, and heating and cooling techniques.

HPMC, hydroxypropylmethylcellulose; HPC, hydroxypropylcellulose; HPMCP, hydroxypropylmethylcellulose phthalate; EC, Ethyl cellulose; MC, methyl cellulose; PVA, polyvinyl alcohol; PVP, polyvinylpyrrolidone; CD, cyclodextrin; RAMEB, methylated-β-cyclodextrin; PEG, polyethylene glycol.

supersaturated formulations by this technique. However, other solvent systems have also been explored to produce supersaturation by CoS mixing. Based on the work performed by Watkinson et al., who observed an exponential increase in the drug solubility with pH,[36] Leveque et al. proposed the use of a combination of buffer solutions with varying pH as a method to produce supersaturated formulations.[37] The authors showed that these supersaturated solutions improved transdermal drug permeation with the added advantages of having pH values similar to that of skin and use of aqueous versus organic solvents.

However, supersaturated systems prepared by the CoS technique are not very stable and stabilization strategies are needed for the effective use of these formulations. Although polymers have been shown to increase the stability of these formulations for up to 1 month without signs of crystallization, long-term stability remains a problem.[38] Kemken et al. suggested the formation of supersaturated formulations *in situ* by the application of subsaturated formulations that become supersaturated during the application period, as an alternative to overcome long-term formulation stability problems. The authors demonstrated that the uptake of water by water-free microemulsions, under occlusive conditions, increased the thermodynamic activity of bupranolol with increased drug permeation *in vivo*.[39]

Loss of Solvent

An alternative technique to produce supersaturated states is based on changes in drug concentration with solvent evaporation. After application of a formulation, the evaporation of any volatile components will increase the drug concentration and produce supersaturated residues as long as the amount of drug exceeds the solubility in the nonvolatile components (or residual phase). This method avoids the long-term stability issues related with supersaturated CoS formulations, as supersaturation is only achieved *in situ*, after application to skin. Volatile components (e.g., ethanol, acetone, isopropanol) are typically used (Table 2.1), as the rapid evaporation will also lead to rapid transitions in residual drug solubility, thus avoiding drug crystallization. Initial studies with supersaturated formulations for transdermal drug delivery exploited solvent loss to increase drug concentration and produce supersaturated states in the residual phase.[40] Since then, little work has been reported using this approach to produce supersaturated states with the exception of the Metered-Dose Transdermal System (MDTS®, Acrux Ltd., Melbourne, Australia). This technology relies on the production of a metastable residue *in situ* by solvent evaporation. Promising results for transdermal drug delivery, *in vitro* and *in vivo*,[41,42] have been reported and several products are now available for clinical use.

Other Techniques

More complex techniques such as *heating and cooling* and production of solid dispersions may also be used to produce supersaturated formulations with increased drug permeation.[43,44]

Stabilization of Supersaturated Systems and Effect of Additives

Stabilization of thermodynamically unstable formulations is necessary for effective permeation enhancement using supersaturated formulations. In many cases, the formation of crystals occurs spontaneously from supersaturated solutions.[45] Application of external forces, such as ultrasound, stirring, or seeding with small particles may also result in the formation of nuclei of critical size and subsequent crystal growth.[46,47] Additives such as hydrophilic polymers are often used to improve formulation stability.[17] Although growth inhibition of crystals by polymers has been extensively reported in the literature (Table 2.1), their mechanism of stabilization is still unknown, and two main theories have been proposed: diffusion theory and surface adsorption theory.

In the context of diffusion theory, it is the increase in viscosity induced by swelling of the hydrophilic polymers that inhibits the crystal growth. In other words, the crystal growth is seen as a reverse diffusion process, where the increase in the solution viscosity will create a stagnant layer around the nuclei, thus delaying the crystal growth.[44]

According to the surface adsorption theory, a molecule has to diffuse onto the crystal surface before incorporation into the crystal site.[48] If a molecule reaches a flat surface of a crystal, it has only one single binding surface, and therefore dissolution is likely to occur. However, when encountering a corner (step and kink sites), more binding sites exist and redissolution is less likely to occur. As a result, the molecule will be incorporated into the crystal.[48] Polymers are believed to stabilize supersaturated solutions by binding to the crystal surface, thus preventing the molecules from binding onto these growth sites.[44,49]

Several authors have stabilized supersaturated states by adding polymers (see Table 2.1). Kondo et al. demonstrated a significant improvement in drug permeation across membranes *in vitro* and *in vivo* when a polymer was added to supersaturated formulations produced by solvent evaporation.[50-52] In another example, using supersaturated solutions prepared by the cosolvent technique, Raghavan et al. suggested that the growth inhibition of hydrocortisone acetate crystals by hydroxypropyl methylcellulose (HPMC) depends on the hydrogen bonding between the drug and the polymer.[53] As a result, it was concluded that crystal growth is inhibited by the adsorption of the polymer onto the crystal surface. The same conclusions were reported for the stabilization of supersaturated solutions of ibuprofen by HPMC.[30] Both studies also reported a change in the crystal size and morphology by the presence of the different polymers, which indicates that the drug–polymer interactions are dependent on the nature of the polymer. Pellett et al. suggested that polymers may also inhibit the polymorphic transitions of drugs to more stable forms.[32] According to the authors, the inhibition of the conversion of the anhydrous form of piroxicam (less soluble) to hydrate form (more soluble) by HPMC was the main mechanism responsible for the stabilization of supersaturated solutions, prepared by mixed cosolvents.

Even in the presence of polymers, some authors suggested that nucleation could be induced by the irregular skin surface or by the presence of desquamated cells that would act as nuclei for crystal growth. However, this is not the case. On the contrary, it was even suggested that supersaturated states may be more stable when applied on the SC than on artificial membranes.[32,54] Pellett et al. suggested that the viscosity of the SC lipids or the presence of natural antinucleant agents in the skin may contribute to the observed efficacy of supersaturated solutions *in vitro* using human skin.[55] In some cases, high drug enhancement flux through human skin (13-fold) was reported, using supersaturated formulations with a DS 18-fold that of saturated solubility and stabilized by PVP.[54]

CHEMICAL PENETRATION ENHANCERS

CPEs are pharmacologically inactive compounds that may partition and diffuse into the membrane and interact with the SC components.[56] Many substances have been identified as drug penetration enhancers, but safety remains the major concern, which limits their clinical use.[57,58] Therefore, researchers have attempted to identify new CPEs that are classified as GRAS (generally recognized as safe).[59,60] Table 2.2 lists the principal properties of an ideal enhancer[59] and Table 2.3 illustrates some of the compounds which are currently in use in transdermal formulations.

Mechanism of Action of Chemical Penetration Enhancers

The intercellular lipids are regarded as the major determinant for the resistance of the skin to passive drug diffusion. Therefore, substances that perturb the highly ordered arrangement of the intercellular lipid bilayers are likely to reduce the diffusional resistance of the SC to most solutes.[4] CPEs are believed to affect permeation by interacting at three main sites (Fig. 2.2) associated with lipid bilayers.[4]

1. Interaction with the polar head groups of the lipids (**Site A**);
2. Interaction in the aqueous domain of the lipid bilayers (**Site B**);
3. Interaction with the lipid alkyl chain (**Site C**).

Table 2.2   Properties of an Ideal Chemical Penetration Enhancer

Ideal chemical penetration enhancer

- Pharmacologically inert
- Nonirritating, nonallergenic, nontoxic
- Nondamaging to viable cells
- Rapid onset of effect with a predictable duration of activity
- Effects are completely and rapidly reversible upon removal
- Effects do not cause the loss of endogenous materials from the body
- Physically and chemically compatible with drugs and excipients in the dosage form
- Cosmetically acceptable when applied to the skin
- Odorless, inexpensive, tasteless, colorless

Source: Adapted from Finnin and Morgan.[59]

Table 2.3   Typical Enhancers Used in Transdermal Delivery

Active	Patch trade name	Enhancer
Fentanyl	Fentalis	Ethanol
	Matrifen	Dipropylene glycol
Nitroglycerin	Minitran	Ethyl oleate
		Glyceryl monolaurate
Estradiol	Estraderm	Isopropyl palmitate
	Estradot	Dipropylene glycol
		Oleyl alcohol
	Fematrix	Diethyltoluamide
	Oestrogel	Ethanol
	Progynova	Ethyl oleate
		Glycerol monolaurate
		IPM
Ethinyl estradiol, norelgestromin	Evra	Lauryl lactate
Oxybutynin	Kentera	Triacetin
Testosterone	Andropatch	Ethanol
		Glycerol monoleate
		Methyl oleate
	Axiron	Octyl salicylate
	Intrinsa	Sorbitan oleate
	Testim	Ethanol
		Pentadecalactone
		PG
	Testogel	Ethanol
		IPM
	Tostran	Ethanol
		Isopropyl alcohol
		OA
		PG

The cornified cell envelope and intercellular junctions are further sites where CPEs can interact.[61] Some CPEs may also cause lipid extraction.[20]

CPEs that interact with the polar head group (**Site A**) by establishing H-bonding and/or ionic forces may disturb the hydration spheres of the lipid bilayers and subsequently disturb the packing order within this polar plane (Fig. 2.2).[4] This perturbation fluidizes the lipid domain and also increases the water volume between layers, thus reducing the diffusional resistance, and therefore promoting the flux of both hydrophilic and lipophilic penetrants.[9] The presence of cholesterol sulfate and the carboxylic acids should permit the expansion (or swelling) of the nearby lipid head groups, thus increasing the area in **Site B** for polar diffusion.[4] For example, Azone® (1-dodecylazacycloheptan-2-one) is an effective skin enhancer at low concentrations (1%–10% w/v).[62] Although its mechanism is not completely understood, *in vitro*

(a)

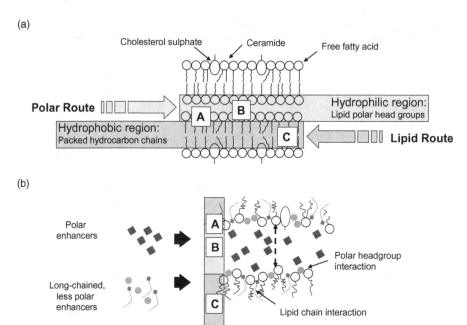

(b)

Figure 2.2 Mechanisms of action of CPEs. (a) Schematic representation of the highly ordered and packed lipid bilayers and the hydrophilic and lipophilic routes of drug penetration through SC with proposed sites of action (**A**, **B**, and **C**) for the permeation enhancers. (b) Action of penetration enhancers: Long chain enhancers include compounds such as Azone, IPM, or OA; circles represent small molecules such as water and squares represent solvents such as PG and dimethyl sulfoxide (DMSO). Adapted from Barry.[4]

permeation, differential scanning calorimetry (DSC), and Fourier transform infrared (FTIR) studies indicated that Azone increases the diffusion coefficient of the drug in the skin by fluidizing the lipid bilayers.[63–65] Structure activity relationships for Azone and analogs suggested that hydrogen bond formation between the polar head group of Azone and ceramides (**Site A**) is important for the enhancement properties observed.[66]

Many CPEs are able to insert directly between the hydrophobic lipid tails (**Site C**). As a result, they are able to disturb the lipid packing, thus increasing lipid fluidity and promoting drug permeation.[4] In some situations, lipid disturbance is also accompanied by some degree of disorder in the polar head group, thus facilitating the permeation of solutes in this region. Several reports suggest that the ability of these CPEs to disturb the packing of the lipid alkyl chains is related to structural features such as their polar head and long saturated alkyl chain (9–14 carbon atoms appear to be optimal),[67,68] For unsaturated long fatty chains, C_{18} appears to be optimal, as for oleic acid (OA).[69] In addition, using a series of isomers of octadecenoic acid, it was found that the *cis* double bound configuration disturbs the intercellular packing more than the *trans* arrangement.[70] The same study also observed that the flux enhancement increases with the distance of the double bond from the carboxylic group. A parabolic relationship between carbon chain length of fatty acids and skin permeation enhancement was found,[71] which represents the balance between partition coefficient/solubility parameter and affinity to the skin.[72] In contrast to Azone, which is homogeneously distributed, FTIR studies using perdeuterated OA indicate that this enhancer forms pools in the skin and the permeant diffuses faster either through these or through the defects between the pools of OA and the structured lipids.[73]

Lastly, CPEs may affect the aqueous domain (**Site B**) by increasing the solubility of this site for the permeant (Fig. 2.2). Solvents such as PG, ethanol, Transcutol® (diethylene glycol monoethyl ether), and N-methyl pyrrolidone are believed to act in this way.[22] These solvents modify the skin permeability by altering the solubility parameter of the skin, in order to match the solubility parameter of the permeant.[22] As a consequence, the partitioning of the drug from the vehicle into the SC increases.[17] Solubility parameters (δ), as defined by Hansen, measure how materials will interact with each other. Materials that have similar solubility parameters are likely to have a high affinity for each other.[74] For example, skin pretreatment with PG ($\delta_{PG} = 28.6$ MPa$^{1/2}$) increases the permeation of metronidazole ($\delta_{Met} = 27.4$ MPa$^{1/2}$), because it shifts the solubility parameter of the skin,[75] estimated to be $\delta_{skin} \sim 20$ MPa$^{1/2}$ to higher and closer values to that of the drug.[17,76] Similarly, Transcutol increased the permeation of some drugs by increasing their SC/vehicle partition coefficients.[65,77]

Mechanisms of Permeation Enhancement: Case Studies

Propylene Glycol

Several biophysical techniques have been used to elucidate the mechanism of PG permeation. DSC studies have shown that the interaction of PG with α-keratin resulted in a smaller and broader transition with increasing concentrations of PG.[78] In addition, slight changes to two other major lipid transitions have also been observed, suggesting that PG may also increase the lipid fluidity.[79,80] As a result, the drug diffusion in the lipid bilayers might also increase. However, it is believed that by competing for the solvation sites of the polar headgroups of the lipid bilayers, PG is in reality increasing the drug partitioning into the SC.[79] Recently, wide- and small-angle X-ray diffraction showed additional interference of PG with the SC lipids.[81] In particular, this study revealed that PG molecules integrate into hydrophilic regions of the packed lipids and increase the distance in the lamellar phase by incorporation between the hydrophilic head groups of the bilayers and in the perpendicular direction to the bilayer (Fig. 2.3).

In the literature, the pre-treatment of skin membranes with PG *in vitro* for 12 hours prior to the application of a solvent deposited dry drug film (100 μL of a 0.3% solution in acetone: ethanol 1:1 v/v), has been shown to increase the penetration of 5-fluorouracil and estradiol by 12- and ninefold, respectively, compared

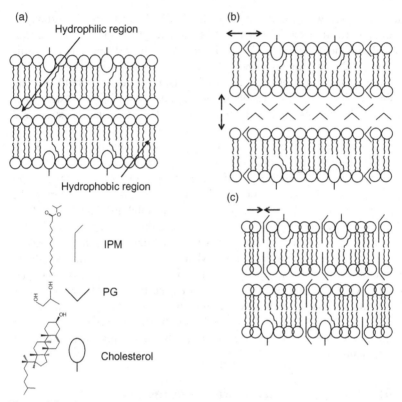

Figure 2.3   Mechanism of action of PG and IPM. (a) Untreated skin; (b) pretreated with PG; and (c) pretreated with IPM. Adapted from Brinkmann and Muller.[80]

with untreated skin.[82] More importantly, PG has shown a synergistic activity with lipophilic enhancers such as terpenes,[79] OA,[81] Azone,[81] and isopropyl myristate (IPM).[83,84] Despite this evidence, a neat PG enhancement effect is still controversial, with some authors suggesting that PG itself is an ineffective chemical penetration enhancer.[77] Møllgaard suggested that the inconsistency in the enhancement activity of PG is the result of different experimental conditions. In particular, the author suggested that PG efficacy is more evident when the SC is not fully hydrated, that is, under nonocclusive conditions.[85]

Isopropyl Myristate

Although IPM has been widely used as a safe permeation enhancer, surprisingly, its mechanism of action has not yet been clarified in detail. Sato et al. suggested that IPM affects the lipids of the SC and the partition coefficient between the SC and vehicle of both drug and solvent.[83] DSC studies showed a decrease in enthalpy and a negative shift in the phase transition temperatures of SC lipids, indicating an integration of IPM within lipid bilayer.[86] These shifts are associated with an increase in the lipid fluidity.[87] However, opposing results were observed with wide angle X-ray diffraction (WAXD) and small angle X-ray diffraction (SAXD) techniques. These studies indicated that IPM slightly increases the short distance of the orthorhombical lipids, while decreasing the hexagonal lipids and keeping the interlamellar distance constant (Fig. 2.3C).[88] The authors suggested that the pre-treatment of skin with IPM resulted in a more densely packed bilayer and a loss of the corneocyte-bonded lipids. In addition, it was also suggested that IPM interacts with the lipids with an anchoring of the isopropyl group in the polar region of the layer.[81] Finally, *in vivo* tape-stripping studies suggested that IPM does not affect the diffusivity of terbinafine in skin in comparison with aqueous solutions.[89]

MISCELLANEOUS PASSIVE PENETRATION STRATEGIES

Ion-Pair Formation

Ion pairs are defined as neutral species formed only by electrostatic attraction between oppositely charged ions[90] that are sufficiently lipophilic to dissolve in a lipoidal medium such as the SC. In theory, ion pair formation offers several advantages over other permeation enhancements strategies, namely enhancement of skin transport of ionic drugs without modification of their structure, and without change in skin barrier function.[91] Hadgraft et al.[92] reported an enhancement in the percutaneous absorption of sodium salicylate using an ethoxylated amine. This approach has also been investigated with varying degrees of success for skin delivery of a range of other molecules including bupranolol, terbutaline, physostigmine, lidocaine, methotrexate, cephalexin, and 5-amino levulinic acid.[91,93–97] Notwithstanding the reports in the literature, there are only a few commercial products which have exploited this strategy, one example being the diethylamine salt of diclofenac, which is marketed as a topical gel.

Eutectic Mixtures

A reduction in the MP of a permeant will have a direct effect on its solubility in skin and thus should increase skin permeability. Manipulation of the MP of a drug may be achieved by formation of a eutectic mixture. In a simple binary eutectic system, the two components inhibit the crystallization process of one another at certain ratios. The overall system has a lower MP than the individual components. A eutectic system is used in the anesthetic cream EMLA (AstraZeneca, Wilmington, DE), which is formed from a mixture of prilocaine and lidocaine and is reported to provide a greater anesthetic response than a noneutectic formulation.[98] The formation of eutectic systems in order to enhance dermal penetration of ibuprofen and propranolol has also been reported by Stott and coworkers.[99,100]

SUMMARY

The routes by which drugs permeate the skin have been considered, as well as the major factors impacting on (trans)dermal delivery. Passive permeation enhancement remains the most widely used approach for (trans)dermal drug delivery. The major approaches that have demonstrated success to date are discussed in some detail. It is important to note that fundamental biophysical studies remain to be conducted on many of the more commonly used penetration enhancers. Strategies less frequently employed have also been discussed and commercial examples have been provided where relevant.

REFERENCES

1. WASHINGTON C, WASHINGTON N. Drug delivery to the skin. In: Wilson CG, Washington N, eds. *Physiological Pharmaceutics: Biological Barriers to Drug Absorption*, 1st ed. Ellis Horwood, Chichester, 1989; 109–120.
2. TROMMER H, NEUBERT RH. Overcoming the stratum corneum: The modulation of skin penetration. A review. *Skin Pharmacol Physiol* 2006; 19: 106–121.
3. SCHEUPLEIN RJ. Permeability of the skin. *Physiol Rev* 1971; 51: 702–747.
4. BARRY BW. Lipid-protein-partition theory of skin penetration enhancement. *J Control Release* 1991; 15: 237–248.
5. ROBERTS MS. Targeted drug delivery to the skin and deeper tissues: Role of physiology, solute structure and disease. *Clin Exp Pharmacol Physiol* 1997; 24: 874–879.
6. ROBERTS MS, CROSS SE, PELLETT MA. Skin transport. In: Walters KA, ed. *Dermatological and Transdermal Formulations*. Marcel Dekker, Inc, New York, 2002; 89–195.
7. ALBERY WJ, HADGRAFT J. Percutaneous absorption: In vivo experiments. *J Pharm Pharmacol* 1979; 31: 140–147.
8. HADGRAFT J. Skin deep. *Eur J Pharm Biopharm* 2004; 58: 291–299.
9. WALKER RB, SMITH EW. The role of percutaneous penetration enhancers. *Adv Drug Deliv Rev* 1996; 18: 295–301.
10. EGELRUD T. Desquamation in the stratum corneum. *Acta Derm Venereol Supp* 2000; 208: 44–45.
11. HADGRAFT J. Structure activity relationships and percutaneous absorption. *J Control Release* 1991; 15: 221–226.
12. CROSS SE, MAGNUSSON BM, WINCKLE G, ANISSIMOV Y, ROBERTS MS. Determination of the effect of lipophilicity on the in vitro permeability and tissue reservoir characteristics of topically applied solutes in human skin layers. *J Invest Dermatol* 2003; 120: 759–764.
13. MICHAELS AS, CHANDRASEKARAN SK, SHAW JE. Drug permeation through human skin: Theory and in vitro experimental measurement. *AIChE J* 1975; 21: 985–996.
14. ALBERY WJ, GUY RH, HADGRAFT J. Percutaneous absorption: Transport in the dermis. *Int J Pharm* 1983; 15: 125–148.
15. CRANK J. The diffusion equations. In: Crank J, ed. *The Mathematics of Diffusion*. Clarendon Press, Oxford, 1975; 1–10.
16. SCHEUPLEIN RJ, BLANK IH, BRAUNER GJ, MacFARLANE DJ. Percutaneous absorption of steroids. *J Invest Dermatol* 1969; 52: 63–70.
17. HADGRAFT J. Skin, the final frontier. *Int J Pharm* 2001; 224: 1–18.
18. VECCHIA BE, BUNGE AL. Evaluating the transdermal permeability of chemicals. In: Guy RH, Hadgraft J, eds. *Transdermal Drug Delivery*, 2nd ed., Revised and Expanded. Marcel Dekker, New York, 2003; 25–55.
19. HADGRAFT J, VALENTA C. pH, pKa and dermal delivery. *Int J Pharm* 2000; 200: 243–247.

20. BARRY BW. Novel mechanisms and devices to enable successful transdermal drug delivery. *Eur J Pharm Sci* 2001; 14: 101–114.
21. MITRAGOTRI S. Breaking the skin barrier. *Adv Drug Deliv Rev* 2004; 56: 555–716.
22. HADGRAFT J. Passive enhancement strategies in topical and transdermal drug delivery. *Int J Pharm* 1999; 184: 1–6.
23. HIGUCHI T. Physical chemical analysis of percutaneous absorption process from creams and ointments. *J Soc Cosmet Chem* 1960; 11: 85–97.
24. DAVIS AF. Topical drug release system. U.S. Patent 4,767,751. 1988.
25. JAMES KC. Solutions and solubility. In: James KC, ed. *Solubility and Related Properties*. Marcel Dekker, New York, 1986; 1–52.
26. DAVIS A, GYURIK RJ, HADGRAFT J, PELLETT MA, WALTERS KA. Formulation strategies for modulating skin permeation. In: Walters KA, ed. *Dermatological and Transdermal Formulations*. Marcel Dekker, New York, 2002; 271–317.
27. YALKOWSKY SH. Solubilization of drugs by cosolvents. In: Yalkowsky SH, Roseman TJ, eds. *Techniques of Solubilization of drugs*. Marcel Dekker, New York, 1981; 91–134.
28. DAVIS AF, HADGRAFT J. Effect of supersaturation on membrane transport: 1. Hydrocortisone acetate. *Int J Pharm* 1991; 76: 1–8.
29. DIAS MMR, RAGHAVAN SL, PELLETT MA, HADGRAFT J. The effect of beta-cyclodextrins on the permeation of diclofenac from supersaturated solutions. *Int J Pharm* 2003; 263: 173–181.
30. IERVOLINO M, CAPPELLO B, RAGHAVAN SL, HADGRAFT J. Penetration enhancement of ibuprofen from supersaturated solutions through human skin. *Int J Pharm* 2001; 212: 131–141.
31. IERVOLINO M, RAGHAVAN SL, HADGRAFT J. Membrane penetration enhancement of ibuprofen using supersaturation. *Int J Pharm* 2000; 198: 229–238.
32. PELLETT MA, CASTELLANO S, HADGRAFT J, DAVIS AF. The penetration of supersaturated solutions of piroxicam across silicone membranes and human skin in vitro. *J Control Release* 1997; 46: 205–214.
33. PELLETT MA, DAVIS AF, HADGRAFT J. Effect of supersaturation on membrane transport: 2. *Piroxicam Int J Pharm* 1994; 111: 1–6.
34. RAGHAVAN SL, KIEPFER B, DAVIS AF, KAZARIAN SG, HADGRAFT J. Membrane transport of hydrocortisone acetate from supersaturated solutions; the role of polymers. *Int J Pharm* 2001; 221: 95–105.
35. RAGHAVAN SL, TRIVIDIC A, DAVIS AF, HADGRAFT J. Effect of cellulose polymers on supersaturation and in vitro membrane transport of hydrocortisone acetate. *Int J Pharm* 2000; 193: 231–237.
36. WATKINSON AC, BRAIN KR, WALTERS KA. The penetration of ibuprofen through human skin in vitro: Vehicle, enhancer and pH effects. In: Brain KR, James V, Walters KA, eds. *Prediction of Percutaneous Penetration*. STS Publishing, Cardiff, 1993; 335–341.
37. LEVEQUE N, RAGHAVAN SL, LANE ME, HADGRAFT J. Use of a molecular form technique for the penetration of supersaturated solutions of salicylic acid across silicone membranes and human skin in vitro. *Int J Pharm* 2006; 318: 49–54.
38. RAGHAVAN SL, SCHUESSEL K, DAVIS A, HADGRAFT J. Formation and stabilisation of triclosan colloidal suspensions using supersaturated systems. *Int J Pharm* 2003; 261: 153–158.
39. KEMKEN J, ZIEGLER A, MÜLLER BW. Influence of supersaturation on the pharmacodynamic effect of bupranolol after dermal administration using microemulsions as vehicle. *Pharm Res* 1992; 9: 554–558.
40. COLDMAN MF, POULSEN BJ, HIGUCHI T. Enhancement of percutaneous absorption by the use of volatile: Nonvolatile systems as vehicles. *J Pharm Sci* 1969; 58: 1098–1102.
41. MORGAN TM, O'SULLIVAN HM, REED BL, FINNIN BC. Transdermal delivery of estradiol in postmenopausal women with a novel topical aerosol. *J Pharm Sci* 1998; 87: 1226–1228.
42. MORGAN TM, PARR RA, REED BL, FINNIN BC. Enhanced transdermal delivery of sex hormones in swine with a novel topical aerosol. *J Pharm Sci* 1998; 87: 1219–1225.
43. HENMI T, FUJII M, KIKUCHI K, YAMANOBE N, MATSUMOTO M. Application of an oily gel formed by hydrogenated soybean phospholipids as a percutaneous absorption-type ointment base. *Chem Pharm Bull* 1994; 42: 651–655.

44. DAVIS AF, HADGRAFT J. Supersaturated solutions as topical drug delivery systems. In: Walters KA, Hadgraft J, eds. *Pharmaceutical Skin Penetration Enhancement*. Marcel Dekker, New York, 1993; 243–267.

45. MA X, TAW J, CHIANG C-M. Control of drug crystallization in transdermal matrix system. *Int J Pharm* 1996; 142: 115–119.

46. MOSER K, KRIWET K, KALIA YN, GUY RH. Stabilization of supersaturated solutions of a lipophilic drug for dermal delivery. *Int J Pharm* 2001; 224: 169–176.

47. CHIANG CM, FLYNN GL, WEINER ND, SZPUNAR GJ. Bioavailability assessment of topical delivery systems: Effect of vehicle evaporation upon in vitro delivery of minoxidil from solution formulations. *Int J Pharm* 1989; 55: 229–236.

48. FRANK FC. The influence of dislocations on crystal growth. *Discuss Faraday Soc* 1949; 5: 48–54.

49. PELLETT MA, RAGHAVAN SL, HADGRAFT J, DAVIS AF. The application of supersaturated systems to percutaneous drug delivery. In: Guy RH, Hadgraft J, eds. *Transdermal Drug Delivery*, 2nd ed. Marcel Dekker, New York, 2003; 305–326.

50. KONDO S, YAMANAKA C, SUGIMOTO I. Enhancement of transdermal delivery by superfluous thermodynamic potential. III. Percutaneous absorption of nifedipine in rats. *J Pharmaco-Biodyn* 1987; 10: 743–749.

51. KONDO S, SUGIMOTO I. Enhancement of transdermal delivery by superfluous thermodynamic potential. I. Thermodynamic analysis of nifedipine transport across the lipoidal barrier. *J Pharmaco-Biodyn* 1987; 10: 587–594.

52. KONDO S, YAMASAKI-KONISHI H, SUGIMOTO I. Enhancement of transdermal delivery by superfluous thermodynamic potential. II. In vitro-in vivo correlation of percutaneous nifedipine transport. *J Pharmaco-Biodyn* 1987; 10: 662–668.

53. RAGHAVAN SL, TRIVIDIC A, DAVIS AF, HADGRAFT J. Crystallization of hydrocortisone acetate: Influence of polymers. *Int J Pharm* 2001; 212: 213–221.

54. MEGRAB NA, WILLIAMS AC, BARRY BW. Oestradiol permeation through human skin and silastic membrane: Effects of propylene glycol and supersaturation. *J Control Release* 1995; 36: 277–294.

55. PELLETT MA, ROBERTS MS, HADGRAFT J. Supersaturated solutions evaluated with an in vitro stratum corneum tape stripping technique. *Int J Pharm* 1997; 151: 91–98.

56. MARJUKKA SUHONEN TA, BOUWSTRA J, URTTI A. Chemical enhancement of percutaneous absorption in relation to stratum corneum structural alterations. *J Control Release* 1999; 59: 149–161.

57. KARANDE P. Principles of penetration. *Nat Rev Drug Discov* 2005; 4: 372–373.

58. KARANDE P, JAIN A, ERGUN K, KISPERSKY V, MITRAGOTRI S. Design principles of chemical penetration enhancers for transdermal drug delivery. *Proc Nat Acad Sci* 2005; 102: 4688–4693.

59. FINNIN BC, MORGAN TM. Transdermal penetration enhancers: Applications, limitations, and potential. *J Pharm Sci* 1999; 88: 955–958.

60. TRAVERSA B. Enhancement of the percutaneous absorption of the opioid analgesic fentanyl. PhD Thesis. Department of Pharmaceutics, Victorian College of Pharmacy, Monash University, Melbourne, 2005.

61. WALTERS KA, ROBERTS MS. The structure and function of skin. In: Walters KA, ed. *Dermatological and Transdermal Formulations*. Marcel Dekker, New York, 2002; 1–39.

62. HADGRAFT J, WILLIAMS DG, ALLAN G. Azone: Mechanisms of action and clinical effect. In: Walters KA, Hadgraft J, eds. *Pharmaceutical Skin Penetration Enhancement*. Marcel Dekker, New York, 1993; 175–197.

63. LAMBERT WJ, HIGUCHI WI, KNUTSON K, KRILL SL. Dose-dependent enhancement effects of Azone on skin permeability. *Pharm Res* 1989; 6: 798–803.

64. HARRISON JE, GROUNDWATER PW, BRAIN KR, HADGRAFT J. Azone(R) induced fluidity in human stratum corneum. A Fourier transform infrared spectroscopy investigation using the perdeuterated analogue. *J Control Release* 1996; 41: 283–290.

65. HARRISON JE, WATKINSON AC, GREEN DM, HADGRAFT J, BRAIN K. The relative effect of Azone and transcutol on permeant diffusivity and solubility in human stratum corneum. *Pharm Res* 1996; 13: 542–546.

66. HADGRAFT J, PECK J, WILLIAMS DG, PUGH WJ, ALLAN G. Mechanisms of action of skin penetration enhancers/retarders: Azone and analogues. *Int J Pharm* 1996; 141: 17–25.
67. AUNGST BJ, ROGERS NJ, SHEFTER E. Enhancement of naloxone penetration through human skin in vitro using fatty acids, fatty alcohols, surfactants, sulfoxides and amides. *Int J Pharm* 1986; 33: 225–234.
68. BOUWSTRA JA, PESCHIER LJC, BRUSSEE J, BODDE HE. Effect of N-alkyl-azocycloheptan-2-ones including Azone on the thermal behaviour of human stratum corneum. *Int J Pharm* 1989; 52: 47–54.
69. WILLIAMS AC, BARRY BW. Penetration enhancers. *Adv Drug Deliv Rev* 2004; 56: 603–618.
70. GOLDEN GM, MCKIE JE, POTTS RO. Role of stratum corneum lipid fluidity in transdermal drug flux. *J Pharm Sci* 1987; 76: 25–28.
71. CHIEN YW, XU H, CHIANG C-C, HUANG Y-C. Transdermal controlled administration of indomethacin. I. Enhancement of skin permeability. *Pharm Res* 1988; 5: 103–106.
72. OGISO T, SHINTANI M. Mechanism for the enhancement effect of fatty acids on the percutaneous absorption of propranolol. *J Pharm Sci* 1990; 79: 1065–1071.
73. ONGPIPATTANAKUL B, BURNETTE RR, POTTS RO, FRANCOEUR ML. Evidence that oleic acid exists in a separate phase within stratum corneum lipids. *Pharm Res* 1991; 8: 350–354.
74. HANSEN C. *Hansen Solubility Parameters: A user's Handbook*. CRC Press, Boca Raton, FL, 2000; 1–24.
75. LIRON Z, COHEN S. Percutaneous absorption of alkanoic acids II: Application of regular solution theory. *J Pharm Sci* 1984; 73: 538–542.
76. WOTTON PK, MOLLGAARD B, HADGRAFT J, HOELGAARD A. Vehicle effect on topical drug delivery. III. Effect of Azone on the cutaneous permeation of metronidazole and propylene glycol. *Int J Pharm* 1985; 24: 19–26.
77. PUGLIA C, BONINA F, TRAPANI G, FRANCO M, RICCI M. Evaluation of in vitro percutaneous absorption of lorazepam and clonazepam from hydro-alcoholic gel formulations. *Int J Pharm* 2001; 228: 79–87.
78. BARRY BW. Mode of action of penetration enhancers in human skin. *J Control Release* 1987; 6: 85–97.
79. BARRY BW, BENNETT SL. Effect of penetration enhancers on the permeation of mannitol, hydrocortisone and progesterone through human skin. *J Pharm Pharmacol* 1987; 39: 535–546.
80. CORNWELL PA, BARRY BW, BOUWSTRA JA, GOORIS GS. Modes of action of terpene penetration enhancers in human skin; Differential scanning calorimetry, small-angle X-ray diffraction and enhancer uptake studies. *Int J Pharm* 1996; 127: 9–26.
81. BRINKMANN I, MULLER-GOYMANN CC. An attempt to clarify the influence of glycerol, propylene glycol, isopropyl myristate and a combination of propylene glycol and isopropyl myristate on human stratum corneum. *Pharmazie* 2005; 60: 215–220.
82. GOODMAN M, BARRY BW. Lipid-protein-partitioning (LPP) theory of skin enhancer activity: Finite dose technique. *Int J Pharm* 1989; 57: 29–40.
83. SATO K, SUGIBAYASHI K, MORIMOTO Y. Effect and mode of action of aliphatic esters on the in vitro skin permeation of nicorandil. *Int J Pharm* 1988; 43: 31–40.
84. SEKI T, SUGIBAYASHI K, JUNI K, MORIMOTO Y. Percutaneous absorption enhancer applied to membrane permeation-controlled transdermal delivery of nicardipine hydrochloride. *Drug Des Deliv* 1989; 4: 69–75.
85. MOLLGAARD B. Synergistic effect in percutaneous enhancement. In: Walters KA, Hadgraft J, eds. *Pharmaceutical Skin Penetration Enhancement*. Marcel Dekker, New York, 1993; 229–242.
86. LEOPOLD CS, LIPPOLD BC. An attempt to clarify the mechanism of the penetration enhancing effects of lipophilic vehicles with differential scanning calorimetry (DSC). *J Pharm Pharmacol* 1995; 47: 276–281.
87. HIRVONEN J, RAJALA R, VIHERVAARA P, LAINE E, PARONEN P, URTTI A. Mechanism and reversibility of penetration enhancer action in the skin. *Eur J Pharm Biopharm* 1995; 40: 81–85.
88. BRINKMANN I, MULLER-GOYMANN CC. Role of isopropyl myristate, isopropyl alcohol and a combination of both in hydrocortisone permeation across the human stratum corneum. *Skin Pharmacol Appl Skin Physiol* 2003; 16: 393–404.

89. ALBERTI I, KALIA YN, NAIK A, BONNY J-D, GUY RH. Effect of ethanol and isopropyl myristate on the availability of topical terbinafine in human stratum corneum, in vivo. *Int J Pharm* 2001; 219: 11–19.

90. KRAUS CA. The ion pair concept: Its evolution and some applications. *J Phys Chem* 1956; 60: 129–141.

91. PARDO A, SHIN Y, COHEN S. Kinetics of transdermal penetration of an organic ion pair. Physostigmine salicylate. *J Pharm Sci* 1992; 81: 990–995.

92. HADGRAFT J, WALTERS KA, WOTTON PK. Facilitated percutaneous absorption: A comparison and evaluation of two in vitro models. *Int J Pharm* 1986; 32: 257–263.

93. LANGGUTH P, MUTSCHLER E. Lipophilization of hydrophilic compounds: Consequences on transepidermal and intestinal transport of trospium chloride. *Arzneimittelforschung* 1987; 37: 1362–1366.

94. GREEN PG, HADGRAFT J, WOLFF M. Physicochemical aspects of the transdermal delivery of bupranolol. *Int J Pharm* 1989; 55: 265–269.

95. KURIHARA-BERGSTROM T, LIN P. Enhanced in vitro skin transport of ionized terbutaline using its sulfate salt form in aqueous isopropanol. *STP Pharma Sci* 1991; 1: 52–59.

96. NASH RA, MEHTA DB, MATIAS JR, ORENTREICH N. The possibility of lidocaine ion pair absorption through excised hairless mouse skin. *Skin Pharmacol* 1992; 5: 160–170.

97. TROTTA M, PATTARINO F, GASCO MR. Influence of counter ions on the skin penetration of methotrexate from water–oil microemulsions. *Pharm Acta Helv* 1996; 71: 135–140.

98. NYQVIST-MAYER AA, BRODIN AF, FRANK SG. Drug release studies on an oil-water emulsion based on a eutectic mixture of lidocaine and prilocaine as the dispersed phase. *J Pharm Sci* 1986; 75: 365–373.

99. STOTT PW, WILLIAMS AC, BARRY BW. Transdermal delivery from eutectic systems: Enhanced permeation of a model drug, ibuprofen. *J Control Release* 1998; 50: 297–308.

100. STOTT PW, WILLIAMS AC, BARRY BW. Mechanistic study into the enhanced transdermal permeation of a model β-blocker, propranolol, by fatty acids: A melting point depression effect. *Int J Pharm* 2001; 219: 161–176.

101. SCHWARB FP, IMANIDIS G, SMITH EW, HAIGH JM, SURBER C. Effect of concentration and degree of saturation of topical fluocinonide formulations on in vitro membrane transport and in vivo availability on human skin. *Pharm Res* 1999; 16: 909–915.

102. MOSER K, KRIWET K, FROEHLICH C, NAIK A, KALIA YN, GUY RH. Permeation enhancement of a highly lipophilic drug using supersaturated systems. *J Pharm Sci* 2001; 90: 607–616.

103. MOSER K, KRIWET K, FROEHLICH C, KALIA YN, GUY RH. Supersaturation: Enhancement of skin penetration and permeation of a lipophilic drug. *Pharm Res* 2001; 18: 1006–1011.

104. MOSER K, KRIWET K, KALIA YN, GUY RH. Enhanced skin permeation of a lipophilic drug using supersaturated formulations. *J Control Release* 2001; 73: 245–253.

105. TANAKA S, TAKASHIMA Y, MURAYAMA H, TSUCHIYA S. Studies on drug release from ointments. V. Release of hydrocortisone butyrate propionate from topical dosage forms to silicone rubber. *Int J Pharm* 1985; 27: 29–38.

106. FANG J-Y, KUO C-T, HUANG Y-B, WU P-C, TSAI Y-H. Transdermal delivery of sodium nonivamide acetate from volatile vehicles: Effects of polymers. *Int J Pharm* 1999; 176: 157–167.

107. LEICHTNAM ML, ROLLAND H, WUTHRICH P, GUY RH. Formulation and evaluation of a testosterone transdermal spray. *J Pharm Sci* 2006; 95: 1693–1702.

108. LEICHTNAM ML, ROLLAND H, WUTHRICH P, GUY RH. Impact of antinucleants on transdermal delivery of testosterone from a spray. *J Pharm Sci* 2007; 96: 84–92.

Chapter 3

Electrical and Physical Methods of Skin Penetration Enhancement

Jeffrey E. Grice, Tarl W. Prow, Mark A.F. Kendall, and Michael S. Roberts

INTRODUCTION

Oral administration of drugs may be unfavorable due to poor bioavailability and variations in metabolism between individuals, while intravenous injection can be poorly tolerated. Consequently, there is increasing research and commercial interest in the transdermal route of drug administration. At the beginning of this century, the transdermal route was vying with oral treatment as the major area of innovation in drug delivery, with a significant proportion of drug delivery candidate products under clinical evaluation in the United States related to transdermal or dermal systems.[1] More recently, in a 2008 review by Prausnitz and Langer,[2] it was estimated that more than 1 billion transdermal patches were being manufactured annually. As well as the pharmaceutical market, cosmetic and cosmeceutical skin care represents a huge worldwide market that is serviced by similar formulation strategies to some of those used in the drug delivery sector.

However, under normal circumstances, where the outer skin layer, the stratum corneum (SC) remains intact, the transdermal route is limited to relatively small molecular weight (MW), neutral, lipophilic molecules. Without manipulation and the use of modern technology to achieve penetration enhancement, many important therapeutic peptides, proteins, vaccines, oligonucleotides, or payload-carrying particles would be unavailable for topical delivery.

The aims of penetration enhancement include:

- to increase the range of penetrants available for transdermal delivery,
- to increase the rate of transdermal delivery for a specific penetrants,

Transdermal and Topical Drug Delivery: Principles and Practice, First Edition. Edited by Heather A.E. Benson, Adam C. Watkinson.

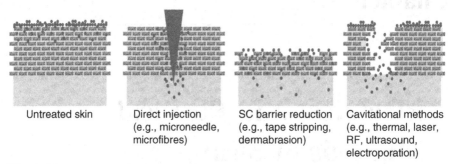

| Untreated skin | Direct injection (e.g., microneedle, microfibres) | SC barrier reduction (e.g., tape stripping, dermabrasion) | Cavitational methods (e.g., thermal, laser, RF, ultrasound, electroporation) |

Figure 3.1 Penetration of topically applied substances through untreated skin and following treatment with direct injection, barrier reduction, and cavitational technologies.

- to target penetrants to specific areas within or beyond the skin, while protecting deeper tissues from damage,
- to achieve these goals with minimal adverse skin reactions.

Strategies for penetration enhancement range from simple occlusion and formulation optimization, to the use of chemical and physical methods/technologies, or combinations of these. This review will focus upon physical manipulations which may be applied to skin before or during topical application. These can include the application of various forms of energy (e.g., heat, sound, light, electrical, magnetic, etc.), or breaching, reducing, or weakening the SC barrier by mechanical means. The various methods will be classified mechanistically, according to their effect on the skin, particularly the SC. Direct injection methods (e.g., microneedles) breach the SC to deliver an active substance at a predetermined depth. Mechanical techniques such as tape stripping or microdermabrasion enhance penetration (in part) by reducing the thickness of the SC barrier, whereas flexing or stretching can cause a general weakening of the barrier. Massage may also promote the follicular delivery route, shown particularly for microparticles, which can be loaded with a drug to create a follicular reservoir.[3] Ablative or cavitational technologies eliminate the SC barrier at discrete sites, forming micropores or microchannels through which diffusion can occur. Finally, there are technologies such as noncavitational ultrasound, dermaportation (magnetophoresis), and iontophoresis designed to enhance penetration by increasing the driving force on a penetrant. Figure 3.1 demonstrates the penetration of topically applied substances through untreated skin and following treatment with direct injection, barrier reduction, and cavitational technologies.

DIRECT INJECTION TECHNIQUES

Microneedles for Vaccine Delivery

Transdermal delivery with microneedles began in the early 1970s with a U.S. patent application from Alza Corp. by Gerstel and Place (US 3,964,482),[4] and applications continue to expand rapidly, with the majority (>60%) of refereed journal articles related to microneedles being published from 2007 to the present. The dramatic increase in microneedle-focused work results both from technological advances in microfabrication technology and increased funding as a result of the successes and potential benefits of the microneedle technology field. While microneedles may be useful for a range of transdermal drug delivery applications, there has been a strong focus on vaccine delivery. Consequently, the remainder of this section will deal with that aspect. The underpinning rationale for the focus of microneedle delivery vaccines stems from the following observations:

1. The skin is abundant in immune cells, and targeting vaccines to these cells provides scope for improved immunogenicity and/or significant dose sparing, compared to the current standard of intramuscular injection[5];

2. Microneedles are effective in delivering these payloads to the skin; and

3. Microneedles can deliver low and high MW substances.

In realizing this potential, there have been great advances in understanding the mechanical interactions of microneedles with skin,[6] as well as vaccine formulation and coating strategies[7–9] and the use of dissolving microneedles.[10–12]

These advances have allowed the application of microneedles to vaccination for all of the key classes of vaccines. Specifically, this scope of vaccination includes:

1. *Conventional Vaccines.* Whole virus and split virus (e.g., for influenza[5,13,14]; Chikengunya virus[15]); virus-like particles (e.g., for human papillomavirus[16]);

2. *DNA Vaccines.* Both plasmid based (e.g., for herpes simplex virus[7,17]) and other formats (e.g., West Nile virus[18]).

The technologies within the microneedle field can be categorized either by the geometry of the device (e.g., either by few or many microneedles; long microneedles or short ones; the shape of the individual microneedles) and/or the vaccine formulation. In considering the formulation of vaccines, approaches have included injecting vaccines through hollow microneedles[19,20] (see Fig. 3.2),

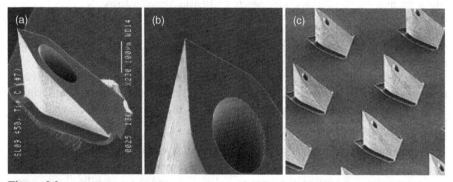

Figure 3.2 Scanning electron micrographs of the MicronJet microneedles (NanoPass Technologies Ltd., Nes Ziona, Israel). (a) A single microneedle. (b) The microneedle tip. (c) A microneedle array during production. Source: Reference 20.

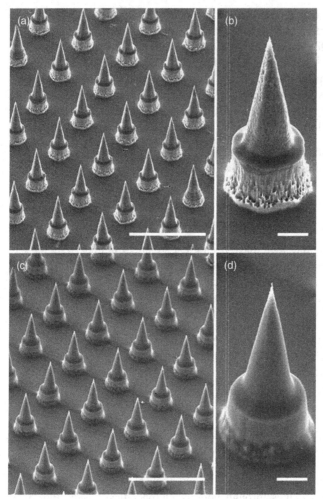

Figure 3.3 Micro-nanoprojection array area showing coated (a, b) and uncoated (c, d) projections prior to insertion into skin. (Bar a, c = 100 mm; b, d = 10 mm). Source: Reference 6.

encapsulation in dissolvable polymer microneedle patches[11] and dry-coated microneedle arrays[6,7,10,14,15,21–24] (see Fig. 3.3).

The field commenced with hollow microneedles, the advantage of this approach being the ability to deliver the same vaccine formulations as delivered by syringe, so there are no major reformulation hurdles to overcome. However, challenges include:

- Maintaining uniform insertion of the needles within the skin. The result of not achieving this aim would be a significant amount of vaccine being released onto the skin surface (i.e., not into the skin) and the variability in delivery associated with this.

- The use of an existing formulation means no improvement in vaccine thermostabilization, that is, if the vaccine is in the same liquid form as used with a needle and syringe, there are no improvements to the existing "cold-chain" requirement for many vaccines.
- The need for an active method for injecting the vaccine through the microneedles, and associated complexity/cost.

These challenges are being addressed by microneedles containing dry-formulated vaccine, which have been more recently developed and indeed have dominated the recent published literature. These devices can be classified as: (1) dry-coated microneedles and (2) dissolving microneedles.

The dry-coated microneedles first have the vaccine formulation modified by excipients such as methylcellulose[7] or carboxymethylcellulose (CMC).[8] Using these solutions, different coating technologies can then be applied. One example is dip coating,[25] which, for the short Nanopatch device projections (~100 μm), has achieved a vaccine yield (i.e., the amount of vaccine delivered into the skin, compared to the amount coated onto the device) of more than 80%. As well, a gas-jet coating approach has been developed as a simple alternative[7], with yields now beginning to approach those achieved by dip coating.[25] Both approaches are conceptually scalable for large volume manufacture at low cost.

When microneedles/micro-nanoprojections are applied to the skin, it has been shown that the dry-coated vaccine becomes wet within the *in vivo* environment, and is released very rapidly (<2 minutes[5]) with high levels of control, both on mass of vaccine and also in direct targeting to skin immune cells.[6,18]

In parallel, dissolving microneedle/micro-nanoprojection devices are also being developed. This approach offers all of the benefits of dry-coated formulation, but because the projections are made from the vaccine itself (plus excipient), there is scope for higher payloads to be delivered. Recent reports of dissolving microneedles[11,12,26] and dissolving Nanopatches—both delivering influenza vaccines—show that successful immunogenicity can be achieved. The Nanopatch has further comparatively favorable attributes of a very rapid release time (just 2 minutes, compared to hours, which is important for vaccination compliance) and confirmed dose sparing.

Research on collective dry-vaccine formulated microneedles has confirmed that enhanced thermostabilization is indeed achieved by these approaches.[27]

And finally—perhaps most importantly for many vaccines—it has been shown that the use of microneedles can indeed exploit the skin immunology for improved immunogenicity, protection, and dose sparing. In one recent, pertinent article, it was shown that a densely packed array (20,000 projections/cm^2) of short projections (~100 μm) bearing an influenza vaccine delivered the vaccine directly to several thousands of epidermal and dermal antigen-presenting cells, in good agreement with predictions from a theoretical probability-based model.[5] And importantly, it was found that that this skin targeting resulted in comparably protective immunity as delivered via needle and syringe into muscle—but with less than 1/100th of the delivered dose. This work, if successfully translated to a human product, could have important implications in improving the reach of vaccines, for example, in the rapid rollout of vaccines in response to a pandemic.

MECHANICAL METHODS

Tape Stripping

One of the simplest mechanical means of enhancing solute penetration in skin is by tape stripping, introduced into transdermal studies in the early 1970s,[28-30] in which the outermost skin layer, the SC, is progressively reduced in thickness by serial application and removal of strips of adhesive tape. From theoretical considerations based on Fick's first law of diffusion, the steady-state flux through a membrane is inversely proportional to the diffusion path length or thickness of the membrane.[31] This is directly applicable to diffusion of solutes through the SC. If the thickness of the SC is reduced by tape stripping, the flux of penetrants applied under similar conditions will therefore be greater. Associated with the increased penetrant flux due to the reduced barrier thickness, there is also increased transepidermal water loss (TEWL) from the internal side of the SC,[32] governed by similar theoretical principles. Not only does tape stripping increase the rate of penetration for a given penetrant, but there is evidence that the MW range of penetrants can be expanded. In tape-stripped murine skin, Tsai et al.[33] showed that the MW cut-off for skin penetration of polyethylene glycol oligomers (300–1000 Da) increased in parallel with barrier disruption, shown by increasing TEWL, as skin was progressively tape-stripped. Tape stripping remains an investigatory tool with little practical use in commercial applications.

Skin Flexing

There are suggestions of increased skin penetration due to regular movement in areas of the body subject to flexing, such as wrists, elbows, and feet. The main interest in this area concerns harmful exposure to particulate material.[34-37] The discovery of soil microparticles in lymph nodes and dermis[34,35] of elephantiasis sufferers in East Africa suggests that organisms may have penetrated bare feet in association with the soil particles. In *in vitro* experiments, Tinkle et al.[37] found evidence that 0.5–1.0 µm fluorescein isothiocyanate (FITC)-coated dextran beads penetrated flexed human skin, while Rouse et al.[36] showed that fullerene-based nanoparticles penetrated flexed pig skin far more readily than unflexed skin.

Skin Stretching

Mechanical devices to stretch skin and hold it under tension, to be used in conjunction with microneedles,[38-40] are the subject of patents for enhancing or sustaining transdermal drug delivery. In addition to microneedles, these devices may be designed to incorporate other technologies to further enhance penetration, such as ultrasound.[39] A recent research study by Abdulmajed and Heard[41] examined the effect of skin stretching on follicular delivery of retinyl ascorbate through porcine ear skin. The authors compared unstretched skin, skin with follicles sealed with superglue, and stretched skin mounted in Franz cells. They concluded that stretching caused enhanced follicular delivery, with a 4-mm (6.7%) stretch resulting in a 20%–40% increase in retinyl ascorbate delivery to the skin. These findings differ from those described in the earlier patent documentation,[40] in which stretching alone failed to enhance drug permeability across the skin. However, the parameter measured in the retinyl ascorbate study[41] was skin content by tape stripping, rather than drug perfusion. Abdulmajed and Heard's findings[41] warrant further investigation of stretching devices for follicular delivery, for which microneedles may not be necessary.

Massage

Two studies suggest that massage may be a useful tool in promoting transdermal delivery. Lademann et al.[3] investigated the transport of nanoparticles into hair follicles of pig skin *in vitro*. When massage was applied, the particles penetrated deeper into the follicles and remained there for up to 10 days. They hypothesized that hair movement created a "nanopump" to drive the particles deeper into the follicle. There was no evidence that particles moved beyond the follicles into deeper tissues. These findings are important as they suggest that coated particles carrying a drug payload could be targeted to the follicles to act as a long-term reservoir for topically applied substances. As the authors point out, the hair follicles are prime targets for drug action because the drug can diffuse out into close proximity to capillaries and Langerhans cells. The Lademann study[3] used a hand-held massage appliance. A Japanese group[42] used a low-frequency massage device which was applied to rats *in vivo*, and incorporated into an *in vitro* diffusion cell containing rat skin. They found some evidence that transdermal delivery of ketoprofen was enhanced *in vivo* and *in vitro* when the substance was applied with massage, but not after massage pre-treatment.

Lademann et al.[43] have suggested an optimum size (300–600 nm) for particles to target follicles, based on the cuticula thickness of hairs, which they suggest act as gears on the pump to drive the particles in. Stretching of skin during massage, as discussed above, may also play a role. Further optimization of follicular delivery may be possible by utilizing different particle forms[44,45] or different vehicles.[46]

Skin Abrasion

Skin abrasion refers to the removal of superficial layers of the skin by various abrasive means. These can include rubbing the skin with sandpaper[47]; motor-driven devices using abrasive wheels, pads, or brushes[48,49]; a "sand-blasting" process using a stream of crystalline particles such as aluminum oxide[50]; or other patented abrasive devices.[51–53] The process has been used for cosmetic skin resurfacing for a number of years[49] but has also been investigated for enhancing the penetration of topically applied substances.[2,54] Skin abrasion has been shown to enhance the skin delivery of a range of hydrophilic molecules (caffeine,[48] acyclovir,[48] 5-fluorouracil (5-FU),[50] vitamin C,[55] 5-aminolevulinic acid[56]), small peptides (angiotensin II,[48] MW 1046 Da), FITC-labeled dextrans[47] (4.3, 9.6, 42.0 kDa), and vaccines.[57,58] The ability to enhance transdermal delivery is highlighted in Figure 3.4, showing delivery of sodium fluorescein through microdermabraded monkey skin and no penetration through untreated skin.[57]

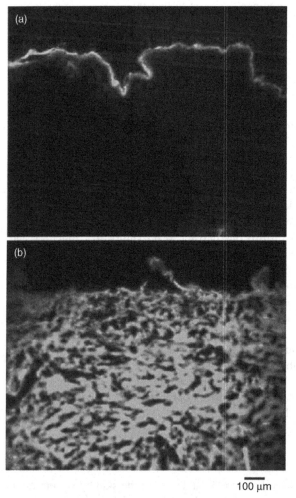

100 μm

Figure 3.4 *In vivo* delivery through microdermabraded skin. Fluorescence images of skin sections obtained from sites topically exposed to sodium fluorescein solution for 2 hours without microdermabrasion treatment (a) and after mobile-mode microdermabrasion at 50 kPa and 50 passes (b). Source: Reference 59.

Karimipour et al.[59] have reported some biochemical and immunohistochemical responses to microdermabrasion in humans. No changes in SC thickness resulted from a single microdermabrasion pass, but elevated transcription factors AP-1 and NF-κB and the cytokines IL-1β and TNF-α were observed. The authors suggest that this represents a dermal remodeling/wound healing cascade, which explains the efficacy of microdermabrasion for cosmetic purposes. Clearly, the process of skin abrasion does more than simply reduce the SC thickness and there may be a link between the expanded range of penetrants and the biochemical changes reported. A study published in 2009 drew attention to the lack of understanding of the cascade of events caused by skin abrasion.[57]

One of the major obstacles to the commercial application of skin abrasion has been the lack of control and reproducibility over the amount of SC that is removed. This was addressed by a Japanese group[60] who adjusted the operating conditions of their microdermabrasion device to control the amount of SC removed from *in situ* skin of sacrificed hairless mice, showing a correlation between this and the rate of skin penetration of a model drug, β-estradiol.[60] Gill et al.[57] suggest that for reproducible results, the entire SC thickness needs to be removed. They demonstrated that complete SC removal could be achieved, with little damage to the viable epidermis, after 30–50 passes of their microdermabrasion device (Megapeel® Gold Series, DermaMed International, Lenni, PA) were applied to skin of Rhesus macaques. The issue of controlled SC removal to give reproducible operator-independent results has also been addressed in a recently patented device.[51]

On the other hand, we applied dermal abrasion to excised human skin using a motor-driven rotating abrasive wheel and showed that most of the SC was removed after only three passes, with residual SC seen histologically only in folds and crevices (unpublished results). Excised human and mouse skin treated in this way showed significantly increased conductance and permeability to salicylic acid. Although our device probably applied more vigorous, less controlled abrasion than the controlled techniques discussed above, these results support the different responses of *in vivo* and *ex vivo* skin to dermal abrasion reported previously by Shim et al.[61] In this work, abdominal skin treated with microdermabrasion and then taken by biopsy showed no change in SC thickness, whereas *ex vivo* skin treated after excision showed reduced SC thickness.

Topical application of vaccines is an expanding field. The active immune cells located in the epidermis, the Langerhans cells, are readily accessible by percutaneous delivery systems and skin abrasion has been investigated as a means of mediating this. In early work, Mikszta et al.[58] used a "microenhancer array" abrasion device containing precise silicon projections to obtain strong reproducible immune responses in mice treated with a naked plasmid DNA. Recently, Gill et al.[57] identified virus-specific antibodies in blood after topical immunization with a live attenuated virus, modified vaccinia Ankara (MVA), was applied to microdermabraded monkey skin.

With advances in control and reproducibility, miniaturization, and incorporation of delivery into the abrasive device, skin abrasion may become an important transdermal delivery system. The potentially wide range of deliverables could find application for home, commercial, or clinical use.

ABLATIVE OR CAVITATIONAL TECHNOLOGIES

Thermal Ablation

Thermal ablation is a process in which microchannels are created by selective removal of SC after focused application of heat.[62] This can be achieved, for example, with a microarray of heating elements[63] or radiofrequency sources[64] to create transient rises in temperature above 100°C. Skin permeability is increased by enhanced diffusion through the microchannels. This mechanism clearly differs from one in which the permeability of intact skin generally increases with temperature.[65–67] Microchannel depths of between 40–50[64] and 70 μm[68] have been reported, indicating that ablation is confined to the upper epidermal layers of the skin. Microchannel surface dimensions are of the same order, depending on the array geometry. The removal of the lipid-rich SC in the microchannel openings creates a pathway through which lipophilic, hydrophilic, and macromolecules could be expected to easily diffuse.

Two systems for thermal ablation are in an advanced stage of development. The PassPort™ system from Altea Therapeutics Corp. (Atlanta, GA, USA) uses an array of resistors as a source of localized heating. On its Web site, Altea lists the substances shown in Table 3.1 as under investigation for delivery with the PassPort system (see http://www.alteatherapeutics.com/mediacoverage/OnDrugDelivery_Final.pdf).

The ViaDerm system[69] (TransPharma Medical Ltd., Lod, Israel) uses an array of radiofrequency (RF) microelectrodes to create microchannels. The system consists of a reusable and rechargeable control unit along with a disposable microelectrode array designed for a single use. TransPharma reports that insulin, human growth hormone, and human PTH (1-34) are the subject of clinical trials with their system.[69]

The scientific literature contains a number of reports of enhanced delivery of hydrophilic molecules, macromolecules, and vaccines using various thermal ablation methods, including those based on the commercial systems. Park et al.[70] designed an apparatus to apply short bursts of heat (at 100–315°C) to human skin *in vitro*. Permeability of calcein (a hydrophilic fluorescent dye with MW of 623 Da) was

Table 3.1   Substances under Trial for Delivery with the Altea PassPort System

Phase I human trials	Pre-clinical trials
Insulin	Influenza hemagglutinin (HA) protein antigen
Interferon-alpha	Avian influenza antigen
Parathyroid hormone	Tetanus protein antigen
Hepatitis B surface antigen	DNA vaccines
Hydromorphone hydrochloride	Erytropoetin
Morphine salts	Apomorphine hydrochloride
	Fentanyl citrate

found to be greatest at the highest temperature (315°C), with a 760-fold increase in transdermal flux compared to untreated skin.

Using an early prototype of the Altea device to deliver replication-defective adenovirus vectors, Bramson et al.[68] found 100-fold increases in reporter gene expression, as well as 10–100-fold greater cellular and humoral immune responses in treated mice, compared to untreated. More recently, Badkar et al.[63] used the PassPort system to create a 2 cm^2 array of microchannels (72/cm^2) on rat skin. Significant delivery of interferon alpha-2B was achieved through the treated skin, with none through untreated skin.

In RF-treated skin using the ViaDerm system, Sintov et al.[64] reported enhanced penetration of the hydrophilic drugs, granisetron hydrochloride, and diclofenac sodium, while Levin et al.[71] demonstrated significant human growth hormone delivery in rats. In addition, growth hormone bioactivity was confirmed by elevated IGF-1 levels in hypophysectomised rats.

Lasers

This technology is similar to thermal ablation in that pulsed laser energy is used to rapidly heat and vaporize the SC at a focused site, with little effect in underlying skin layers. The resulting microchannels formed through the SC lead to increased skin permeability. This was shown in an early study using a UV laser (193 nm, 14-ns pulsewidth) to treat excised human skin, where significant increases in tritiated water permeability and reductions in skin resistance were seen.[72] More recent work using infrared (IR) or visible wavelength lasers has shown increased permeability to a range of small lipophilic and hydrophilic compounds.[55,56,73–76] Control of the degree of ablation can be achieved by setting the laser parameters, including wavelength and pulse energy, frequency, and width. For example, a recent study by Gomez et al.[74] used a Q-switched Nd:YAG laser, emitting radiation at 1064, 532 (second harmonic), and 355 nm (third harmonic) to treat excised rabbit ear skin before 5-FU permeation. They concluded that visible radiation enhanced 5-FU delivery with the least risk of skin damage. IR radiation at 1064 nm penetrated more deeply, affecting collagen fibers, while UV radiation caused more alteration to lipid structures but was more difficult to control.

Some commercial applications of laser ablation technology have been explored, with early patents for controlled SC ablation by laser techniques[77,78] and one device currently marketed, a hand-held "laser-assisted drug delivery" (LAD) device developed by the Australian company Norwood Abbey Ltd. (Frankston, Victoria, Australia). This device uses an Er:YAG laser to deliver radiation at 2940 nm and has been approved by regulatory bodies of Australia (Therapeutic Goods Association) and the United States (Food and Drug Administration) for delivery of 4% lidocaine cream as a topical anesthetic. In human trials[73] with 4% lidocaine cream, 60% reductions in pain compared to appropriate controls were reported. As well, the time to reach equivalent levels of anesthesia was reduced from 60 to 5 minutes. For more details on Norwood Abbey, see http://www.norwoodabbey.com.au/technology.htm.

Intense laser pulses can also be used to generate high-amplitude pressure waves (photomechanical waves), which permeabilize the skin by creating hydrophilic channels without cavitation. Examples of pressure wave-mediated delivery include insulin,[79] allergens,[80] nanoparticles,[81] and gene transfer.[82]

Ultrasound

Sonophoresis (or phonophoresis) is the term used to describe enhanced transdermal delivery following application of ultrasound energy to the skin. Some early studies in this area used high frequency ultrasound of around 1–3 MHz,[83] whereas low frequency ultrasound (<100 kHz, usually 20 kHz) is now more commonly used.[84] Low frequency ultrasound at 20 kHz was reported to be up to 1000 times more efficient at enhancing drug delivery than higher frequencies (1–3 MHz).[84,85]

In simple terms, the mechanism is believed to involve cavitation due to rapid expansion and contraction of gas bubbles within the lipid bilayers of the SC. This results in the formation of aqueous channels through which compounds of various sizes, charges, and lipophilicities may permeate. These channels are formed in discrete areas, termed localized transport regions (LTRs)[86] (see Fig. 3.5). More complex investigations of the mechanisms of transdermal sonophoresis, including mathematical modeling of cavitational bubble growth and channel creation, have recently been reported and the interested reader is referred to these.[87,88]

Rather than being transient, these channels appear to remain open for extended periods of time. In a recent study[89] where 55 kHz ultrasound was applied to the forearm skin of healthy adults with a commercial device (SonoPrep® Ultrasonic skin permeation system, Sontra Medical Corp., Franklin, MA), enhanced permeability (by skin impedance measurement) was seen for up to 48 hours following treatment, particularly with occlusion.

There are numerous reports of enhanced delivery of drugs, macromolecules, oligonucleotides, DNA, and vaccines by sonophoresis, and these are summarized in some excellent recent reviews.[84,86,90,91] Lanke et al.[92] found that sonophoresis could

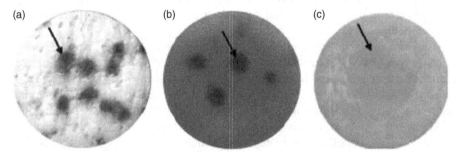

(a)   (b)   (c)

Figure 3.5   Representative images of LTR formation in (a) full-thickness pig skin with sulforhodamine B (SRB), (b) full-thickness human cadaver skin with SRB, and (c) full-thickness hairless rat skin with fluorescein isothiocyanate dextran (FITC-dextran 40). In a–c, the black arrow points to a representative LTR in each skin sample. Source: Reference 88.

successfully deliver low molecular weight heparin (LMWH, 3000 Da) to a depth of 150 µm below the SC surface of hairless rat skin, with a similar flux to that seen with iontophoresis. These data are shown in Figure 3.6, compared to the results with microneedles, which directly injected the LMWH to a depth of 500 µm.

An important potential use of sonophoresis is the transdermal delivery of insulin in the treatment of insulin-dependent diabetes mellitus. Several studies have demonstrated the feasibility of this approach. In early work from Tachibana,[93] rabbits were exposed to porcine insulin under ultrasound (105 KHz, 5-second pulses at 5-second intervals for 90 minutes) and significant plasma insulin rises and falls in blood glucose compared to controls were seen. In work by Boucaud et al.,[94] insulin delivered to rats with ultrasound (20 KHz for 15 minutes) lowered blood glucose to levels comparable with those after subcutaneous injections (0.5 U). Importantly, blood glucose fell only when insulin was delivered with ultrasound and not after pre-treatment. Later reports[95,96] better defined the ultrasound delivery parameters and refined the sonication apparatus for *in vivo* application. Other recent work[97] on insulin delivery in rats showed that blood glucose could be lowered to a greater extent with sonophoresis than with a 0.25 U/kg subcutaneous injection, a standard insulin dose in people with diabetes. The authors suggested that a similar drop in blood glucose achieved with sonophoresis in humans after a comparable insulin dose would be sufficient to treat frank diabetes.[97]

Vaccine delivery is another application for which ultrasound has been investigated. In two reports of sonophoresis-assisted delivery of tetanus toxoid, activation of Langerhans cells[98] and strong antibody titers[98,99] were achieved without the need for other powerful adjuvants. Sonophoresis itself was regarded as an effective physical adjuvant, lessening the need for irritants, toxins, or abrasion for this purpose and could therefore be developed as another alternative for needle-free, painless immunization.

Electroporation

The use of electroporation for transdermal delivery involves the application of high voltage pulses to the skin, leading to the creation of aqueous pores or pathways through the SC. The pores are small (<10 nm), sparse (0.1% of surface area), and transient (from microseconds to seconds)[100] and congregated in discrete local transport regions. Transport through the pores is believed to occur by passive diffusion, electrophoretic forces on charged molecules, and electroosmotic effects.[101]

Delivery of small molecules with a range of lipophilicities and charges, including fentanyl,[102] mannitol,[103] timolol,[104] tetracaine,[105] methotrexate,[106] 5-ALA,[107] vitamin C,[108] and tea catechins[109] has been successfully enhanced in early *in vitro* skin studies with electroporation. Hydrophilic molecules tended to show greater degrees of enhancement.[100] An interesting application is electrochemotherapy, in which anticancer drugs with poor skin permeability, such as bleomycin and cisplatin, were administered safely and efficiently by electroporation for treatment of cutaneous and subcutaneous tumors.[110]

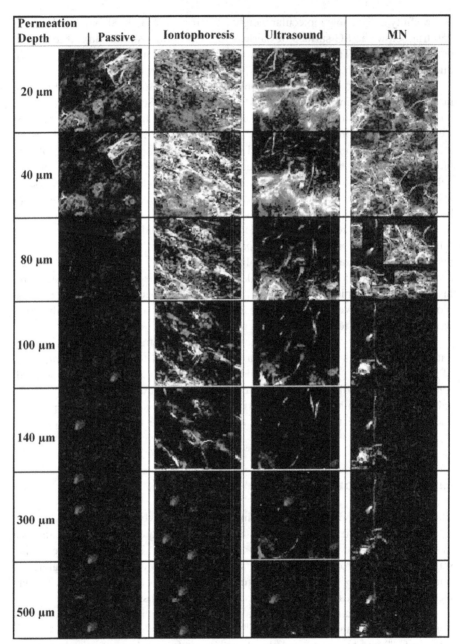

Figure 3.6   Confocal microscopic images (×10 objective) of the permeation of FITC-labeled heparin across hairless rat skin at various depths from the surface of the SC. Heparin transported across microchannel can be seen as bright areas up to a depth of 500 μm. Source: Reference 94.

In addition to drugs, electroporation has been successful for delivery of macromolecules, including peptides, vaccines, and DNA.[2] Tokumoto et al.[111] used electroporation (150 or 300 V, 10 pulses, 10 milliseconds) to achieve high plasma levels of human insulin in rats, where passive delivery was not possible. When electroporation was combined with iontophoresis, a synergistic plasma insulin response was obtained. The potential for vaccine delivery was demonstrated by Zhao et al.,[112] where a K^b-binding ovalbumin (OVA)-peptide SIINFEKL delivered by electroporation to mouse skin induced a peptide-specific cytotoxic T lymphocyte response, which was equivalent to that generated by intradermal injection. There is also considerable interest in the use of electroporation for gene transfer, with recent reports of successful delivery of plasmid DNA by electroporation, following intradermal delivery,[113–116] including a Phase I trial of interleukin-12 plasmid electroporation in metastatic melanoma patients.[113] This work was performed with a Medpulser DNA delivery device using electroporation technology from Inovio Biomedical Inc., San Diego, CA.

A major concern over the use of electroporation is the pain and muscle stimulation and the possibility of tissue damage[101] that may be associated with pulses in the order of hundreds of volts. A microelectrode array designed for painless electroporation, which successfully delivered toluidine blue O in mouse skin, gave no pain perception in humans after 60 pulses of 1 millisecond at 150 V.[117] A less robust alternative to electroporation, low voltage electropulsation operating at 30 V, has recently been reported[118] to enhance the transport of salicylic acid, lidocaine hydrochloride, and FITC-dextran (10 kDa) *in vitro*.

INCREASED DRIVING FORCE TECHNOLOGIES

Dermaportation

Magnetic fields have been used to treat musculoskeletal injuries for many years, while more recently, other therapeutic targets such as wound healing, nerve regeneration, and graft management have been promoted.[119] Some mechanistic support for the efficacy of magnetic fields in wound healing comes from recent work by Vianale et al.[120] They found that extremely low frequency magnetic fields enhanced keratinocytes cell growth and reduced inflammation by inhibition of the NF-κB signaling pathway. In the transdermal area, Murthy et al.[121,122] reported that static magnetic fields enhanced penetration of topically applied substances, in a process they termed magnetophoresis. Here, they sandwiched permanent flat magnets $(1 \times 10^{-4} T)$ with transdermal patches and applied them to human skin *in vitro*, conscious guinea pigs, and human volunteers. The presence of the magnetic fields enhanced benzoic acid and terbutaline sulfate flux *in vitro*, with the effect on terbutaline sulfate being of a similar magnitude to that caused by chemical enhancement with 4% isopropyl myristate alone.[122] Terbutaline sulfate penetration was also enhanced in the guinea pigs, shown by increased preconvulsive times following histamine hydrochloride aerosol treatment,[122] and in humans, where terbutaline sulfate elimination half-lives were significantly prolonged compared to oral administration.[122] The authors[122] suggested that the magnetic field increased the driving force on diamagnetic substances through the skin. They also hypothesized that the field could cause a temporary alteration in skin structure, although they presented no evidence for this.

There has been little interest in magnetophoresis until recently, when an Australian company, OBJ Ltd., developed a technology described as dermaportation, which applies pulsatile electromagnetic fields to target tissues, unlike the static fields used in Murthy's work.[121,122] Research into dermaportation and other magnetic enhancement techniques is being carried out at Curtin University, Western Australia. Dermaportation has been reported to enhance penetration of 5-aminolevulinic acid[123] and a dipeptide, Ala-Trp,[124] through human epidermis *in vitro*. Like Murthy et al.,[121,122] Namjoshi et al.[124] suggest that the mechanism of enhancement involves both a direct magnetic repulsion on the penetrants and increased permeability due to a rearrangement of the SC lipid bilayers. Recent work by Krishnan et al.[125] showing that dermaportation caused enhanced naltrexone penetration though human epidermal membranes, but not through silicone membranes, provides some evidence to support a direct effect of pulsed magnetic fields on skin. Moreover, imaging by multiphoton microscopy and fluorescence lifetime imaging (MPM-FLIM) showed that 10-nm gold nanoparticles applied to excised human skin penetrated through the SC into the viable epidermis.[125] The authors suggested that the pulsed magnetic fields facilitate the movement of the nanoparticles through the skin, through channels greater than their 10 nm diameter. Curtin et al. have also been investigating the effect of passive magnetic fields generated by a flexible magnetic film. In preliminary work,[126] they applied magnetic films over a moisturizing urea gel with appropriate controls and reported enhanced *in vitro* penetration of urea in human epidermal membranes and increased epidermal hydration *in vivo*. This technology shows promise if these preliminary findings can be confirmed.

Magnetic technologies potentially offer several advantages for penetration enhancement in a commercial setting. Technologies like those being developed by OBJ Ltd. and studied by Curtin et al. require very little energy to generate the electromagnetic fields and could be miniaturized and easily incorporated into skin patches. Electromagnetic fields are unlikely to cause skin irritation.

However, to be commercially viable, it must be demonstrated that these magnetic technologies are effective for a broad range of molecules, particularly larger MW species such as therapeutic peptides. The mechanism(s) by which the reported effects occur must also be elucidated. Evidence for alteration in lipid arrangements might come from Fourier transform infrared (FTIR) spectroscopy,[127] while confocal or multiphoton microscopy (MPM)[128] offer the possibility of studying changes in skin morphology and metabolic processes.

Iontophoresis

Iontophoresis uses small electric currents to drive ionic molecules across membranes and can be used as a noninvasive method of enhancing transdermal drug delivery.

It is particularly effective for water-soluble ionic drugs such as peptides, which are very poorly absorbed by the skin under normal conditions. Three main mechanisms affect iontophoretic skin transport:

a. Electrorepulsion of charged solutes by the electrode

b. Electroosmotic effects on unionized, polar species

c. Permeabilization of the skin by the electric current

The technique has been summarized in a recent book chapter[129] and a comprehensive review of clinical applications of iontophoresis appears in the following chapter of this book. The reader is directed toward these sources.

SKIN AND PENETRANT IMAGING

Various experimental techniques have been used to visualize the penetration of applied solutes, as well as to image the effect of the physical enhancement technologies on the skin itself.

Stained histological sections have proved useful to show reductions in SC thickness following dermal abrasion.[55,56] Histological evidence suggests that low frequency ultrasound does little physical damage to skin and underlying tissues,[85,130] although localized transport pathways were recognized in hematoxylin–eosin (H&E)-stained porcine skin, with evidence of antisense oligonucleotide penetration in those regions. Sintov et al.[64] took histological sections of porcine skin treated with radiofrequency energy in a 200 electrode/cm^2 array and showed that localized microchannels were created, extending into the superficial dermis.

Confocal laser scanning microscopy[128] and MPM[131](also known as multiphoton tomography) can provide morphological and biochemical information about skin by detecting autofluorescence from endogenous skin fluorophores. In addition, the penetration of fluorescent or fluorescently labeled solutes can be visualized. Using these techniques, "slices" of skin parallel to the surface can be scanned at various depths, with little damage to the tissue, particularly with MPM. They are useful for *in vitro* as well as *in vivo* imaging. Park et al.[70] used confocal microscopy to image lipids stained with Nile red to show structural changes caused by heat in pig skin. The effect of ultrasound treatment was demonstrated by confocal imaging of FITC-labeled dextrans at different skin depths by Morimoto et al.[132] Confocal imaging was also used to track the penetration of quantum dots,[133] FITC-labeled fullerene particles,[36] and macromolecules[134] promoted by various physical enhancement techniques. Kushner et al.[135] examined the effect of low frequency ultrasound and chemical enhancers on *ex vivo* human skin with MPM imaging of the penetration of fluorescent hydrophilic and lipophilic penetrants. They were able to discriminate between autofluorescence and penetrant fluorescence by splitting the signals into two separate channels. Fluorescence lifetime imaging (FLIM)[136,137] is a novel imaging technique used in conjunction with fluorescence microscopy to provide information about the state or environment of a particular fluorophore, which may be useful in assessing the effects of physical treatments.

Confocal Raman spectroscopy is a recent addition to the available imaging technologies. This allows real-time, noninvasive *in vivo* imaging of penetrants and skin components, based on their specific IR–Raman signature and can be used for quantitative estimation of skin penetrants. The technique expands the range of substances that can be detected, beyond that available with fluorescence confocal or multiphoton techniques. Melot et al.[138] recently used the technique to study the effect of penetration enhancers on trans-retinol delivery to skin. It has also been used to examine SC barrier properties, including quantitative measures of SC thickness and hydration levels after treatment with topical moisturizers.[139]

REFERENCES

1. BARRY BW. Novel mechanisms and devices to enable successful transdermal drug delivery. *Eur J Pharm Sci* 2001; 14(2): 101–114.
2. PRAUSNITZ MR, LANGER R. Transdermal drug delivery. *Nat Biotechnol* 2008; 26(11): 1261–1268.
3. LADEMANN J, et al. Nanoparticles—An efficient carrier for drug delivery into the hair follicles. *Eur J Pharm Biopharm* 2007; 66(2): 159–164.
4. GERSTEL MS, PLACE VA. Drug delivery device. Patent. [3,964,482]. 1976.
5. FERNANDO GJ, et al. Potent immunity to low doses of influenza vaccine by probabilistic guided micro-targeted skin delivery in a mouse model. *PLoS ONE* 2010; 5(4): e10266.
6. CRICHTON ML, et al. The effect of strain rate on the precision of penetration of short densely-packed microprojection array patches coated with vaccine. *Biomaterials* 2010; 31(16): 4562–4572.
7. CHEN X, et al. Dry-coated microprojection array patches for targeted delivery of immunotherapeutics to the skin. *J Control Release* 2009; 139(3): 212–220.
8. GILL HS, PRAUSNITZ MR. Coated microneedles for transdermal delivery. *J Control Release* 2007; 117(2): 227–237.
9. GILL HS, PRAUSNITZ MR. Coating formulations for microneedles. *Pharm Res* 2007; 24(7): 1369–1380.
10. RAPHAEL AP, et al. Targeted, needle-free vaccinations in skin using multilayered, densely-packed dissolving microprojection arrays. *Small* 2010; 6(16): 1785–1793.
11. SULLIVAN SP, et al. Dissolving polymer microneedle patches for influenza vaccination. *Nat Med* 2010; 16(8): 915–920.
12. SULLIVAN SP, MURTHY N, PRAUSNITZ MR. Minimally invasive protein delivery with rapidly dissolving polymer microneedles. *Adv Mater* 2008; 20(5): 933–938.
13. QUAN FS, et al. Stabilization of influenza vaccine enhances protection by microneedle delivery in the mouse skin. *PLoS ONE* 2009; 4(9): e7152.
14. KOUTSONANOS DG, et al. Transdermal influenza immunization with vaccine-coated microneedle arrays. *PLoS ONE* 2009; 4(3): e4773.
15. PROW TW. Toxicity of nanomaterials to the eye. *Wiley Interdiscip Rev Nanomed Nanobiotechnol* 2010; 2(4): 317–333.
16. CORBETT HJ, et al. Skin vaccination against cervical cancer associated human papillomavirus with a novel micro-projection array in a mouse model. *PLoS ONE* 2010; 5(10): e13460.
17. KASK AS, et al. DNA vaccine delivery by densely-packed and short microprojection arrays to skin protects against vaginal HSV-2 challenge. *Vaccine* 2010; 28(47): 7483–7491.
18. PROW TW, et al. Nanopatch-targeted skin vaccination against west nile virus and chikungunya virus in mice. *Small* 2010; 6(16): 1776–1784.
19. MOREFIELD GL, et al. An alternative approach to combination vaccines: Intradermal administration of isolated components for control of anthrax, botulism, plague and staphylococcal toxic shock. *J Immune Based Ther Vaccines* 2008; 6: 5–15.

20. VAN DAMME P, et al. Safety and efficacy of a novel microneedle device for dose sparing intradermal influenza vaccination in healthy adults. *Vaccine* 2009; 27(3): 454–459.

21. ANDRIANOV AK, et al. Poly[di(carboxylatophenoxy)phosphazene] is a potent adjuvant for intradermal immunization. *Proc Natl Acad Sci USA* 2009; 106(45): 18936–18941.

22. GILL HS, et al. Cutaneous vaccination using microneedles coated with hepatitis C DNA vaccine. *Gene Ther* 2010; 17(6): 811–814.

23. JIN CY, et al. Mass producible and biocompatible microneedle patch and functional verification of its usefulness for transdermal drug delivery. *Biomed Microdevices* 2009; 11(6): 1195–1203.

24. KIM YC, et al. Enhanced memory responses to seasonal H1N1 influenza vaccination of the skin with the use of vaccine-coated microneedles. *J Infect Dis* 2010; 201(2): 190–198.

25. CHEN C, et al. Site-selectively coated, densely-packed microprojection array patches for targeted delivery of vaccines to skin. *Adv Funct Mater* 2010.

26. LEE JW, PARK JH, PRAUSNITZ MR. Dissolving microneedles for transdermal drug delivery. *Biomaterials* 2008; 29(13): 2113–2124.

27. CHEN C, KENDALL MA. Enhanced Thermostabilization for Dry-Vaccine Formulated Microneedles. *J Control Release* 2011. Submitted.

28. HOJYO-TOMOKA MT, KLIGMAN AM. Does cellophane tape stripping remove the horny layer? *Arch Dermatol* 1972; 106(5): 767–768.

29. KAMMERAU B, ZESCH A, SCHAEFER H. Absolute concentrations of dithranol and triacetyl-dithranol in the skin layers after local treatment: *In vivo* investigations with four different types of pharmaceutical vehicles. *J Invest Dermatol* 1975; 64(3): 145–149.

30. WEIGAND DA, GAYLOR JR. Removal of stratum corneum *in vivo*: An improvement on the cellophane tape stripping technique. *J Invest Dermatol* 1973; 60(2): 84–87.

31. HIGUCHI TJ. Physical chemical analysis of percutaneous absorption process from creams and ointments. *J Soc Cosmet Chem* 1960; 11: 85–87.

32. KALIA YN, PIROT F, GUY RH. Homogeneous transport in a heterogeneous membrane: Water diffusion across human stratum corneum *in vivo*. *Biophys J* 1996; 71(5): 2692–2700.

33. TSAI JC, et al. Tape stripping and sodium dodecyl sulfate treatment increase the molecular weight cutoff of polyethylene glycol penetration across murine skin. *Arch Dermatol Res* 2003; 295(4): 169–174.

34. BLUNDELL G, HENDERSON WJ, PRICE EW. Soil particles in the tissues of the foot in endemic elephantiasis of the lower legs. *Ann Trop Med Parasitol* 1989; 83(4): 381–385.

35. CORACHAN M, et al. Podoconiosis in Aequatorial Guinea. Report of two cases from different geological environments. *Trop Geogr Med* 1988; 40(4): 359–364.

36. ROUSE JG, et al. Effects of mechanical flexion on the penetration of fullerene amino acid-derivatized peptide nanoparticles through skin. *Nano Lett* 2007; 7(1): 155–160.

37. TINKLE SS, et al. Skin as a route of exposure and sensitization in chronic beryllium disease. *Environ Health Perspect* 2003; 111(9): 1202–1208.

38. CORMIER MJN, et al. Skin treatment apparatus for sustained transdermal delivery. Patent. [WO 2001/041864]. 2001.

39. TOKUMOTO S, MATSUDO T, KUWAHARA T. Transdermal drug administration apparatus having microneedles. Patent. [U.S. 2009/0030365]. 2009.

40. TRAUTMAN JC, et al. Device and method for enhancing microprotrusion skin piercing. Patent. [WO 2001/041863]. 2001.

41. ABDULMAJED K, HEARD CM. Topical delivery of retinyl ascorbate. 3. Influence of follicle sealing and skin stretching. *Skin Pharmacol Physiol* 2008; 21(1): 46–49.

42. SAKURAI H, TAKAHASHI Y, MACHIDA Y. Influence of low-frequency massage device on transdermal absorption of ionic materials. *Int J Pharm* 2005; 305(1–2): 112–121.

43. LADEMANN J, et al. Determination of the cuticula thickness of human and porcine hairs and their potential influence on the penetration of nanoparticles into the hair follicles. *J Biomed Opt* 2009; 14(2): 021014.

44. JUNG S, et al. Innovative liposomes as a transfollicular drug delivery system: Penetration into porcine hair follicles. *J Invest Dermatol* 2006; 126(8): 1728–1732.

45. Tabbakhian M, et al. Enhancement of follicular delivery of finasteride by liposomes and niosomes 1. *In vitro* permeation and *in vivo* deposition studies using hamster flank and ear models. *Int J Pharm* 2006; 323(1–2): 1–10.

46. Grice JE, et al. Relative uptake of minoxidil into appendages and stratum corneum and permeation through human skin *in vitro*. *J Pharm Sci* 2010; 99(2): 712–718.

47. Wu XM, Todo H, Sugibayashi K. Effects of pre-treatment of needle puncture and sandpaper abrasion on the *in vitro* skin permeation of fluorescein isothiocyanate (FITC)-dextran. *Int J Pharm* 2006; 316(1–2): 102–108.

48. Akomeah FK, et al. Effect of abrasion induced by a rotating brush on the skin permeation of solutes with varying physicochemical properties. *Eur J Pharm Biopharm* 2008; 68(3): 724–734.

49. Gold MH. Dermabrasion in dermatology. *Am J Clin Dermatol* 2003; 4(7): 467–471.

50. Lee WR, et al. Microdermabrasion as a novel tool to enhance drug delivery via the skin: An animal study. *Dermatol Surg* 2006; 32(8): 1013–1022.

51. Lastovich AG, et al. Microabrader with controlled abrasion features. Patent. [U.S. 7,422,567]. 2008.

52. Mikszta JA, et al. Topical delivery of vaccines. Patent. [6,595,947 B1]. 2003.

53. Sage BH, Bock CR. Method and device for abrading skin. Patent [U.S. 6,835,184 B1]. 2004.

54. Brown MB, et al. Transdermal drug delivery systems: Skin perturbation devices. *Methods Mol Biol* 2008; 437: 119–139.

55. Lee WR, et al. Lasers and microdermabrasion enhance and control topical delivery of vitamin C. *J Invest Dermatol* 2003; 121(5): 1118–1125.

56. Fang JY, et al. Enhancement of topical 5-aminolaevulinic acid delivery by erbium:YAG laser and microdermabrasion: A comparison with iontophoresis and electroporation. *Br J Dermatol* 2004; 151(1): 132–140.

57. Gill HS, et al. Selective removal of stratum corneum by microdermabrasion to increase skin permeability. *Eur J Pharm Sci* 2009; 38(2): 95–103.

58. Mikszta JA, et al. Improved genetic immunization via micromechanical disruption of skin-barrier function and targeted epidermal delivery. *Nat Med* 2002; 8(4): 415–419.

59. Karimipour DJ, et al. Microdermabrasion: A molecular analysis following a single treatment. *J Am Acad Dermatol* 2005; 52(2): 215–223.

60. Fujimoto T, Shirakami K, Tojo K. Effect of microdermabrasion on barrier capacity of stratum corneum. *Chem Pharm Bull (Tokyo)* 2005; 53(8): 1014–1016.

61. Shim EK, et al. Microdermabrasion: A clinical and histopathologic study. *Dermatol Surg* 2001; 27(6): 524–530.

62. Arora A, Prausnitz MR, Mitragotri S. Micro-scale devices for transdermal drug delivery. *Int J Pharm* 2008; 364(2): 227–236.

63. Badkar AV, et al. Transdermal delivery of interferon alpha-2B using microporation and iontophoresis in hairless rats. *Pharm Res* 2007; 24(7): 1389–1395.

64. Sintov AC, et al. Radiofrequency-driven skin microchanneling as a new way for electrically assisted transdermal delivery of hydrophilic drugs. *J Control Release* 2003; 89(2): 311–320.

65. Akomeah F, et al. Effect of heat on the percutaneous absorption and skin retention of three model penetrants. *Eur J Pharm Sci* 2004; 21(2–3): 337–345.

66. Blank IH, Scheuplein RJ, MacFarlane DJ. Mechanism of percutaneous absorption. 3. The effect of temperature on the transport of non-electrolytes across the skin. *J Invest Dermatol* 1967; 49(6): 582–589.

67. Ribaud C, et al. Organization of stratum corneum lipids in relation to permeability: Influence of sodium lauryl sulfate and preheating. *Pharm Res* 1994; 11(10): 1414–1418.

68. Bramson J, et al. Enabling topical immunization via microporation: A novel method for pain-free and needle-free delivery of adenovirus-based vaccines. *Gene Ther* 2003; 10(3): 251–260.

69. Levin G. Advances in radio-frequency transdermal drug delivery. *Pharm Technol* 2008. Available at http://pharmtech.findpharma.com/pharmtech/author/authorInfo.jsp?id=43941.

70. Park JH, et al. The effect of heat on skin permeability. *Int J Pharm* 2008; 359(1–2): 94–103.

71. Levin G, et al. Transdermal delivery of human growth hormone through RF-microchannels. *Pharm Res* 2005; 22(4): 550–555.

72. JACQUES SL, et al. Controlled removal of human stratum corneum by pulsed laser. *J Invest Dermatol* 1987; 88(1): 88–93.

73. BARON ED, et al. Laser-assisted penetration of topical anesthetic in adults. *Arch Dermatol* 2003; 139(10): 1288–1290.

74. GOMEZ C, et al. Laser treatments on skin enhancing and controlling transdermal delivery of 5-fluorouracil. *Lasers Surg Med* 2008; 40(1): 6–12.

75. LEE WR, et al. Topical delivery of methotrexate via skin pretreated with physical enhancement techniques: Low-fluence erbium:YAG laser and electroporation. *Lasers Surg Med* 2008; 40(7): 468–476.

76. LEE WR, et al. Transdermal drug delivery enhanced and controlled by erbium:YAG laser: A comparative study of lipophilic and hydrophilic drugs. *J Control Release* 2001; 75(1–2): 155–166.

77. JACQUES SL, et al. Controlled removal of human stratum corneum by pulsed laser to enhance percutaneous transport. Patent. [U.S. 4,775,361]. 1988.

78. MARCHITTO KS, FLOCK ST. Laser assisted pharmaceutical delivery and fluid removal. Patent. [U.S. 6,315,772 B1]. 2001.

79. LEE S, et al. Photomechanical transdermal delivery of insulin *in vivo*. *Lasers Surg Med* 2001; 28(3): 282–285.

80. GONZALEZ S, et al. Rapid allergen delivery with photomechanical waves for inducing allergic skin reactions in the hairless guinea pig animal model. *Am J Contact Dermat* 2001; 12(3): 162–165.

81. LEE S, et al. Photomechanical delivery of 100-nm microspheres through the stratum corneum: Implications for transdermal drug delivery. *Lasers Surg Med* 2002; 31(3): 207–210.

82. OGURA M, et al. *In vivo* targeted gene transfer in skin by the use of laser-induced stress waves. *Lasers Surg Med* 2004; 34(3): 242–248.

83. MITRAGOTRI S, et al. A mechanistic study of ultrasonically-enhanced transdermal drug delivery. *J Pharm Sci* 1995; 84(6): 697–706.

84. SMITH NB. Perspectives on transdermal ultrasound mediated drug delivery. *Int J Nanomedicine* 2007; 2(4): 585–594.

85. MITRAGOTRI S, BLANKSCHTEIN D, LANGER R. Transdermal drug delivery using low-frequency sonophoresis. *Pharm Res* 1996; 13(3): 411–420.

86. KUSHNER J, BLANKSCHTEIN D, LANGER R. Heterogeneity in skin treated with low-frequency ultrasound. *J Pharm Sci* 2008; 97(10): 4119–4128.

87. LAVON I, et al. Bubble growth within the skin by rectified diffusion might play a significant role in sonophoresis. *J Control Release* 2007; 117(2): 246–255.

88. UEDA H, et al. Acoustic cavitation as an enhancing mechanism of low-frequency sonophoresis for transdermal drug delivery. *Biol Pharm Bull* 2009; 32(5): 916–920.

89. GUPTA J, PRAUSNITZ MR. Recovery of skin barrier properties after sonication in human subjects. *Ultrasound Med Biol* 2009; 35(8): 1405–1408.

90. OGURA M, PALIWAL S, MITRAGOTRI S. Low-frequency sonophoresis: Current status and future prospects. *Adv Drug Deliv Rev* 2008; 60(10): 1218–1223.

91. RAO R, NANDA S. Sonophoresis: Recent advancements and future trends. *J Pharm Pharmacol* 2009; 61(6): 689–705.

92. LANKE SS, et al. Enhanced transdermal delivery of low molecular weight heparin by barrier perturbation. *Int J Pharm* 2009; 365(1–2): 26–33.

93. TACHIBANA K. Transdermal delivery of insulin to alloxan-diabetic rabbits by ultrasound exposure. *Pharm Res* 1992; 9(7): 952–954.

94. BOUCAUD A, et al. Effect of sonication parameters on transdermal delivery of insulin to hairless rats. *J Control Release* 2002; 81(1–2): 113–119.

95. PARK EJ, WERNER J, SMITH NB. Ultrasound mediated transdermal insulin delivery in pigs using a lightweight transducer. *Pharm Res* 2007; 24(7): 1396–1401.

96. SMITH NB, LEE S, SHUNG KK. Ultrasound-mediated transdermal *in vivo* transport of insulin with low-profile cymbal arrays. *Ultrasound Med Biol* 2003; 29(8): 1205–1210.

97. PARK EJ, DODDS J, SMITH NB. Dose comparison of ultrasonic transdermal insulin delivery to subcutaneous insulin injection. *Int J Nanomedicine* 2008; 3(3): 335–341.

98. TEZEL A, et al. Low-frequency ultrasound as a transcutaneous immunization adjuvant. *Vaccine* 2005; 23(29): 3800–3807.

99. DAHLAN A, et al. Transcutaneous immunisation assisted by low-frequency ultrasound. *Int J Pharm* 2009; 368(1–2): 123–128.

100. DENET AR, VANBEVER R, PREAT V. Skin electroporation for transdermal and topical delivery. *Adv Drug Deliv Rev* 2004; 56(5): 659–674.

101. HUI SW. Overview of drug delivery and alternative methods to electroporation. *Methods Mol Biol* 2008; 423: 91–107.

102. VANBEVER R, LEBOULENGE E, PREAT V. Transdermal delivery of fentanyl by electroporation. I. Influence of electrical factors. *Pharm Res* 1996; 13(4): 559–565.

103. VANBEVER R, LEROY MA, PREAT V. Transdermal permeation of neutral molecules by skin electroporation. *J Control Release* 1998; 54(3): 243–250.

104. DENET AR, PREAT V. Transdermal delivery of timolol by electroporation through human skin. *J Control Release* 2003; 88(2): 253–262.

105. HU Q, et al. Enhanced transdermal delivery of tetracaine by electroporation. *Int J Pharm* 2000; 202(1–2): 121–124.

106. WONG TW, et al. Pilot study of topical delivery of methotrexate by electroporation. *Br J Dermatol* 2005; 152(3): 524–530.

107. JOHNSON PG, HUI SW, OSEROFF AR. Electrically enhanced percutaneous delivery of delta-aminolevulinic acid using electric pulses and a DC potential. *Photochem Photobiol* 2002; 75(5): 534–540.

108. ZHANG L, et al. Electroporation-mediated topical delivery of vitamin C for cosmetic applications. *Bioelectrochem Bioenerg* 1999; 48(2): 453–461.

109. FANG JY, et al. Transdermal delivery of tea catechins by electrically assisted methods. *Skin Pharmacol Physiol* 2006; 19(1): 28–37.

110. SERSA G, et al. Electrochemotherapy in treatment of tumours. *Eur J Surg Oncol* 2008; 34(2): 232–240.

111. TOKUMOTO S, HIGO N, SUGIBAYASHI K. Effect of electroporation and pH on the iontophoretic transdermal delivery of human insulin. *Int J Pharm* 2006; 326(1–2): 13–19.

112. ZHAO YL, et al. Induction of cytotoxic T-lymphocytes by electroporation-enhanced needle-free skin immunization. *Vaccine* 2006; 24(9): 1282–1290.

113. DAUD AI, et al. Phase I trial of interleukin-12 plasmid electroporation in patients with metastatic melanoma. *J Clin Oncol* 2008; 26(36): 5896–5903.

114. FERRARO B, et al. Intradermal delivery of plasmid VEGF(165) by electroporation promotes wound healing. *Mol Ther* 2009; 17(4): 651–657.

115. HELLER R, et al. Electrically mediated delivery of plasmid DNA to the skin using a multi electrode array. *Hum Gene Ther* 2010; 21(3): 357–362.

116. MAZERES S, et al. Non invasive contact electrodes for *in vivo* localized cutaneous electropulsation and associated drug and nucleic acid delivery. *J Control Release* 2009; 134(2): 125–131.

117. WONG TW, et al. Painless electroporation with a new needle-free microelectrode array to enhance transdermal drug delivery. *J Control Release* 2006; 110(3): 557–565.

118. SAMMETA SM, VAKA SR, MURTHY SN. Transdermal drug delivery enhanced by low voltage electropulsation (LVE). *Pharm Dev Technol* 2009; 14(2): 159–164.

119. BASSETT CA. Beneficial effects of electromagnetic fields. *J Cell Biochem* 1993; 51(4): 387–393.

120. VIANALE G, et al. Extremely low frequency electromagnetic field enhances human keratinocyte cell growth and decreases proinflammatory chemokine production. *Br J Dermatol* 2008; 158(6): 1189–1196.

121. MURTHY SN. Magnetophoresis: An approach to enhance transdermal drug diffusion. *Pharmazie* 1999; 54(5): 377–379.

122. MURTHY SN, HIREMATH SR. Physical and chemical permeation enhancers in transdermal delivery of terbutaline sulphate. *AAPS Pharm Sci Tech* 2001; 2(1): E-TN1.

123. NAMJOSHI S, et al. Liquid chromatography assay for 5-aminolevulinic acid: Application to *in vitro* assessment of skin penetration via Dermaportation. *J Chromatogr B Analyt Technol Biomed Life Sci* 2007; 852(1–2): 49–55.

124. NAMJOSHI S, et al. Enhanced transdermal delivery of a dipeptide by dermaportation. *Biopolymers* 2008; 90(5): 655–662.
125. KRISHNAN G, et al. Enhanced skin permeation of naltrexone by pulsed electromagnetic fields in human skin *in vitro*. *J Pharm Sci* 2010; 99(6): 2724–2731.
126. BENSON HA, et al. Enhanced skin permeation and hydration by magnetic field array: Preliminary in-vitro and in-vivo assessment. *J Pharm Pharmacol* 2010; 62(6): 696–701.
127. DIAS M, et al. *In vivo* infrared spectroscopy studies of alkanol effects on human skin. *Eur J Pharm Biopharm* 2008; 69(3): 1171–1175.
128. ALVAREZ-ROMAN R, et al. Visualization of skin penetration using confocal laser scanning microscopy. *Eur J Pharm Biopharm* 2004; 58(2): 301–316.
129. KANIKKANNAN N, et al. Iontophoresis. In: Walters KA, Roberts MS, eds. *Dermatologic, Cosmeceutic, and Cosmetic Development*. Informa Healthcare, New York, 2008; 517–535.
130. TEZEL A, MITRAGOTRI S. Interactions of inertial cavitation bubbles with stratum corneum lipid bilayers during low-frequency sonophoresis. *Biophys J* 2003; 85(6): 3502–3512.
131. TSAI TH, et al. Multiphoton microscopy in dermatological imaging. *J Dermatol Sci* 2009; 56(1): 1–8.
132. MORIMOTO Y, et al. Elucidation of the transport pathway in hairless rat skin enhanced by low-frequency sonophoresis based on the solute-water transport relationship and confocal microscopy. *J Control Release* 2005; 103(3): 587–597.
133. PALIWAL S, MENON GK, MITRAGOTRI S. Low-frequency sonophoresis: Ultrastructural basis for stratum corneum permeability assessed using quantum dots. *J Invest Dermatol* 2006; 126(5): 1095–1101.
134. WEIMANN LJ, WU J. Transdermal delivery of poly-l-lysine by sonomacroporation. *Ultrasound Med Biol* 2002; 28(9): 1173–1180.
135. KUSHNER J, et al. Dual-channel two-photon microscopy study of transdermal transport in skin treated with low-frequency ultrasound and a chemical enhancer. *J Invest Dermatol* 2007; 127(12): 2832–2846.
136. GALLETLY NP, et al. Fluorescence lifetime imaging distinguishes basal cell carcinoma from surrounding uninvolved skin. *Br J Dermatol* 2008; 159(1): 152–161.
137. ROBERTS MS, et al. *In vitro* and *in vivo* imaging of xenobiotic transport in human skin and in the rat liver. *J Biophotonics* 2008; 1(6): 478–493.
138. MELOT M, et al. Studying the effectiveness of penetration enhancers to deliver retinol through the stratum cornum by *in vivo* confocal Raman spectroscopy. *J Control Release* 2009; 138(1): 32–39.
139. CROWTHER JM, et al. Measuring the effects of topical moisturizers on changes in stratum corneum thickness, water gradients and hydration *in vivo*. *Br J Dermatol* 2008; 159(3): 567–577.

Chapter 4

Clinical Applications of Transdermal Iontophoresis

Dhaval R. Kalaria, Sachin Dubey, and Yogeshvar N. Kalia

THE "HOW" AND "WHY" OF IONTOPHORESIS

Transdermal iontophoresis involves the application of a small electric potential to facilitate the transport of polar and charged hydrosoluble permeants across the skin and it has been successfully used to enhance the delivery of low molecular weight (MW) therapeutics, peptides, and proteins.[1-3] The first reports describing the use of an electric current to deliver medicinal agents into the body date back to Pivati in 1747.[4] During the 18th and 19th centuries, Rossi, Palaprat, Wagner, and Morton tried to deliver various molecules using electric currents.[5] At the turn of the 20th century, Le Duc confirmed that strychnine could be driven across skin with the aid of an electric current.[6]

In addition to expanding the range of therapeutics that can be administered transdermally,[7] the key advantage of iontophoresis is that modulation of the applied current enables precise control over the rate and profile of drug delivery.[8] Thus, it is possible to achieve complex delivery kinetics, for example, pulsatile or on-demand bolus inputs that otherwise require the use of an infusion pump. Drug input can also be titrated—for example, in therapies that require a gradual "ramping" of the dose—and the clinician can provide individualized therapy by reprogramming the device. Despite the numerous reports describing iontophoretic drug delivery *in vitro* and *in vivo* either in animals or in humans, prefilled iontophoretic systems have only become available in the last few years. This can be attributed to advances made on three fronts: (1) progress in microelectronics and engineering processes that has enabled the development of miniaturized and cost-effective delivery systems[9]; therefore, iontophoretic systems can no longer be considered as cumbersome machines but as portable user-friendly devices readily capable of replacing more invasive systems; (2) patient compliance and the financial success of passive transdermal

Transdermal and Topical Drug Delivery: Principles and Practice, First Edition. Edited by Heather A.E. Benson, Adam C. Watkinson.

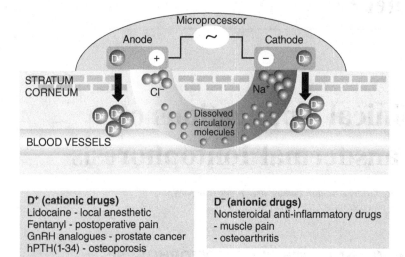

D+ (cationic drugs)
Lidocaine - local anesthetic
Fentanyl - postoperative pain
GnRH analogues - prostate cancer
hPTH(1-34) - osteoporosis

D- (anionic drugs)
Nonsteroidal anti-inflammatory drugs
- muscle pain
- osteoarthritis

Figure 4.1 A schematic representation of an iontophoretic patch system. At the heart of the system is a microprocessor that controls device function and drug delivery. The patch contains active and return electrode compartments.

patches stimulating the pharmaceutical industry to look more closely at the transdermal route; and (3) rational drug design and recombinant DNA technology yielding increasing numbers of therapeutically important peptides and proteins where iontophoresis can provide a method for their controlled noninvasive delivery.

An iontophoretic system comprises a microprocessor, a power source, and two electrode compartments—anodal and cathodal (Fig. 4.1). The drug formulation is placed in the donor compartment based on the net charge of the therapeutic agent; for example, a cationic drug is placed in the anodal compartment. Once the current is applied, the ions migrate out from the device and into the skin under the influence of the electric field. The electrical circuit is completed by the movement of endogenous counterions, primarily chloride and sodium ions, moving out from the skin and into the anodal and cathodal chambers, respectively.

In addition to the duration and intensity of current application, other formulation conditions also impact upon drug delivery.[2] These include: (1) drug content that will influence drug concentration in the skin; (2) the pH, which determines the degree of drug ionization; and (3) the patch application area, which can be tailored as per clinical needs. Here, we provide a brief review of preliminary clinical studies that describe promising clinical applications of iontophoresis.

TOPICAL APPLICATIONS

Anesthetics: Providing Fast Onset of Action

Lidocaine, when delivered parenterally, is a fast-acting effective anesthetic; however, the injection can be painful. For some patients, the pain and fear associated with injection reduces the likelihood that they will seek medical care, pursue diagnostic testing, or receive appropriate immunization or parenteral medications.[10] In children, needlesticks can arouse more fear than major surgeries and other more invasive procedures.[11] Topical formulations such as EMLA® cream (AstraZeneca, Wilmington, DE), a eutectic mixture of lidocaine and prilocaine, have been used to provide local anesthesia; however, they suffer from a slow onset of action (1–2 hours) and the shallow depth of anesthesia achieved (~3–5 mm).[12] These failings led to the investigation and development of fast-acting iontophoretic systems for topical lidocaine delivery.

Several clinical trials have shown the efficacy of lidocaine iontophoresis in dermal anesthesia.[13–17] Two studies suggested that lidocaine iontophoresis was superior to eutectic lidocaine and prilocaine cream for topical anesthesia before intravenous (IV) cannulation.[18,19] All of the above studies used electrodes from commercial suppliers such as Iomed Inc. (Salt Lake City, UT) and Dupel® Iontophoresis System (Empi Co., St. Paul, MN). Treatment was initiated with a current of 1.0 mA and gradually increased to a maximum of 4.0 mA as tolerated by the subject; the total amount of charge delivered was 20, 30, or 40 mA/min.

These first-generation iontophoretic devices were less convenient as they were neither prefilled with drug nor preprogrammed, and required a higher iontophoretic dose than necessary for effective topical anesthesia, thereby increasing the risk of adverse events.[20] The LidoSite™ Topical System (lidocaine topical anesthetic system) developed by Vyteris, Inc. (Fair Lawn, NJ) and approved by the U.S. Food and Drug Administration (FDA) in 2005 is a small, easy-to-use, preprogrammed iontophoretic lidocaine delivery system composed of a drug-filled patch connected to a controller (Fig. 4.2). The patch is a single-use disposable drug product, which contains a 5-cm² circular drug reservoir (anode) that delivers lidocaine and

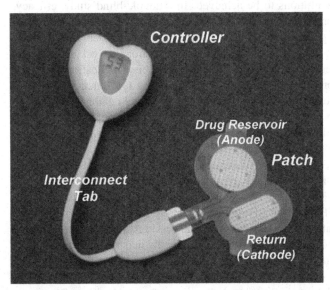

Figure 4.2 The LidoSite topical lidocaine delivery system comprises a reusable controller and single-use disposable patches.

epinephrine to the skin, and a 2.5-cm^2 oval return reservoir (cathode) containing electrolytes. The controller can be reused up to 100 times and applies a current of 1.77 mA for 10 minutes (i.e., 17.7 mA/min). It is designed to achieve local anesthesia before medical interventions such as insertion of IV catheters, needlesticks for blood withdrawal, and other dermatological applications.

Phase I clinical studies showed that 10 minutes of iontophoresis was sufficient to anesthetize the skin to a depth of at least 6 mm (often 10 mm or more), which is more than adequate for needlesticks and dermatological procedures. Neither lidocaine nor epinephrine was detected in the systemic circulation. Phase II studies demonstrated the suitability of the device for pediatric patients requiring venipuncture, while Phase III clinical studies established that patients (adults and children) receiving lidocaine from the LidoSite system reported significantly less pain upon venipuncture or IV cannulation than the corresponding control subjects.[2,21] Furthermore, adult and pediatric patients treated with LidoSite experienced little or no pain during surgical procedures, such as incisional or excisional treatment of superficial skin lesions.

Pain Management and Delivery of Nonsteroidal Anti-Inflammatory Agents: Targeted Pain Relief to Reduce the Risk of Systemic Side-Effects

Transdermal delivery of nonsteroidal anti-inflammatory drugs (NSAIDs) is of considerable interest since it reduces the risk of gastrointestinal (GI)-related side effects commonly encountered when these agents are administered by the oral route. In addition to minimizing systemic exposure, it also enables targeted delivery and allows high local concentrations to be achieved. In a double-blind study, efficacy, and tolerability of pirprofen and "lysine soluble aspirin" (lysine acetylsalicylate) were delivered by iontophoresis to 80 patients suffering from a variety of rheumatic conditions. Treatment lasted 2 weeks with five administrations a week each lasting 20 minutes (direct current mean intensity, 2–3 mA). After five applications, patients showed significant improvement in pain at rest and during movement; there were no significant differences between pirprofen and aspirin. Final results were good or excellent in ~75% of the patients treated and functional improvement was satisfactory in about 80%. Furthermore, only local penetration of the drug in the inflamed area was noted without high systemic levels.[22]

Ketoprofen[23] and ketorolac[24] have also been successfully delivered by iontophoresis to human volunteers; the latter was reported to be efficient in treating pain due to rheumatic disease. Ketoprofen was delivered using the Dupel iontophoretic system with a current of 4 mA for 40 minutes; ketorolac was delivered using silver electrodes with a current of 2 mA for five treatment sessions with 20 minutes every day. Diclofenac iontophoresis has also been used clinically in patients suffering from arthritis and epicondylitis.[25] They received 20 treatments of 30-minutes duration with a current intensity 4–8 mA; however, other studies have reported side effects, including a systemic adverse reaction[26] and allergic contact dermatitis.[27] Cutaneous bioavailability (BA) of piroxicam following passive and iontophoretic delivery from a commercially available gel formulation was compared in healthy volunteers.[28] Cathodal iontophoresis was employed using silver electrodes with a current of 0.3 mA/cm^2 for 125 minutes. Quantification of drug levels in the stratum corneum revealed that the amount of piroxicam delivered via passive and iontophoresis was 5.4 ± 2.0 and 48.6 ± 18.8 μg/cm^2, respectively.

Iontophoresis was used to deliver dexamethasone in 25 patients (double-blind study) with Achilles tendon injury.[29] Patients received four 20-minute treatments at intervals of 3–4 days using iontophoresis in a 2-week period and were evaluated before treatment and at a series of time points post-treatment (after 2 and 6 weeks, 3 and 6 months, and 1 year). Several significant improvements in terms of physical activity were noticed in the treatment group as compared to the control group. Nirschl et al. conducted a double-blind placebo-controlled study into the iontophoretic delivery of dexamethasone sodium phosphate in 199 patients with acute epicondylitis.[30] Each patient received 40 mA/min of either the active or placebo treatment on six occasions. Patients received current up to 4.0 mA, depending on their sensitivity, and once the preset dose of 40 mA/min was delivered, the current automatically ramped down to 0 mA. Iontophoretic treatment was well tolerated by most patients and was effective in reducing epicondylitis symptoms at short-term follow-up.

Dermatological Applications: Improving Local BA

Following idoxuridine iontophoresis into 14 recurrent herpes labialis lesions in six patients, the subjects reported immediate relief from discomfort and swelling, rapid appearance and coalescence of vesicles, minimal or no spread of the lesions, and accelerated healing with minimal or no scab formation.[31]

In a recent study, iontophoretic application of 5% aciclovir cream was tested in a multicenter, placebo-controlled trial for the episodic treatment of herpes labialis among 200 patients with an incipient cold sore outbreak at the erythema or papular/edema lesion stage.[32] The study was performed with a portable, hand-held iontophoretic device with treatment for 20 minutes. The median classic lesion healing time was shortened by 35 hours in the active treatment group with respect to the control (113 vs. 148 hours). Furthermore, in the subgroup of patients that presented lesions in the erythema stage, the median classic lesion healing time was shortened by up to 3 days for the aciclovir group, compared with the control group (49 vs. 120 hours). In addition, it was reported that the aciclovir-treated group tended to have more aborted lesions than the control group (46% vs. 24%). It was concluded that single-dose topical iontophoresis of aciclovir was a convenient and effective treatment for cold sores.

In a double-blind, placebo-controlled clinical study, Gangarosa et al. compared iontophoresis of vidarabine monophosphate (Ara-AMP) and aciclovir for efficacy against herpes orolabialis.[33] A group of 27 human volunteers with vesicular orolabial herpes were divided into three equal subgroups that received either vidarabine monophosphate (Ara-AMP) or aciclovir or NaCl. Results showed that Ara-AMP-treated lesions yielded lower viral titers after 24 hours compared with lesions treated with NaCl or aciclovir. There was also a significant decrease in the duration of virus shedding and the time to dry crust in the Ara-AMP-treated group as compared to the two other groups.

Twenty-six patients with biopsy-proven Bowen's disease received eight iontophoretic treatments of 5-fluorouracil (5-FU) over a period of 4 weeks.[34] A commercially available portable iontophoretic device, Phoresor II (Iomed Inc.), was used with a treatment regimen of 4 mA for 10 minutes twice a week for 4 weeks. Three months after the last treatment, local excisions were done and in the treated group only one patient out of 26 displayed any histological evidence of bowenoid changes, thus proving the efficacy of the treatment.[34] However, a case report described a cutaneous allergic reaction upon 5-FU iontophoresis, although the conclusion was derived from only one patient.[35]

Aminolevulinic acid (ALA) is a precursor of the endogenous fluorescent photosensitizer protoporphyrin IX (PpIX), which is used in the treatment of a range of cancers.[36] However, the therapeutic potential of this molecule is limited by its high polarity; simple cream formulations require several hours of application in order to penetrate into the skin.[37] Rhodes et al., studied ALA pharmacokinetics following iontophoretic delivery of a 2% ALA solution in the upper inner arm of healthy volunteers. Using the Phoresor II system, an iontophoretic current of 0.2 mA was applied on a circular surface of 1 cm diameter and its permeation quantified by measurement of PpIX fluorescence and phototoxicity. Studies revealed that ALA delivery was sufficient to induce tumor necrosis.[37] Gerscher et al. used the same conditions to compare the pharmacokinetics and phototoxicity from ALA as well as two ester derivatives in healthy human volunteers; it was reported that ALA-n-hexyl ester iontophoresis resulted in greater PpIX formation and lower phototoxicity relative to the other ester (ALA-n-butyl) and the parent molecule. A linear correlation between the logarithm of prodrug dose and PpIX fluorescence was observed for the three compounds[38]; a similar relationship was also observed with ALA-n-pentyl ester.[39]

Cisplatin has been iontophoresed into basal and squamous cell carcinomas (BCC/SCC).[40–42] Chang et al. studied 15 BCC or SCC lesions in 12 patients; 1 mg/mL of cisplatin was applied at a current of 0.5–1.0 mA for a period of 20–30 min on a lesion area of 2.9 cm × 2.0 cm. The response was good, as 11 out of the 15 lesions showed either a complete or a 50% decrease in lesion area after iontophoresis.[40] Subsequently, this protocol was successfully applied (four cycles) to a 67-year old man with BCC.[42] Iontophoretic delivery of cisplatin also produced partial remission when applied to patients with BCC or SCC lesions on the eyelids and periorbital tissues.[41]

Recalcitrant psoriasis in a 46-year-old male with well-defined bilateral psoriatic plaques on the palms was treated by methotrexate iontophoresis (0.6 mA/cm^2 for 15 minutes) with aluminum foil electrodes supported by an adhesive polyethylene sheet; treatment was performed once a week for a total of 4 weeks.[43] It was suggested that the lesion on the right palm, treated with topical methotrexate iontophoresis, showed >75% improvement by the end of 4 weeks (the left palm lesion served as a control and did not receive any treatment).

Iontophoretic delivery of 1 % vinblastine solution at 4 mA for 10–90 minutes was used to treat patients with Kaposi's sarcoma[44]; all 31 lesions treated showed partial to complete clearing and symptomatic improvement.

Diagnostic Application

The diagnosis of cystic fibrosis by pilocarpine iontophoresis was one of the earliest clinical applications of this technology.[45] Cystic fibrosis is a hereditary systemic disorder of the mucus-producing exocrine glands that affects the pancreas, bronchi, intestine, and liver. The perspiration contains an abnormal concentration of sodium and chloride ions[46] and assay of the latter is the basis for the diagnostic test.[47] The collection of sweat for diagnostic purposes is facilitated by the iontophoretic delivery of pilocarpine, a small, positively charged cholinergic agent that induces sweating. The diagnostic test was first introduced by Gibson and Cooke and received FDA approval in 1983, and several commercial iontophoretic systems for the diagnosis of cystic fibrosis have been developed[48,49] (CF Indicator®, Scandipharm, Birmingham, AL; Webster Sweat Inducer, Wescor Inc., Logan, UT). It has since become a standard screening test and is commonly used by pediatricians.[50]

SYSTEMIC APPLICATIONS

Opioids: Using Iontophoresis to Provide Fast-Acting Systemic Pain Relief

Several opioid analgesics are good candidates for iontophoresis from both physico-chemical and pharmacological standpoints. They are usually ionized at physiological pH, possess moderate MW (<500 Da), and are frequently highly potent. These characteristics, when combined with the ability of iontophoresis to provide fast controlled input kinetics, make a compelling argument for the development of ion-tophoretic systems for relief from acute pain.

An early study investigated the efficacy of morphine iontophoresis in a group of postsurgery patients initially placed on IV meperidine; they were divided into two subgroups, one of which received iontophoretic morphine for a period of 6 hours at the current required to deliver an equianalgesic dose of meperidine while the control group received buffer.[51] The patient-controlled analgesia (PCA) option remained available to both sets of patients and the results demonstrated that the iontophoretic group made fewer requests for PCA than the control group. Minimally effective concentrations (~20 ng/mL) were achieved in the blood within 30 minutes of commencing iontophoresis and levels capable of providing consistent pain relief (~40 ng/mL) were achieved during current application. Patients in the iontophoretic group displayed a red wheal and flare under and around the anodal compartment that was attributed to local histamine release provoked by morphine.

Fentanyl is one of the most widely studied opioids when it comes to transdermal iontophoresis. In addition to its physicochemical properties, it is extremely potent— between 100- and 500-fold superior to morphine depending on the assay; moreover, it does not induce histamine release. Its physicochemical and pharmacological properties together with its pharmacokinetics—short half-life, high first-pass effect— makes it an ideal candidate for transdermal administration.[52] Although passive transdermal fentanyl patches have been marketed for nearly 20 years for the treatment of chronic pain, they cannot provide a rapid bolus drug input for relief from acute pain.[53] The feasibility of using iontophoresis to deliver fentanyl was demonstrated *in vitro* and *in vivo*[54–56] and led to the development of the Ionsys™ system (using E-TRANS® electrotransport technology; Alza Corporation, Mountain View, CA)—a preprogrammed, self-contained, on-demand drug delivery system that is activated by the patient and can deliver 80 doses of 40 μg of fentanyl in a 24-hour period.[9] Figures 4.3 and 4.4 show a photograph and an exploded view, respectively, of the E-TRANS fentanyl system. The system is composed of two primary components; the upper component houses the battery and electronic hardware responsible for monitoring the system. The lower component is composed of two hydrogel reservoirs. One is the anode containing active fentanyl hydrochloride. The other hydrogel reservoir (cathode) contains only inactive substances. The system is held in place by a polyisobutylene skin adhesive.[57]

Based on pharmacokinetic studies, a current of 170 μA was selected to deliver each 40-μg dose over 10 minutes.[58,59] The maximum number of 80 doses was shown to be sufficient to achieve effective analgesia and if a patient required additional analgesia, a new system could be applied to a different skin site. The size, shape, and materials of the system allowed the patient comfortable, unrestricted movement during wear (typically on the upper arm and the chest). In addition to the fundamental electronic design parameters of current intensity and duration and the number of

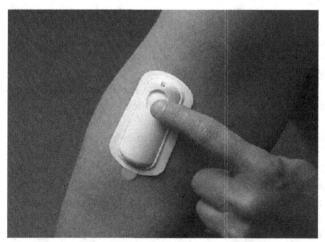

Figure 4.3 The fully integrated fentanyl ITS can be applied to the patient's upper arm and drug delivery initiated using the controller button.

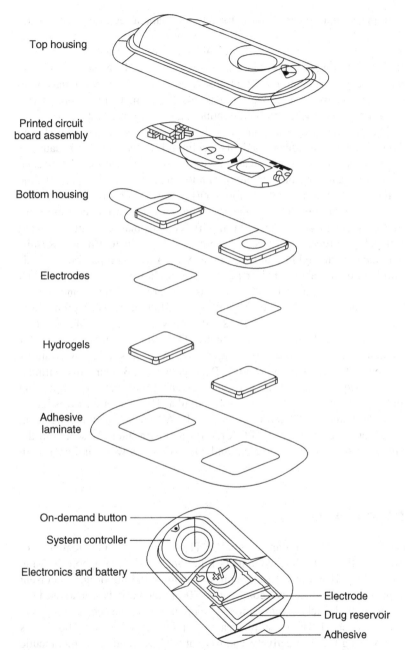

Top housing

Printed circuit
board assembly

Bottom housing

Electrodes

Hydrogels

Adhesive
laminate

On-demand button

System controller

Electronics and battery

Electrode

Drug reservoir

Adhesive

Figure 4.4 A detailed view inside the E-TRANS iontophoretic drug delivery system showing the major components: top housing, printed circuit board assembly that forms the controller, a bottom housing containing reservoirs for placement of electrodes and hydrogels, and an adhesive laminate. The E-TRANS technology was used to develop the Ionsys™ fentanyl ITS.

doses allowed per system, other important safety and patient feedback features are included in the system design.[9] Clinical studies showed that the Ionsys system was well tolerated by patients with postoperative pain and was equivalent to an IV morphine pump demonstrating the importance of this device in medical care.[60–64] Viscusi et al. compared the fentanyl iontophoretic transdermal system (ITS) with placebo in postoperative pain management among 484 patients. Supplemental IV fentanyl was available to patients upon request in both treatment groups for the first 3 hours after enrollment. The main efficacy end point was the patient global assessment (PGA) of the method of pain control; fewer patients receiving ITS discontinued because of inadequate analgesia compared with placebo and it was concluded that ITS was an excellent method of pain control.[60] In another multicenter study in 504 patients, the ITS (40 μg fentanyl [10-minute infusion/lockout], up to 6 doses/h) was compared with intravenous patient-controlled analgesia (IV PCA) with morphine (1 mg morphine bolus [5-minute lockout], up to 10 mg/h) for pain management following abdominal or pelvic surgery—PGA scores were used to evaluate efficacy. Results demonstrated that the fentanyl ITS and morphine IV PCA were comparable methods of pain control following abdominal or pelvic surgery; however, the fentanyl ITS was rated superior to morphine IV PCA for ease of care by patients and nurses. Overall discontinuation rates were not significantly different between groups and commonly occurring adverse events were similar between groups.[61] Ahmad et al. compared the efficacy and safety of the fentanyl ITS with morphine IV PCA for pain management following gynecologic surgery—PGA success ratings were statistically equivalent between the two groups.[62] Pain intensity at 3 hours, discontinuations due to inadequate analgesia, and the percentage of patients requesting supplemental opioids in the first 3 hours were similar. Hartrick et al. investigated the efficacy of the fentanyl ITS and morphine IV PCA for acute pain management in patients after orthopedic surgery.[63] PGA ratings and pain intensity scores in the first 24 hours were statistically equivalent and adverse events were similar in both the groups.

Antimigraine Drugs

The pharmacokinetics of alniditan, a novel $5HT_{1D}$ agonist for the treatment of migraine, were studied in healthy volunteers following anodal iontophoresis using 10-cm^2 hydrophilic polyurethane foam patches containing 0.5 mg drug.[65] A current of 0.2 mA/cm^2 was applied for two consecutive 30-minute periods (separated by a 90-minute interval) and patches were removed 90 minutes after the end of the second current application period. The mean plasma concentrations at 30 and 150 minutes were 4.49 and 5.37 ng/mL, respectively, and were at the lower end of the therapeutic range (5–20 ng/mL). Moreover, the plasma concentration achieved after 30 minutes of iontophoretic delivery was equivalent to simulated subcutaneous administration of 0.5 mg dose.

Siegel et al. investigated sumatriptan iontophoresis in healthy volunteers[66]; of the six treatment groups, two received oral sumatriptan (50 mg) and 6 mg subcutaneous injection, respectively. The remaining iontophoretic treatment groups (10 cm^2 patches) received (1) 1.0 mA for 1.5 hours for a theoretical dose of 1.5 mg (treatment 3); (2) 0.5 mA for 3 hours for a theoretical dose of 1.5 mg (treatment 4); (3) two patches at 1.0 mA for 3 hours for a theoretical dose of 6 mg (treatment 5); and (4) two patches at 1.0 mA for 6 hours for a theoretical dose of 12 mg sumatriptan (treatment 6). The areas under the curve (AUC)$_{0-24}$ for treatments 3 and 4 were ~19% of the oral and 26% of the injection; C$_{max}$ was 31% of oral and 14% of injection for treatment 3 and 20% of oral and 9% of injection for treatment 4. Treatment 5 yielded an AUC$_{0-24}$ value, which was approximately 88% of the 50 mg oral preparation and 122% of the 6 mg injection. Treatment 6 yielded an AUC$_{0-24}$ that was approximately 187% of the 50 mg oral preparation and 259% of the 6 mg injection; C$_{max}$ was 109% of oral and 49% of injection for treatment 5 and 131% of oral and 59% of the injection for treatment 6. Treatments 5 and 6 maintained sumatriptan levels above 10 ng/mL for 4 and 7 hours, respectively, as compared to approximately 3 hours for oral and 1.5 hours for injectable. Thus, transdermal iontophoresis was capable of maintaining therapeutic sumatriptan levels for four times longer than the 6.0 mg injection and twice as long as the 50 mg oral preparation, offering substantially longer duration of treatment than either preparation. The T$_{max}$ for oral and injection formulations was 1.31 and 0.28 hours, respectively, while the maximum serum concentration was reached in approximately 1.5 hours for all patch formulations and was sustained until patch removal. Although this was comparable to oral administration, the iontophoretic system should ideally approach the fast onset of the subcutaneous injection.

Drugs for Treatment of Neurodegenerative Diseases

Kankkunen et al. investigated the iontophoretic delivery of a reversible acetylcholinesterase inhibitor, tacrine, in healthy adult volunteers.[67] They performed two experiments: the first using commercially available Iogel® electrodes (Chattanooga Group, Chattanooga, TN), while the second employed a novel two-compartment electrode system in which the drug reservoir was separated from the electrode by a membrane to maximize the transport efficiency by avoiding competition from other ions. A 0.4 mA/cm^2 current was applied for 3 hours using patches with an active surface area of 10 cm^2. The tacrine plasma concentrations measured after iontophoresis using the "in-house" electrodes (14.9 ± 2.6 ng/mL) compared favorably with those achieved with the Iogel electrodes (21.3 ± 5.9 ng/mL). Both values lie within the range of blood levels seen following oral administration of tacrine.

Van der Geest et al. iontophoresed R-apomorphine, a potent dopamine agonist, in patients with idiopathic Parkinson's disease.[68,69] Two different current intensities of 0.25 and 0.375 mA/cm^2 were applied for 1 hour using patches having a surface area of 10 cm^2. Although measurable plasma apomorphine concentrations of 1.3 ± 0.6 and 2.5 ± 0.7 ng/mL, at 0.25 and 0.375 mA/cm^2, respectively, were achieved, these levels were subtherapeutic. Furthermore, qualitative clinical improvement could only be confirmed in one patient treated with the higher current density; however, the study was not blinded so a placebo effect cannot be excluded.

Li et al. combined transdermal iontophoretic delivery of R-apomorphine with surfactant pre-treatment in patients with advanced Parkinson's disease.[70] Iontophoretic patches were applied in 16 patients for 3.5 hours, with 0.5 hour of passive delivery followed by 3 hours of current application at a current density of 0.25 mA/cm^2. Eight patients were treated with a surfactant formulation consisting of laureth-3 ethyloxylene ether, laureth-7 ethyloxylene ether, and sodium sulfosuccinate (in a molar ratio of 0.7:0.3:0.05, respectively) with a concentration of 5% w/w prior to iontophoresis. The surfactant formulation (20 µL/cm^2) was applied nonocclusively at the anode site on the dorsal forearm of patients for 1 hour before patch placement. The patients treated with the surfactant formulations showed a higher BA and steady-state input rate compared to the control group (patients receiving iontophoresis without surfactant), with BA at 13.2 ± 1.4 and 10.6 ± 0.8% and flux at 98.3 ± 12.1 and 75.3 ± 6.6 nmol/cm^{2}h, respectively. Clinical improvement was observed in five out of eight patients in the study group and in three out of eight patients in the control group. No clinically relevant systemic adverse effects were observed.

Antiemetics

Cormier et al. investigated metoclopramide iontophoresis in the presence and absence of hydrocortisone in humans in order to determine whether codelivery of hydrocortisone was effective in inhibiting local skin reactions.[71] Each volunteer was subjected to two identical treatments (metoclopramide alone and in combination with hydrocortisone) one after the other with a wash-out period of 1 week. A current of 500 µA was used for all the studies. There was no statistically significant difference in AUC, plasma concentration, and half-life of metoclopramide with or without hydrocortisone. A steady-state flux of ~100 µg/cm^{2}h was achieved after 1-hour transport. Furthermore, hydrocortisone iontophoresis was successful in suppressing local site reactions.

NONINVASIVE DELIVERY OF PEPTIDES AND PROTEINS

Peptides and proteins are generally inactive orally because of their susceptibility to chemical and enzymatic degradation in the GI tract. They are usually potent and can have complex secretion profiles in the body (e.g., the variation in basal and postprandial insulin levels); an ideal delivery system should be able to provide controlled drug inputs as required. In addition to being ideally suited to the delivery of polar and charged molecules with good aqueous solubility, transdermal iontophoresis permits tight control over drug transport rates and enables complex input kinetics to be used. It follows that there have been several reports into the iontophoretic delivery of peptide hormones, including luteinizing-hormone-releasing hormone (LHRH),[72,73] calcitonin,[74,75] growth-hormone-releasing hormone,[76] human parathyroid hormone,[77] and insulin[78,79] using different iontophoretic systems.

Investigation into the effect of formulation parameters on the iontophoretic delivery of leuprolide, an LHRH superagonist, in human volunteers showed that steady-state serum concentrations could be achieved within 30 minutes; anodal delivery from a 10 mg/mL formulation in acetate buffer using a current of 0.2 mA was able to reach mean steady-state serum concentration of 0.8 ng/mL.[80] An earlier double-blind, randomized, crossover study in 13 healthy men investigating leuprolide iontophoresis (5 mg; 0.2 mA, 70 cm[2]) showed that the patches, though large, were well tolerated and luteinizing hormone (LH) concentration was increased from a baseline of 11.3 ± 3.1 mIU/mL to 56.4 ± 49.6 mIU/mL at 4 hours.[81] Another study compared LH pharmacodynamics after iontophoretic delivery with subcutaneous injection in a group of 18 human volunteers.[82] The applied dose was kept constant at 5 mg/mL, and using a current of 0.22 μA it was observed that the time to first response was shorter for subcutaneous injection (73 ± 74 and 147 ± 108 minutes, respectively) and the AUC for the first 150 minutes was greater for subcutaneous delivery (3655 ± 2246 and 8666 ± 4067 mIU min/mL, respectively). No major adverse effects were observed at the application site following iontophoresis, thus it might be possible to increase the current intensity in order to reduce the lag time.

A crossover study comparing intramuscular (IM) bolus, 6-hour IV infusion, and 6-hour iontophoretic delivery (200 μA/cm[2]) of a calcitonin analog (MW ~3 kDa) was performed in healthy human volunteers.[83] The plasma levels observed following iontophoresis closely mimicked those seen after IM injection with similar AUC and inter-individual variability. On termination of the current at 6 hours, a fairly rapid decline in the plasma levels was observed. After 6 hours, the skin sites were observed for any topical effects, which suggested a slight pink coloration on skin that eventually disappeared after 24 hours.

CONCLUSION

The results to date demonstrate that iontophoresis is a drug delivery platform that has been used to administer a variety of therapeutic agents with many different clinical applications. Moreover, it is the only transdermal delivery technology that has managed to produce FDA-approved products; although both systems (LidoSite and Ionsys) contain low MW therapeutics, the technique is uniquely suited to the delivery of peptides and proteins. Physicochemical properties and drug pharmacokinetics obviously put a limit on the number of drug candidates that can be delivered by transdermal iontophoresis. In the most favorable conditions (for compounds with low MW and multiple charges), the maximum amount of drug that can be delivered per day from a reasonably sized patch will probably be in the range of 20–30 mg. However, technical feasibility alone cannot drive a molecule to the market—drug candidates have to address an unmet clinical need. Furthermore, several issues, including cost of therapy and the risk of skin irritation, may also limit potential applications. Nevertheless, transdermal iontophoresis is a promising technique that requires a greater focus on research directed toward formulation development in an effort to design efficient iontophoretic patch systems, particularly with a view to the delivery of biotechnology-derived therapeutics. Stability of the drug along with other patch components for periods up to 18 months will be critical as well as challenging. The delivery of peptides and proteins, which are susceptible to degradation in aqueous solution, may require the development of dry patches where the biomolecule is hydrated immediately prior to use.[84-88] Thus, the development of future iontophoretic systems will require a multidisciplinary effort from fields such as pharmaceutics, material sciences, and electrochemistry in order to take a promising candidate from bench to bedside.

REFERENCES

 1. LICHT S. History of electrotherapy. In: Stilwell GK, ed. *Therapeutic Electricity and Ultraviolet Radiation*, 3rd ed. Williams & Wilkins, Baltimore, MD, 1983; 1–64.
 2. KALIA YN, NAIK A, GARRISON J, et al. Iontophoretic drug delivery. *Adv Drug Deliv Rev* 2004; 56: 619–658.
 3. CÁZARES-DELGADILLO J, NAIK A, GANEM-RONDERO A, et al. Transdermal delivery of cytochrome C—A 12.4kDa protein—Across intact skin by constant-current iontophoresis. *Pharm Res* 2007; 24: 1360–1368.
 4. WATKINS AL. *A Manual of Electrotherapy*, 2nd ed. Lea and Febiger, Philadelphia, 1968.
 5. BANGA AK. Percutaneous absorption and its enhancement. In: Banga AK, ed. *Electrically Assisted Transdermal and Topical Drug Delivery*. Taylor & Francis, Bristol, PA, 1998; 1–12.
 6. LE DUC S. *Electric Ions and Their Use in Medicine*. Rebman, Liverpool, 1908.
 7. ABLA N, NAIK A, GUY RH, KALIA YN. Iontophoresis: Clinical applications and future challenges. In: Smith EW, Maibach HI, eds. *Percutaneous Penetration Enhancers*, 2nd ed. Taylor & Francis, Bristol, PA, 2005; 177–219.
 8. NAIK A, KALIA YN, GUY RH. Transdermal drug delivery: Overcoming the skin's barrier function. *Pharm Sci Technol Today* 2000; 3: 318–326.
 9. SUBRAMONY JA, SHARMA A, PHIPPS JB. Microprocessor controlled transdermal drug delivery. *Int J Pharm* 2006; 317: 1–6.
10. HOLMES HS. Choosing a local anesthetic. *Dermatol Clin* 1994; 12: 817–823.
11. MENKE EM. School-aged children's perception of stress in the hospital. *Child Health Care* 1981; 9: 80–86.
12. WAHLGREN CF, QUIDING H. Depth of cutaneous analgesia after application of a eutectic mixture of the local anesthetics lidocaine and prilocaine (EMLA cream). *J Am Acad Dermatol* 2000; 42: 584–588.
13. ZEMPSKY WT, PARKINSON TM. Lidocaine iontophoresis for topical anesthesia before dermatologic procedures in children: A randomized controlled trial. *Pediatr Dermatol* 2003; 20: 364–368.
14. ZEMPSKY WT, ANAND KJ, SULLIVAN KM, et al. Lidocaine iontophoresis for topical anesthesia prior to intravenous line placement in children. *J Pediatr* 1998; 32: 1061–1063.
15. WALLACE MS, RIDGEWAY B, JUN E, et al. Topical delivery of lidocaine in healthy volunteers by electroporation, electroincorporation, or iontophoresis: An evaluation of skin anesthesia. *Reg Anesth Pain Med* 2001; 26: 229–238.
16. ROSE JB, GALINKIN JL, JANTZEN EC, et al. A study of lidocaine iontophoresis for pediatric venipuncture. *Anesth Analg* 2002; 94: 867–871.
17. KIM MK, KINI NM, TROSHYNSKI TJ, et al. A randomized clinical trial of dermal anesthesia by iontophoresis for peripheral intravenous catheter placement in children. *Ann Emerg Med* 1999; 33: 395–399.
18. SQUIRE SJ, KIRCHHOFF KT, HISSONG K. Comparing two methods of topical anesthesia used before intravenous cannulation in pediatric patients. *J Pediatr Health Care* 2000; 14: 68–72.
19. MILLER KA, BALAKRISHNAN G, EICHBAUER G, et al. 1% lidocaine injection, EMLA cream, or "Numby Stuff" for topical analgesia associated with peripheral intravenous cannulation. *J Am Assoc Nurse Anesth* 2001; 69: 185–187.

20. ZEMPSKY WT, ASHBURN MA. Iontophoresis: Noninvasive drug delivery. *Am J Anesthesiol* 1998; 25: 158–162.

21. ZEMPSKY WT, SULLIVAN J, PAULSON DM, et al. Evaluation of a low-dose lidocaine iontophoresis system for topical anaesthesia in adults and children: A randomized, controlled trial. *Clin Ther* 2004; 26: 1110–1119.

22. GARAGIOLA U, DACATRA U, BRACONARO F, et al. Iontophoretic administration of pirprofen or lysine soluble aspirin in the treatment of rheumatic diseases. *Clin Ther* 1988; 10: 553–558.

23. PANUS PC, CAMPBELL J, KULKARNI SB, et al. Transdermal iontophoretic delivery of ketoprofen through human cadaver skin and in humans. *J Control Release* 1997; 44: 113–121.

24. SAGGINI R, ZOPPI M, VECCHIET F, et al. Comparison of electromotive drug administration with ketorolac or with placebo in patients with pain from rheumatic disease: A double-masked study. *Clin Ther* 1996; 18: 1169–1174.

25. VECCHINI L, GROSSI E. Ionization with diclofenac sodium in rheumatic disorders: A double-blind placebo-controlled trial. *J Int Med Res* 1984; 12: 346–350.

26. MACCHIA L, CAIAFFA MF, DI GIOIA R, et al. Systemic adverse reaction to diclofenac administered by transdermal iontophoresis. *Allergy* 2004; 59: 367–368.

27. FOTI C, CASSANO N, CONSERVA A, et al. Allergic contact dermatitis due to diclofenac applied with iontophoresis. *Clin Exp Dermatol* 2004; 29: 91.

28. CURDY C, KALIA YN, NAIK A, et al. Piroxicam delivery into human stratum corneum *in vivo*: Iontophoresis versus passive diffusion. *J Control Release* 2001; 76: 73–79.

29. NEETER C, THOMEE R, SILBERNAGEL KG, et al. Iontophoresis with or without dexamethasone in the treatment of acute Achilles tendon pain. *Scand J Med Sci Sports* 2003; 13: 376–382.

30. NIRSCHL RP, RODIN DM, OCHIAI DH, et al. Iontophoretic administration of dexamethasone sodium phosphate for acute epicondylitis. *Am J Sports Med* 2003; 31: 189–195.

31. GANGAROSA LP, MERCHANT HW, PARK NH, et al. Iontophoretic application of idoxuridine for recurrent herpes labialis: Report of preliminary clinical trials. *Methods Find Exp Clin Pharmacol* 1979; 1: 105–109.

32. MORREL EM, SPRUANCE S, GOLDBERG DI. Topical iontophoretic acyclovir cold sore study group, topical iontophoretic administration of acyclovir for the episodic treatment of herpes labialis: A randomized, double-blind, placebo-controlled clinic-initiated trial. *Clin Infect Dis* 2006; 43: 460–467.

33. GANGAROSA LP, HILL JM, THOMPSON BL, et al. Iontophoresis of vidarabine monophosphate for herpes orolabialis. *J Infect Dis* 1986; 154: 930–934.

34. WELCH ML, GRABSKI WJ, McCOLLOUGH ML, et al. 5-fluorouracil iontophoretic therapy for Bowen's disease. *J Am Acad Dermatol* 1997; 36: 956–958.

35. ANDERSON LL, WELCH ML, GRABSKI WJ. Allergic contact dermatitis and reactivation phenomenon from iontophoresis of 5-fluorouracil. *J Am Acad Dermatol* 1997; 36: 478–479.

36. PENG Q, WARLOE T, BERG K, et al. 5-Aminolevulinic acid based photodynamic therapy. *Cancer* 1997; 79: 2282–2308.

37. RHODES LE, TSOUKAS MM, ANDERSON RR, et al. Iontophoretic delivery of ALA provides a quantitative model for ALA pharmacokinetics and PpIX phototoxicity in human skin. *J Invest Dermatol* 1997; 108: 87–91.

38. GERSCHER S, CONNELLY JP, GRIFFITHS J, et al. Comparison of the pharmacokinetics and phototoxicity of protoporphyrin IX metabolized from 5-aminolevulinic acid and two derivatives in human skin *in vivo*. *Photochem Photobiol* 2000; 72: 569–574.

39. GERSCHER S, CONNELLY JP, BEIJERSBERGEN VAN HENEGOUWEN GM, et al. A quantitative assessment of protoporphyrin IX metabolism and phototoxicity in human skin following dose-controlled delivery of the prodrugs 5-aminolaevulinic acid and 5-aminolaevulinic acid-n-pentylester. *Br J Dermatol* 2001; 144: 983–990.

40. CHANG BK, GUTHRIE TH, HAYAKAWA K, et al. A pilot study of iontophoretic cisplatin chemotherapy of basal and squamous cell carcinomas of the skin. *Arch Dermatol* 1993; 129: 425–427.

41. LUXENBERG MN, GUTHRIE TH. Chemotherapy of basal cell and squamous cell carcinoma of the eyelids and periorbital tissues. *Ophthalmology* 1986; 93: 504–510.

42. BACRO TR, HOLLADAY EB, STITH MJ, et al. Iontophoresis treatment of basal cell carcinoma with cisplatin: A case report. *Cancer Detect Prev* 2000; 24: 610–619.
43. TIWARI SB, KUMAR BCR, UDUPA N, et al. Topical methotrexate delivered by iontophoresis in the treatment of recalcitrant psoriasis—a case report. *Int J Dermatol* 2003; 42: 157–159.
44. SMITH KJ, KONZELMAN JL, LOMBARDO FA, et al. Iontophoresis of vinblastine into normal skin and for treatment of Kaposi's sarcoma in human immunodeficiency virus-positive patients. *Arch Dermatol* 1992; 128: 1365–1370.
45. GANGAROSA S, HILL JM. Modern iontophoresis for local drug delivery. *Int J Pharm* 1995; 123: 159–171.
46. HUANG YY, WU SM, WANG CY, et al. Response surface method as an approach to optimization of iontophoretic transdermal delivery of pilocarpine. *Int J Pharm* 1996; 129: 41–50.
47. GIBSON LE, COOKE RE. A test for the concentration of electrolytes in sweat in cystic fibrosis of the pancreas utilizing pilocarpine by iontophoresis. *Pediatrics* 1959; 23: 545–549.
48. FOGT EJ, NORENBERG MS, UNTEREKER DF, et al. Fluid absorbent quantitative test device. U.S. patent 4,444,193, 1984.
49. YEUNG WH, PALMER J, SCHIDLOW D, et al. Evaluation of a paper-patch test for sweat chloride determination. *Clin Pediatr* 1984; 23: 603–607.
50. SINGH P, MAIBACH HI. Iontophoresis in drug delivery: Basic principles and applications. *Crit Rev Ther Drug Carrier Syst* 1994; 11: 161–213.
51. ASHBURN MA, STEPHEN RL, ACKERMAN E, et al. Iontophoretic delivery of morphine for postoperative analgesia. *J Pain Symptom Manage* 1992; 7: 27–33.
52. CHELLY JE, GRASS J, HOUSEMAN TW, et al. The safety and efficacy of a fentanyl patient-controlled transdermal system for acute postoperative analgesia: A multicenter, placebo-controlled trial. *Anesth Analg* 2004; 98: 427–433.
53. SCOTT ER, PHIPPS JB, GYORY JR, et al. Electrotransport system for transdermal delivery. A practical implementation of iontophoresis. In: Wise DL, ed. *Handbook of Pharmaceutical Controlled Release Technology*. Marcel Dekker, New York, NY, 2000; 617–659.
54. THYSMAN S, TASSET C, PRÉAT V. Transdermal iontophoresis of fentanyl: Delivery and mechanistic analysis. *Int J Pharm* 1994; 101: 105–113.
55. THYSMAN S, PRÉAT V. *In vivo* iontophoresis of fentanyl and sufentanil in rats: Pharmacokinetics and acute antinociceptive effects. *Anesth Analg* 1993; 77: 61–66.
56. ASHBURN MA, STREISAND J, ZHANG J, et al. The iontophoresis of fentanyl citrate in humans. *Anesthesiology* 1995; 82: 1146–1153.
57. HENDRON CM. Iontophoretic drug delivery system: Focus on fentanyl. *Pharmacotherapy* 2007; 27: 745–754.
58. GUPTA SK, SOUTHAM M, SATHYAN G, et al. Effect of current density on pharmacokinetics following continuous or intermittent input from a fentanyl electrotransport system. *J Pharm Sci* 1998; 87: 976–981.
59. GUPTA SK, SATHYAN G, PHIPPS JB, et al. Reproducible fentanyl doses delivered intermittently at different time intervals from an electrotransport system. *J Pharm Sci* 1999; 88: 835–841.
60. VISCUSI ER, REYNOLDS L, TAIT S, et al. An iontophoretic fentanyl patient-activated analgesic delivery system for postoperative pain: A double-blind, placebo-controlled trial. *Anesth Analg* 2006; 102: 188–194.
61. MINKOWITZ HS, RATHMELL JP, VALLOW S, et al. Efficacy and safety of the fentanyl iontophoretic transdermal system (ITS) and intravenous patient-controlled analgesia (IV PCA) with morphine for pain management following abdominal or pelvic surgery. *Pain Med* 2007; 8: 657–668.
62. AHMAD S, DAMARAJU CV, HEWITT DJ. Fentanyl HCl iontophoretic transdermal system versus intravenous morphine pump after gynecologic surgery. *Arch Gynecology Obstet* 2007; 276: 251–258.
63. HARTRICK CJ, BOURNE MH, GARGIULO K, et al. Fentanyl iontophoretic transdermal system for acute-pain management after orthopedic surgery: A comparative study with morphine intravenous patient-controlled analgesia. *Reg Anesth Pain Med* 2006; 31: 546–554.
64. VISCUSI ER, REYNOLDS L, CHUNG F, et al. Patient-controlled transdermal fentanyl hydrochloride vs intravenous morphine pump for postoperative pain. *J Am Med Assoc* 2004; 291: 1333–1341.

65. JADOUL A, MESENS J, CAERS W, et al. Transdermal permeation of alniditan by iontophoresis: *In vitro* optimization and human pharmacokinetic data. *Pharm Res* 1996; 13: 1348–1353.
66. SIEGEL SJ, NEILL CO, DUBÉ ML, et al. Unique iontophoretic patch for optimal transdermal delivery of sumatriptan. *Pharm Res* 2006; 24: 1919–1926.
67. KANKKUNEN T, SULKAVA R, VUORIO M, et al. Transdermal iontophoresis of tacrine *in vivo*. *Pharm Res* 2002; 19: 704–708.
68. VAN DER GEEST R, DANHOF M, BODDÉ HE. Iontophoretic delivery of apomorphine: *In vitro* optimization and validation. *Pharm Res* 1997; 14: 1798–1803.
69. DANHOF M, VAN DER GEEST R, VAN LAAR T, et al. An integrated pharmacokinetic–pharmacodynamic approach to optimization of R-apomorphine delivery in Parkinson's disease. *Adv Drug Deliv Rev* 1998; 33: 253–263.
70. LI GL, DE VRIES JJ, VAN STEEG TJ, et al. Transdermal iontophoretic delivery of apomorphine in patients improved by surfactant formulation pre-treatment. *J Control Release* 2005; 101: 199–208.
71. CORMIER M, CHAO ST, GUPTA SK, et al. Effect of transdermal iontophoresis codelivery of hydrocortisone on metoclopramide pharmacokinetics and skin-induced reactions in human subjects. *J Pharm Sci* 1999; 88: 1030–1035.
72. HEIT MC, WILLIAMS PL, JAYES FL, et al. Transdermal iontophoretic peptide delivery: *In vitro* and *in vivo* studies with luteinizing hormone releasing hormone. *J Pharm Sci* 1993; 82: 240–243.
73. RAIMAN J, KOLJONEN M, HUIKKO K, et al. Delivery and stability of LHRH and Nafarelin in human skin: The effect of constant/pulsed iontophoresis. *Eur J Pharm Sci* 2004; 21: 371–377.
74. THYSMAN S, HANCHARD C, PREAT V. Human calcitonin delivery in rats by iontophoresis. *J Pharm Pharmacol* 1994; 46: 725–730.
75. MORIMOTO K, IWAKURA Y, NAKATANI E, et al. Effects of proteolytic enzyme inhibitors as absorption enhancers on the transdermal iontophoretic delivery of calcitonin in rats. *J Pharm Pharmacol* 1992; 44: 216–218.
76. KUMAR S, CHAR H, PATEL S, et al. *In vivo* transdermal iontophoretic delivery of growth hormone releasing factor GRF (1–44) in hairless guinea pigs. *J Control Release* 1992; 18: 213–220.
77. SUZUKI Y, NAGASE Y, IGA K, et al. Prevention of bone loss in ovariectomized rats by pulsatile transdermal iontophoretic administration of human PTH (1-34). *J Pharm Sci* 2002; 91: 350–361.
78. SIDDIQUI O, SUN Y, LIU JC, et al. Facilitated transdermal transport of insulin. *J Pharm Sci* 1987; 76: 341–345.
79. KARI B. Control of blood glucose levels in alloxan-diabetic rabbits by iontophoresis of insulin. *Diabetes* 1986; 35: 217–221.
80. LU MF, LEE D, CARLSON R, et al. The effects of formulation variables on iontophoretic transdermal delivery of leuprolide to humans. *Drug Dev Ind Pharm* 1993; 19: 1557–1571.
81. MEYER BR, KREIS W, ESCHBACH J, et al. Successful transdermal administration of therapeutic doses of a polypeptide to normal human volunteers. *Clin Pharmacol Ther* 1988; 44: 607–612.
82. MEYER BR, KREIS W, ESCHBACH J, et al. Transdermal versus subcutaneous leuprolide: A comparison of acute pharmacodynamic effect. *Clin Pharmacol Ther* 1990; 48: 340–345.
83. GREEN PG. Iontophoretic delivery of peptide drugs. *J Control Release* 1996; 41: 33–48.
84. EVERS HCA, BROBERG FB, DENUZZIO JD, et al. User activated iontophoretic device and method for using same, World Patent Application 93/18727, 1993.
85. KONNO Y, MITONI M, SONOBE T, et al. Plaster structural assembly for iontophoresis. U.S. Patent 4,842,577, 1989.
86. HAAK RP, GYORY JR, THEEUWES F, et al. Iontophoretic delivery device and methods of hydrating same. U.S. Patent 5,288,289, 1994.
87. HAAK RP, GYORY JR, THEEUWES F, et al. Iontophoretic delivery device and methods of hydrating same. U.S. Patent 5,320,598, 1994.
88. GYORY JR, PERRY JR. Iontophoretic delivery device and methods of hydrating same. U.S. Patent 5,310,404, 1994.

Chapter 5

In Vitro Skin Permeation Methodology

Barrie Finnin, Kenneth A. Walters, and Thomas J. Franz

INTRODUCTION

Final international acceptance of the Organisation for Economic Cooperation and Development (OECD) 428 "Guideline for the Testing of Chemicals: Skin Absorption *In Vitro* Method" and the associated Guidance 28 in 2004 marked an important point in the regulatory acceptance of *in vitro* methods for examination of skin permeation and distribution.[1,2] These set out a detailed framework of the numerous issues that should be addressed in study design if meaningful data are to be obtained. However, they allow significant variations in protocol design that, although to some extent are desirable in terms of ensuring that a particular study uses conditions that are relevant and appropriate to the use of the data, some experts believe that this results in a guideline and guidance that are actually too imprecise to ensure that study data are consistent and reproducible. The latter view can be effectively countered by the argument that a "one size fits all" protocol cannot be appropriate for all test substances and exposure scenarios. It is important to appreciate that the OECD has provided *guidelines* and not a specific *protocol* that can be instantly applied without extensive preexperimental consideration of the nature of the test material, exposure scenario, and the objectives of the study. It is also important to appreciate that in the "reporting" section, OECD 428 includes an extensive list of required experimental detail, together with the requirement to *justify the test system*. Comprehensive justification of the test system includes a wide range of parameters, including species, membrane type, receptor fluid, integrity testing, test vehicle, dose applied, time points and experimental duration, terminal washing procedures, extraction methods, and assay validation. Only prestudy performance of such a justification procedure in the design of a specific experimental protocol can ensure that production of relevant data is possible.

Transdermal and Topical Drug Delivery: Principles and Practice, First Edition. Edited by Heather A.E. Benson, Adam C. Watkinson.
© 2012 John Wiley & Sons, Inc. Published 2012 by John Wiley & Sons, Inc.

In addition, demonstration of relevant experimental proficiency in the area, as shown by the ability to accurately reproduce data generated in competent laboratories, is essential. The wide variability in the data generated in the multicenter study on permeation of methyl paraben through the same silicone membrane (thereby excluding biological variation) demonstrated very clearly that imprecise specification and control of experimental conditions and procedures had a very marked effect on the results.[3] A similar European multicenter study compared the permeation of three reference compounds (caffeine, testosterone, and benzoic acid) through human skin *in vitro*.[4] Although in the latter study the authors concluded that the *in vitro* skin permeation methodology was relatively robust, not all variables were controlled. They attributed the observed variation to human variability in dermal absorption and the skin source.

In this chapter we discuss some of the more important aspects of *in vitro* skin penetration and permeation measurements, we point out some factors that could critically affect variability within and between experiments, and we propose a more rigorous guideline to enable interlaboratory studies that may provide more consistent results.

METHODOLOGY

Diffusion Cell Design

Diffusion cell design is primarily dictated by the objectives of the experiment and the preference of the investigator. Three basic types exist: (1) two-chambered (horizontal), (2) one-chambered static (vertical), and (3) one-chambered flow-through (vertical) (Fig. 5.1).

Early studies in the field of percutaneous absorption were largely directed at understanding the underlying mechanism and, typically, a technique commonly used in the physical sciences was employed to study the process.[5] Skin was clamped between two horizontally positioned chambers, each filled with an "infinite" amount of aqueous (in most cases) solution, and the rate of movement of test article from outside to inside measured. Application of an "infinite" dose led to the development of a steady-state rate of absorption and enabled use of a simple, long-established method of data analysis, the calculation of the permeability coefficient (K_P). One cannot underestimate the importance of these seminal studies as the data obtained are the foundation on which much of our current understanding of the permeability of skin rests.

As the focus in the field moved from mechanism to practical issues related to human pharmacology and toxicology, limitations of the two-chamber cell became obvious. *In vitro* studies, whose objective is to obtain data accurately reflecting the living state, need to be conducted in such a manner that all critical parameters associated with the situation being modeled are precisely duplicated. Since the skin normally functions in the dry environment of air, the most serious objection to the use of the two-chamber cell is that the stratum corneum (SC) is in contact with an

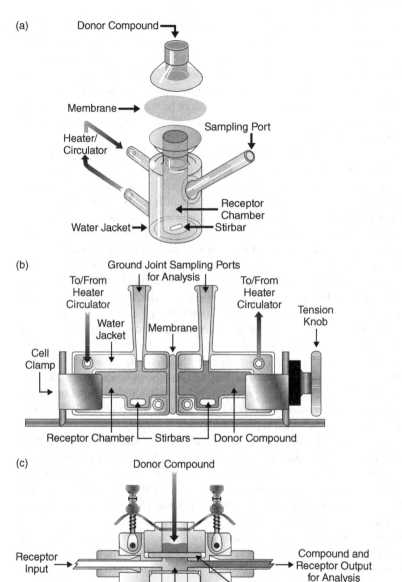

(a) Donor Compound

Membrane

Sampling Port

Heater/
Circulator

Receptor
Chamber

Water Jacket — Stirbar

(b) Ground Joint Sampling Ports
for Analysis

To/From
Heater
Circulator

To/From
Heater
Circulator

Tension
Knob

Water
Jacket

Membrane

Cell
Clamp

Receptor Chamber — Stirbars — Donor Compound

(c) Donor Compound

Receptor
Input

Compound and
Receptor Output
for Analysis

Receptor Chamber

Membrane

Figure 5.1 Diffusion cell designs. (a) Franz cell. (b) Side-by-side cell. (c) Flow-through cell.
Images adapted courtesy of PermeGear (http://www.permegear.com).

aqueous solution or other solvent for prolonged periods of time. Although this situation may be a relevant model for certain situations encountered by living man (e.g., swimming/bathing) and of importance to those in the field of toxicology and risk assessment, its use to those interested in topical or transdermal drug delivery is limited.

The static vertical cell was specifically developed to study percutaneous absorption under conditions that simulate those most commonly encountered in everyday life.[6,7] In this cell the skin is clamped between a lower (dermal) chamber containing the receptor solution and an upper (epidermal) "chimney" that is open to the ambient laboratory environment. It was designed to both duplicate the physical conditions existing in and around the SC (temperature, relative humidity) as well as to allow the flexibility to apply either a finite or an infinite dose of any formulation type, including transdermal devices.

The exposed epidermal surface allows easy access for dosing of liquid formulations or the chimney top can be temporarily removed for dosing of semisolid formulations that require thorough spreading to assure equal distribution to the entire exposed surface area. It also allows for the conduct of a surface wash where such is required to duplicate a specific *in vivo* scenario or to assess unabsorbed test article.

The dermal surface is bathed by some form of aqueous solution, buffered isotonic saline being the most frequent choice, and its temperature regulated by thermostatically controlled water circulating through a jacket surrounding the chamber in order to maintain the skin surface at 32°C. In cells without a jacket, a heating block or water bath can be used for temperature control. Homogeneous temperature distribution in the dermal bathing solution is maintained by a Teflon-covered magnetic stirring bar, driven by an external magnet mounted on a timing motor. Absorption is measured by periodically sampling the dermal bathing solution. Though some prefer to remove only an aliquot for analysis and, therefore, determine the cumulative amount of test compound as it penetrates, this has the potential to lead to loss of sink conditions as the experiment proceeds and possible underestimation of the amount absorbed. An alternative procedure is to remove the receptor solution in its entirety at each sampling time and replace with fresh solution.

The third type of diffusion cell design is the one-chamber flow-through type introduced by Bronaugh and Stewart.[8] Like the static cell, the basic philosophy of duplicating *in vivo* conditions is followed, but it has the advantage of automating the sampling procedure by continually pumping receptor fluid through the dermal chamber and collecting the effluent in a fraction collector. The one-chambered flow-through and static cells have been found to yield similar results.

An important consideration in the use of flow-through cells is the relationship between receptor volume, flow rate, and analytical sensitivity. If the *in vitro* kinetics are to accurately match those existing *in vivo*, the flow rate must be sufficient to totally replace the receptor volume many times during each sampling interval, yet not generate such a large volume of solution that the test compound is diluted beyond the lower limit of quantitation. This is best achieved by the use of a small receptor compartment (<0.5 mL). The small volume also obviates the need for stirring as the perfusing fluid itself serves this function.

No matter what type of cell is used it is important that the material from which the cell is made not adsorb the test article under study. In this regard, glass or Teflon (DuPont, Wilmington, DE) is the most frequently used material because of their inertness to most chemicals. Plexiglas (Dow Chemical) was found not to be a suitable alternative.[8] Glass also facilitates visual inspection of the underside of the skin to ensure the absence of bubbles. One commercially available flow-through cell is made of Teflon but has a glass window in the bottom (PermeGear Inc., Hellertown, PA).

Variations of the vertical cell are numerous but all retain the core design. At the chimney–skin–reservoir interface one has the choice between a flat ground-glass surface and an o-ring seal. The sampling port may be found near the top or bottom of the receptor chamber. Automatic sampling systems have been developed. There are vertical cells with and without water jackets. A cell has been designed to mount fingernails in place of skin. Sizes of cells, based on the available skin-dosing surface area, can be found ranging from as small as 0.25 cm^2 to as large as 12.5 cm^2. In addition, innovative chimney designs have emerged for unique study designs, such as to allow for vapor or gas exposure, recovery of volatile compounds, or the use of caps or closures for occlusion.[9]

Receptor Chamber and Medium

The receptor or acceptor solution must have adequate solubility for the compound under study so that sink conditions are sustained throughout the length of the study, allowing the rate of absorption to proceed as it would normally under *in vivo* conditions with a functioning circulatory system. For water-soluble compounds, isotonic saline or buffered isotonic saline (pH ~7.4) are considered the rational choice for the maintenance of a physiological environment. Preservatives are not always necessary but are used by many to prevent microbial buildup, particularly where experiments are of long duration or where one wants to exclude a microbial contribution to skin metabolism. It must be established that the preservative used does not interfere with the assay of the compound under study or the barrier function of the skin.

Studies in which maintenance of skin viability is essential so that simultaneous measurement of metabolic activity and absorption can be assessed require the use of special receptor solutions. Eagle's minimal essential medium (MEM), HEPES-buffered Hanks' balanced salt solution (HHBSS), and Dulbecco modified phosphate-buffered saline (DMPBS) are all capable of maintaining the viability of fresh, dermatomed rat skin for a period of 24 hours.[10]

Measurement of the absorption of highly water-insoluble compounds requires modification of the usual saline receptor; however, this must be done without damaging the integrity of the SC barrier. Additionally, since absorption into the systemic circulation *in vivo* can take place in capillary beds that sit very close to the dermal–epidermal junction, the great bulk of the highly aqueous dermis (1–2 mm) present in full-thickness skin can represent an "artificial" barrier to lipophilic molecules. To avoid this problem dermatomed skin or isolated epidermis must be used.

Bronaugh and Stewart examined the effectiveness of different receptor solutions on the permeation of two highly water-insoluble compounds, cinnamyl anthranilate (0.23 mg/L) and acetyl ethyl tetramethyl tetralin (AETT) (0.012 mg/L), in dermatomed rat skin (350 μm).[11] *In vitro* absorption was found to be 8–90 times lower than that determined *in vivo* when a saline receptor was used, with the discrepancy

Table 5.1   *In vitro* Absorption Through Dermatomed Rat Skin, in Comparison to *In Vivo* Absorption (IVIV Ratio), when Using Different Receptor Media to Solubilize Highly Water-Insoluble Cinnamyl Anthranilate and Acetyl Ethyl Tetramethyl Tetralin (AETT)

	Solubility (mg/L)	IVIV ratio	Cortisone K_p ($\times 10^5$)
Cinnamyl anthranilate	0.23		
Saline		0.13	7.1 ± 0.5
3% BSA		0.27	5.4 ± 0.2
1.5% PEG-20 oleyl ether		0.34	6.1 ± 0.5
6% PEG-20 oleyl ether		0.61	7.0 ± 0.9
20% PEG-20 oleyl ether		0.40	9.3 ± 0.9
50:50 methanol:water		0.59	17.2 ± 0.2^a
AETT	0.012		
Saline		0.01	6.3 ± 0.3
1.5% PEG-20 oleyl ether		0.12	4.9 ± 0.2
6% PEG-20 oleyl ether		0.32	7.0 ± 0.9^b
40% ethanol:water		0.32	21.7 ± 3.3^a

Cortisone flux was used as a control to monitor barrier integrity (mean ± standard error).

[a] Statistically significant increase over normal saline receptor.

[b] Value not measured, assumed to be identical to that determined above in cinnamyl anthranilate experiment.

Source: Data adapted from Reference 11.

being greater for the compound with the lower water solubility. The use of various concentrations of the nonionic surfactant polyethylene glycol (PEG)-20-oleyl ether (Volpo 20, Oleth 20) in water improved *in vitro/in vivo* correlation considerably without altering barrier function, as determined by simultaneous measurement of cortisone absorption (Table 5.1). However, the *in vitro* values were still 30%–60% below those seen *in vivo*. Other receptor solutions that they tried were either ineffective (rabbit serum, MEM, 3% bovine serum albumin, or 6% Poloxamer 188) or resulted in barrier damage (50:50 methanol:water, saline plus 1.5% or 6% Octoxynol 9). Volpo 20 was itself ineffective when used with full-thickness skin, but could be used at a lower concentration when thinner dermatomed skin was used (200 μm vs. 300 μm).[12]

Scott and Ramsey examined the permeation of the water-insoluble insecticide cypermethrin (0.009 mg/L) in rat epidermal membranes and found that 50% aqueous ethanol was the only receptor solution that yielded *in vitro* results in agreement with *in vivo*.[13] Although some absorption was detectable with Volpo 20, the values were much lower. Cypermethrin absorption was undetectable with either Volpo 20 or 50% aqueous ethanol when used with full-thickness rat skin. When human skin was used, no absorption could be measured through full-thickness skin with any receptor and, even with epidermal membranes, absorption was only detectable with 50% aqueous ethanol. However, there is no human *in vivo* data for cypermethrin with which the

Table 5.2 *In vitro* Absorption of Three Doses of Fluazifop-Butyl through Isolated Human Epidermis, in Comparison to *In Vivo* Absorption, When Using Different Receptor Media to Solubilize the Highly Water-Insoluble Pesticide (1.0 mg/L)

Dose	*In vitro*			*In vivo*
	TCM	6% Volpo 20	Aq. EtOH	
2.5	0.01 ± 0.002	0.01 ± 0.002	0.06 ± 0.05	0.20 ± 0.04
25	0.58 ± 0.04	0.12 ± 0.07	0.69 ± 0.30	0.84 ± 0.19
250	0.70 ± 0.40	0.90 ± 0.30	6.0 ± 3.2	4.09 ± 0.89

All values in $\mu g/cm^2$, mean ± standard deviation.

TCM, tissue culture medium (Medium 199 containing Earle's salts, bovine serum albumin, and antibiotics); Volpo 20, 6% PEG-20 oleyl ether in saline; Aq. EtOH, 50:50 ethanol:water.

Source: Data adapted from References 14 and 15.

in vitro results can be compared. The use of organic solvents, such as ethanol, is potentially problematic since they may alter barrier function. If an organic solvent is to be added to the receptor phase to increase test article solubility, absence of a change in barrier integrity should be documented at the conclusion of the study. Simultaneous measurement of the absorption of a control compound with the test article is one approach to consider (e.g., see Table 5.1).

Ramsey et al. measured the *in vitro* absorption of the water-insoluble pesticide fluazifop-butyl (1.0 mg/L) through human epidermal membranes and found substantial agreement with the *in vivo* results with only one of three receptor solutions examined.[14,15] Of the three solutions used—50% aqueous ethanol, 6% Volpo 20 in saline, and tissue culture medium (Medium 199 with Earle's salts) supplemented with bovine serum albumin—only the results obtained with 50% aqueous ethanol were in reasonable agreement with the results obtained in living man (Table 5.2). However, there was no documentation that the barrier was not altered by the ethanol.

The definition of water insoluble becomes somewhat arbitrary in relation to *in vitro* absorption studies, particularly since the rate of absorption can be very low for many compounds and solubility in the grams per liter range is not needed. For example, testosterone, an important and well-studied compound in this field, has a water solubility of only ~11 mg/L,[11] yet its *in vitro* absorption through dermatomed human skin (350 μm) into isotonic saline has been shown to closely mirror that observed *in vivo* when using drug doses of only 1–3 $\mu g/cm^2$.[16]

The consensus of international experts in the field of percutaneous absorption is that a receptor solution in which the maximum solubility of the test compound is 10 times greater than that needed under experimental conditions is sufficient to maintain sink conditions and minimize back diffusion.[2] Permeation through the skin is often so low, frequently of the order of nanograms per square centimeter per hour, that even isotonic saline can be a sufficiently adequate receptor for some compounds traditionally considered to be water insoluble. Current literature data suggest that the major problem arises when dealing with compounds whose water solubility is in the range of 1 mg/L and below. Determining solubility and stability of the compound of interest in the selected receptor solution(s) should be a primary consideration prior to study conduct.

Selection, Variation, and Preparation of Skin Membranes

A major potential variant in the design of *in vitro* skin permeation experiments is the nature of the skin membrane. Animal skin has been widely used as a substitute for human skin (see e.g., Bronaugh et al.[17]) but, although some animal models are still occasionally promoted (e.g., Barbero and Frasch[18]), such models are generally believed to give unreliable results (see Eppler et al.[19]). On the basis that the most reliable model for human skin penetration and permeation *in vivo* is human skin *in vitro*, this membrane will be the subject of the following discussion.

Intra- and Intersubject Variation

Southwell et al.[20] investigated the *in vitro* and *in vivo* variation in the permeability of human skin between different specimens (interdonor) and the same specimens (intradonor). Based on the permeation characteristics of a series of compounds, they concluded that *in vitro* interspecimen variation was 66% and intraspecimen variation was 43%. Benfeldt and colleagues[21] reported *in vivo* intersubject variabilities of 61% when evaluating the bioequivalence of lidocaine using microdialysis, and 68% for ketoprofen permeation from a topical gel.[22] The degree of variability in skin permeation is a concern during *in vitro* experiments. Experimenters attempt to reduce variability by using skin from the same body area across donors and test groups (i.e., abdominal skin is compared to abdominal skin, rather than breast or leg skin). Williams et al.[23] examined the permeation of 5-fluorouracil (644 determinations from 71 specimens) and estradiol (221 determinations from 28 specimens) through human abdominal skin. Here, where site variability was excluded, the data were log-normally distributed.

Donor Age Effects

Full-term infants possess a SC with reasonable barrier properties,[24] albeit with an immature immune system, and the epidermis continues to develop through the first year of life.[25] The effect of age on percutaneous absorption has been examined *in vivo* in man with variable results. Several reports have demonstrated that transepidermal water loss is less in older skin (>65 years) than younger skin.[26,27] Roskos et al.[28] postulated that reduced hydration levels and lipid content of older skin may be responsible for the demonstrated reduction in skin permeability where the permeants were hydrophilic in nature (no reduction was seen for model hydrophobic compounds; Table 5.3). A study on the bioavailability of transdermal fentanyl in

Table 5.3   Age-Related Differences in Percutaneous Absorption

Permeant	log P[a]	% applied dose permeated over 7 days[b]	
		22–40 years	>65 years
Testosterone	3.32	19.0 ± 4.4	16.6 ± 2.5
Estradiol	2.49	7.1 ± 1.1	5.4 ± 0.4
Hydrocortisone	1.61	1.5 ± 0.6	0.54 ± 0.15
Benzoic acid	1.83	36.2 ± 4.6	19.5 ± 1.6
Acetylsalicylic acid	1.26	31.2 ± 7.3	13.6 ± 1.9
Caffeine	0.01	48.2 ± 4.1	25.2 ± 4.8

[a] Octanol:water partition coefficient of the permeant.
[b] Compounds (4 $\mu g/cm^2$) were applied in 20 μL acetone to ventral forearm (n = 3–8).
Source: Reference 28.

cancer patients indicated that permeation of the drug across the skin was significantly reduced in patients over 75 years of age compared to those less than 65 years of age.[29]

A number of physiological changes that may be responsible for age-related alterations in skin permeability have been suggested. These include an increase in the size of individual SC corneocytes throughout life, increased dehydration of the outer layers of the SC with age, decreased epidermal turnover, and decreased microvascular clearance (for reviews, see Grove[30]; Roskos et al.[31]; Farage et al.[32]). Elias and Ghadially[33] described a biochemical basis for aberrant barrier homeostasis in aged skin based on a reduction in SC lipids and an abnormality in cholesterol synthesis brought on by malfunctioning cytokine signaling pathways. This was confirmed by Jensen et al.,[34] who found reduced activities of the ceramide-generating enzymes, sphingomyelinase and ceramide synthase, in the inner epidermis of aged skin. More recently, however, Elias et al. have reported that the abnormal barrier homeostasis may be due to defective SC acidity.[35] Human subjects aged 13–21 years were found to have a skin surface pH of about 4.9, whereas in individuals aged 51–80 years, skin surface pH was measured at about 5.3. It is difficult, however, to anticipate what effect such a small change in SC pH would have on skin permeation. Certainly, given the lipid nature of the SC, there is a relationship between the degree of a compound's ionization and its permeation rate (e.g., see Sridevi and Diwan[36] and Huang et al.[37]), but such a small change in pH is unlikely to significantly affect the rate of permeation of most compounds. Any alterations in permeation rates would more likely be a consequence of the effect of the small pH increase on the formation of the lipid barrier.

Sauermann et al.[38] used confocal laser scanning microscopy to evaluate differences between young (18–25 years) and old (>65 years) skin. Although there was no statistical difference in SC thickness between the two groups, the basal layer of older skin was significantly thinner than that in the younger group, and the number of dermal papillae per unit area was reduced in the older population, resulting in a flattened epidermal–dermal junction. Once again, it is difficult to hypothesize what effect the flattening of the epidermal–dermal junction could have on skin permeation. This is somewhat confounded by a lack of understanding of the exact nature of the function of the dermal rete ridges (dermal papillae). For the most part, in biological systems the major function of microscopic ridge and villi-type structures is to increase surface area to facilitate nutrient exchange, and it is tempting to suggest that a flattening of the rete ridges in the elderly dermis could lead to a decrease in the area available for permeated material to partition from the viable epidermis into the dermis with a consequential reduction in percutaneous absorption.

One other aspect of aging that will have considerable implications in percutaneous absorption involves skin blood flow. It is well documented that older men and women have an impaired vasodilation response to hyperthermia.[39] On average, healthy aged humans show a 25%–50% reduction in skin blood flow compared with healthy younger adults. It has been suggested that the rate of clearance of a solute from the skin via the dermal capillary network can affect the rate of permeation across the skin.[40] Perhaps predictably, a reduction in skin blood flow attenuates the clearance of permeated molecules from the dermis, resulting in a decrease in the concentration gradient of the permeant across the skin, with a consequential reduction in the rate of permeation.

When using excised human skin for *in vitro* skin permeation experiments, however, physiological factors such as skin blood flow and age-related changes such as dermal thinning are unlikely to generate any differences in the rate and extent of the measured skin permeation. It is unsurprising, therefore, that when comparing the barrier function of older (>65 years) skin with that of younger adults, the data are equivocal. Most studies conclude that there is no discernible dependence of skin permeability on age, sex, or storage conditions.[23,41,42] It is important to appreciate, however, that when interpreting data from *in vitro* studies and attempting to relate these to the *in vivo* situation, there are trends indicating that skin blood flow is reduced with age and that the dermis becomes thinner.

Racial Differences

Several authors have shown that there are differences in the permeability characteristics of skin of different racial groups. In general, it has been noted that white skin is slightly more permeable than black skin,[43,44] which correlates with observations that black skin has both more cell layers within the SC [45] and a higher lipid content,[46] and that there are racial differences in hair follicle distribution.[47] A study of Caucasian, Hispanic, Black, and Asian skin ranked them in order of permeability to methyl nicotinate as Black < Asian < Caucasian < Hispanic.[48] On the other hand, no racial difference in the *in vivo* percutaneous absorption of diflorasone diacetate was observed.[49] Similarly, Lotte et al.[50] found no statistical differences in the penetration or permeation of benzoic acid, caffeine, or acetylsalicylic acid into and through Asian, Black, and Caucasian skin (Table 5.4). Rawlings[51] provided a comprehensive review of ethnic differences in skin structure and function.

Table 5.4 Race-Related Differences in Percutaneous Absorption

Permeant	Race	Amount of permeant recovered (nmol/cm^2)	
		Urine at 24 hours	SC at 30 minutes[a]
Benzoic acid	Caucasian	9.0 ± 1.5	6.8 ± 1.0
	Black	6.4 ± 0.9	6.1 ± 1.0
	Asian	9.7 ± 1.2	8.1 ± 1.5
Caffeine	Caucasian	5.9 ± 0.6	5.5 ± 0.6
	Black	4.5 ± 1.0	5.8 ± 1.0
	Asian	5.2 ± 0.8	6.1 ± 0.9
Acetylsalicylic acid	Caucasian	6.2 ± 1.9	11.9 ± 1.9
	Black	4.7 ± 0.9	9.0 ± 1.7
	Asian	5.4 ± 1.7	10.1 ± 1.7

[a] Amount in SC determined by tape stripping ($n = 6$–9).
Source: Reference 50.

Storage Conditions

In the conduct of *in vitro* experiments, it is inevitable that some form of skin storage will be necessary. Human skin is sourced from cadavers or, preferably, from cosmetic reduction surgery. While it is occasionally possible to transport tissue directly from the operating theatre to the diffusion cell without freezing, under most circumstances the skin will be frozen prior to processing. Although some authors concluded that freezing had no measurable effect on permeability,[52,53] Wester et al.[54] cautioned against the use of frozen stored human skin for studies in which cutaneous metabolism may be a contributing factor. There are indications that storing animal skin in a frozen state may decrease barrier properties on thawing.[55,56] Nonetheless, provided human skin is not overly hydrated when frozen, it is unlikely that subsequent permeation characteristics will be significantly different from nonfrozen skin.

Membrane Preparation

Different methods can be used to prepare human skin for *in vitro* experimentation. Under most circumstances one of the following three membranes will be used in the diffusion cell: (1) full-thickness skin, incorporating the SC, viable epidermis, and dermis; (2) dermatomed skin, in which the lower dermis has been removed; and (3) epidermal membranes, comprising the viable epidermis and the SC (prepared by heat separation).

The choice of membrane is, for the most part, dependent upon the aqueous or lipid solubility characteristics of the permeant. Although *in vivo* the presence of blood flow will remove a considerable amount of the permeant reaching the dermis, *in vitro*, in the absence of blood flow, the relatively aqueous nature of the dermis will reduce the penetration of lipophilic compounds. Therefore, the use of heat-separated epidermal membranes is more appropriate for permeants that are highly water insoluble, and such membranes or dermatomed skin are appropriate for permeants that are poorly water soluble. It is important to appreciate that the preparation of epidermal membranes is time consuming and the necessary processing increases the possibility of damage to the skin membrane. Careful consideration of the most appropriate type of skin preparation is required and this should address the physicochemical nature of the penetrating species, the data required, tissue availability, and the timescales involved. To prepare heat-separated epidermal membranes, full-thickness skin is immersed in water at 60°C for ~45 seconds. Following removal from the water, the epidermis is gently removed using a pair of blunt curved forceps.[57]

The Permeation Experiment

Membrane Integrity

When the membrane has been selected and placed in position in or on the diffusion cell, there may be a requirement to assess membrane integrity to ensure that the data subsequently derived using the test material are reliable. Although simple visual examination of specimens will give a qualitative indication of skin integrity, quantitative evaluation may be obtained by the measurement of skin conductance, transepidermal water loss, or the flux of a marker compound such as tritiated water. Those skin samples that are found to be outside the "normal" range of values for such measurements are discarded.

Application of Test Material

For the test material, a suitable application procedure should be followed. Here it is necessary to consider the intrinsic purpose of the study. For example, risk assessment involving the study of the skin penetration of an ingredient in a cosmetic should be performed with the material in the marketed formulation and with a regime that mimics as closely as possible the "in use" situation (e.g., Walters et al.[58]). Similarly, a pharmaceutical product application should be conducted as recommended for therapeutic effect. The in use scenario often implies that the permeant is applied as a *finite* dose and may show marked depletion in donor concentration over the course of the experiment. On the other hand, the application of a transdermal therapeutic system under in use conditions may produce *infinite* dose conditions, in which there is sufficient permeant on the donor side to make any changes in donor concentration throughout the experiment negligible. In the finite dose situation, depletion of the permeant from the donor side usually results in a reduction in the rate of permeation and an eventual plateau in the cumulative permeation profile (Fig. 5.2). For permeants applied in semisolid formulations, various guidelines suggest application weights of 2–5 mg/cm² of formulation. Liquid formulations are normally applied at 5 µL/cm². For applications by weight, the precise amount applied is determined

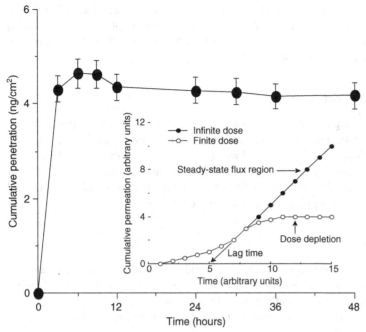

Figure 5.2   Permeation profile for a highly volatile compound permeating through human skin *in vitro*. The compound was applied at finite dose levels and permeation was significantly reduced by evaporation following 6 hours exposure. Inset shows sample cumulative permeation patterns following finite and infinite dosing regimes. With infinite dose, permeation normally reaches a steady-state flux region, whereas in finite dosing the permeation profile normally exhibits a plateauing effect as a result of donor depletion.

by difference, and it is advisable for all test materials to be applied by the same operator.

Duration of Experiment

Most investigators agree that for the duration of the permeation experiments, 24 or 48 hours is sufficient. However, for the evaluation of permeation from long-term transdermal delivery systems, it may be necessary to extend the experiment to 72 hours or longer. For longer-term experiments it is advisable to incorporate antimicrobial agents into the receptor phase. Investigators should, however, be aware of possible barrier degradation over extended time frames.

Sample Interval

Sample intervals should be frequent enough to allow assessment of lag-time, steady-state, or pseudo-steady-state flux. For a compound with unknown permeation characteristics, it may be necessary to run pilot experiments with samples taken at 2-hour intervals for the duration of the experiment. Early sample points (1–4 hours) can be important in identifying diffusion cells with damaged skin membranes that often show abnormal permeability values.

Number of Replicates

Because there is a high intra- and intersubject variability in human skin permeability, the number of replicates for each dosage regimen is recommended to be 12 (e.g., four donors with three replicates per donor or three donors with four replicates per donor), and comparisons between groups should use matched skin samples. Fewer replicates may be employed if cost, time, or skin availability are a problem, provided that the limitations of replicate reduction are recognized.

Temperature

Skin permeation experiments are normally conducted with a skin temperature of 32°C and this is achieved by maintaining the receptor solutions at 35–37°C, either by immersing cells in a water bath, heating block, or by using jacketed cells perfused with water at the correct temperature. Infrared surface thermometers have proven to be exceptionally useful for measuring skin surface temperature.

Analysis of Data

The OECD Guideline 428[1] has little to say about the way in which data from *in vitro* permeation studies should be analyzed. The guideline states:

> The analysis of receptor fluid, the distribution of the test substance chemical in the test system and the absorption profile with time, should be presented. When finite dose conditions of exposure are used, the quantity washed from the skin, the quantity associated with the skin (and in the different skin layers if analysed) and the amount present in the receptor fluid (rate, and amount or percentage of applied dose) should be calculated. Skin absorption may sometimes be expressed using receptor fluid data alone. However, when the test substance remains in the skin at the end of the study, it may need to be included in the total amount absorbed (see Guidance Document, paragraph 66). When infinite dose conditions of exposure are used the data may permit the calculation of a permeability constant (Kp). Under the latter conditions, the percentage absorbed is not relevant.

For infinite-dose studies, the objective will be to obtain constants that can define the kinetics of permeation. The constants most often used are the permeability coefficient K_p and the lag time t_{lag}. The profile expected from infinite dose studies is illustrated in Figure 5.3. After an initial lag period, the cumulative amount of chemical appearing in the receptor fluid will increase linearly with time; in other words, the flux across the skin will reach a steady state. The t_{lag} can be determined from extrapolation of the linear portion of the plot to the *x*-axis. While the K_p can be

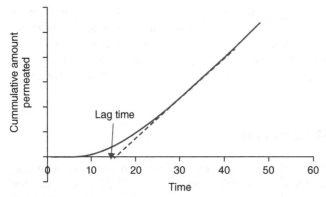

Figure 5.3   Typical plot of the cumulative amount of a chemical permeating the skin during an *in vitro* permeation study with an infinite dose. The rate of permeation increases gradually to eventually reach a steady state. Extrapolation of the steady state portion of the plot yields the lag time (t_{lag}).

determined from the slope of the terminal portion of the plot of cumulative amount penetrated versus time, because of the difficulty in determining when steady state has been reached, this method is often inaccurate.

The mathematical expression for the amount of permeant Q transported through a homogeneous membrane and appearing in the receptor chamber following the application of a "infinite" dose is given in Equation 5.1:

$$Q_{(t)} = A.P.h.C.\left[D.\frac{t}{h^2} - \frac{1}{6} - \frac{2}{\pi^2} \sum_{n=1}^{\infty} \frac{(-1)^n}{n^2} .\exp\left(\frac{-D.n^2.\pi^2.t}{h^2} \right) \right], \qquad (5.1)$$

where $Q(t)$ is the quantity of penetrant that has reached the receptor solution at a particular time t, A is the surface area of skin available for diffusion, P is the partition coefficient between the membrane and the donor vehicle, h is the membrane thickness, C is the concentration of the permeant in the donor solution, and D is the diffusion coefficient of the permeant in the membrane. Because of the difficulty in measuring the path length (h), the equation can be simplified by replacing the terms $P.h$ and D/h^2 with two new constants P_1 and P_2, as shown in Equation 5.2:

$$Q_{(t)} = A.P_1.C\left[P_2.t - \frac{1}{6} - \frac{2}{\pi^2} \sum_{n=1}^{\infty} \frac{(-1)^n}{n^2} .\exp\left(-P_2.n^2.\pi^2.t \right) \right]. \qquad (5.2)$$

The data obtained from the permeation study can be fitted to this equation using suitable nonlinear least squares methods and the values of P_1 and P_2 obtained.[59,60]

The permeability coefficient is then given by Equation 5.3:

$$K_p = P_1.P_2 \qquad (5.3)$$

The lag time (t_{lag}) is given by Equation 5.4:

$$t_{lag} = \frac{1}{6.P_2}. \qquad (5.4)$$

The mathematical expressions for fitting data from finite-dose permeation experiments are far more complex and are not amenable to routine use. In many cases, the important information required from such experiments is the total amount of substance penetrating through a given area in a given time. Thus the quantity of substance permeating after 24 or 48 hours is commonly used for comparison purposes.

Impact of Skin Metabolism

It has long been known that the skin, and the epidermis in particular, contains enzymes capable of metabolizing xenobiotic compounds.[61-63] The impact of this for *in vitro* skin perfusion methodology is twofold. First, this technique has been used to study some of the metabolic processes and to isolate the location of the metabolic activity. Second, and perhaps more importantly, it is necessary to understand the contribution that metabolism may play in the observed permeation rates and the ability to extrapolate from these *in vitro* studies to likely behavior *in vivo*.

Because of the complication associated with the lack of an intact circulation, and questions of maintenance of viability, the use of skin permeation for studying skin metabolism has limitations and other methods are likely to be more easily interpreted. These methods have been reviewed elsewhere.[64-66]

The use of *in vitro* skin permeation studies for evaluating the contribution of metabolism during absorption to exposure to chemicals is recognized in the OECD 428 "Guideline for the Testing of Chemicals Skin Absorption: *In Vitro* Method."[1] The guideline states: "When metabolically active systems are used, metabolites of the test chemical may be analysed by appropriate methods. At the end of the experiment the distribution of the test chemical and its metabolites are quantified, when appropriate." The guideline further states: "If metabolism is being studied, the receptor fluid must support skin viability throughout the experiment" and "When skin metabolism is being investigated, freshly excised skin should be used as soon as possible, and under conditions known to support metabolic activity. As a general guidance freshly excised skin should be used within 24 hrs, but the acceptable storage period may vary depending on the enzyme system involved in metabolisation and storage temperatures."

Nature of Enzymes

The nature of xenobiotic metabolizing enzymes that has been shown to be present in the skin is very diverse and includes both Phase I and Phase II enzymes,[67-69] as well as proteolytic enzymes.[70] These are the subject of recent reviews.[64,65,71]

Understanding the extent of xenobiotic metabolism in the skin is important for assessing potential toxicity and the impact on drug delivery; both reduced delivery because of metabolism of the drug and improved delivery because of conversion of prodrugs into their active forms. The importance of accounting for "first-pass" skin metabolism to assessing the potential toxicity of hair dyes has been pointed out by Nohynek et al.[72] Kao and Hall[73] demonstrated first-pass metabolism of steroids using mouse skin in perfusion chambers. They concluded that both diffusional and metabolic processes are important in determining the fate of topically applied steroids.

Prodrugs

The potential to use the metabolic activity of the skin to convert lipophilic prodrugs into more hydrophilic drugs was recognized by Bucks.[74] The approach to improve transdermal delivery with the use of prodrugs has been recently reviewed.[75]

Detection of Metabolism

It is obviously important to detect metabolism occurring during any *in vitro* diffusion study. Understanding the metabolism of a substance at other sites, particularly the liver, may alert one to the need to look for metabolism in the skin. The basic safeguards to ensure that significant metabolism is not missed include the use of specific assays, examination for the presence of known metabolites, and performance of mass balance at the end of a diffusion study to ensure that all of the applied substance can be accounted for.

An important use of *in vitro* permeation studies is to predict *in vivo* permeation. When there is significant metabolism of the substance concerned in the skin, this introduces a number of complications. The difficulty in quantitatively determining the contribution of metabolism during passage through the skin by measurements of permeation *in vitro* was illustrated by the studies of Potts et al.,[76,77] where major differences between *in vitro* and *in vivo* conditions were observed. The proportion of a diester of salicylic acid converted into salicylic acid was influenced by the rate of permeation. As might be predicted, the longer the ester remained in the skin the greater the extent of metabolic conversion. Choi et al.[78] found that proteolytic enzyme activities as measured by permeation studies with hairless mouse skin was different to that observed with skin homogenates.

An important complication introduced by metabolism of a substance is dose dependency. While this can be addressed with suitable modeling, as discussed later, nonlinear processes are always more difficult to extrapolate than linear systems.

Site of Metabolism

The relevance of a particular *in vitro* method will be influenced by the site of enzymic conversion. Skin obtained from cadavers and from plastic surgery is routinely treated with antiseptics and is likely to be devoid of the normal microflora. The ability of microorganisms on the skin to metabolize drugs has been demonstrated.[79,80] On the basis of a model that was elaborated to probe the possible effect of metabolism by skin microflora on topical bioavailability, Denyer et al.[81] concluded that such metabolism could have a significant effect, particularly for thin film application.

The results obtained with full-thickness skin, dermatomed skin, or epidermal membrane may be impacted by the location of the enzymes. Most metabolic activity has been assigned to the epidermis. Lui et al.,[82] on the basis of analysis of data from diffusion and metabolism of β-estradiol in hairless mouse skin, suggest that the enzyme responsible for the metabolism is likely to be uniformly distributed in the epidermis rather than being spread through both the epidermis and the dermis or specifically located in the basal cell layer of the epidermis. This finding is consistent with a study where the aminopeptidase activity in human skin was visualized using confocal laser scanning microscopy and was found to be spread throughout the viable epidermis.[78] Enzyme activity was much lower in both the dermis and the SC. Although, for a number of compounds, most activity resides in the hair follicles and the sebaceous glands,[83,84] in some cases activity has been observed in sole of foot, which is devoid of appendages.[85] Lodén[86] showed that the degree of metabolism of diisopropyl fluorophospate during permeation of human skin *in vitro* was much higher when full-thickness skin was used in comparison to epidermal membranes.

One of the difficulties in quantitatively assessing the contribution of metabolism in *in vitro* permeation studies is the potential for enzymes to leach into the receptor fluid and metabolism may continue after permeation. This phenomenon has been observed in a number of studies.[76,84]

Factors Affecting Enzymic Activity

- Species differences: Reviewed elsewhere.[65]
- Exposure to inducing agents prior to obtaining skin samples.[87]
- Source of skin
  - cadaver versus fresh
  - site[61,88,89]
  - age
- Skin preparation: When mouse skin was treated at 54°C to facilitate isolation of the epidermis, there was significant loss of aryl hydrocarbon hydroxylase activity.[87] Wester et al.[54] showed that heat separation of the epidermis of human cadaver skin at 60°C for 1 minute reduced enzymic activity.
- Storage: Freezing and storage frozen at *20°C for 6 weeks was shown not to affect esterase activity in rat skin,[90] but on the other hand, Wester et al.[54] found that freezing of human cadaver skin dramatically reduced viability. Higo et al.[69] found that while storage of hairless mouse skin at 4°C did not alter barrier function, the metabolism of nitroglycerin was decreased fivefold. Wester et al.[54] measured the viability of human cadaver skin stored refrigerated and concluded that viability was maintained for 18 hours, but decreased threefold by day 2. The level of viability was maintained for 8 days and then decreased a further 50% by day 13. Another factor that is an important consideration with excised skin is the presence of necessary cofactors. Hsia et al.[85] found that cadaver skin lost the ability to metabolize hydrocortisone

several hours after death. This activity could be restored by including a generating system for cofactors.

- Receptor fluid: The choice of receptor fluid to not only maintain sink conditions but also to maintain skin viability and enzyme activity is obviously important. The effect of receptor solution composition on skin viability in flow-through diffusion cells has been studied.[10] The use of Eagle's MEM, HHBSS, or DMPBS supported skin viability more than phosphate-buffered saline. Storm et al.[91] showed that the use of MEM as a receptor fluid increased the metabolism of nitroglycerin by rat skin *in vitro* compared to phosphate-buffered saline. The possible effect of additives in the receptor fluid necessary to increase solubility of the penetrant or prevent microbial growth needs to be recognized.

Modeling

Numerous models have been developed in an attempt to describe the kinetics of permeation across skin *in vitro* and that allow for simultaneous diffusion and metabolism. The extent of metabolism within the skin during absorption will be determined not only by the metabolic activity but also the residence time within the skin. Fox et al.[92] have developed a model using a computational approach that is particularly suited to steady-state data for simultaneous diffusion and metabolism in biological membranes. Hadgraft[93] developed a mathematical model to show the effect of metabolism within the epidermis and the relative effects of enzyme location within in a particular part of the epidermis.

A method for analysis of *in vitro* permeation data involving simultaneous diffusion and metabolism has been proposed and evaluated by following penetration and metabolism of ethyl nicotinate through hairless rat skin *in vitro*. The maximum metabolic rate, V_{max}, and the Michaelis constant, k_m, were determined using tissue homogenates.[94]

A model to describe diffusion and concurrent metabolism through stripped human skin *in vitro* was elaborated by Boderke et al.,[95] who validated the model by measuring the permeation and concurrent metabolism of a peptidomimetic compound. The degree of metabolism was decided by the residence time in the tissue and their analysis showed that the impact of tissue thickness was greater than the diffusion rate of the compound.

The diffusion of estradiol esters and their metabolism to estradiol in hairless mouse skin has been modeled.[88] The model obtained fitted the experimental data at earlier time points but there was a deviation at later time points that was attributed to decreased metabolic activity in the skin as it aged.

CONCLUDING REMARKS

While the important elements of *in vitro* skin permeation methodology have been outlined in the OECD guidelines,[1,2] it is clear that the details of the method adopted in specific instances need to be tailored to the circumstance. The purpose of performing the *in vitro* study must be taken into account. For example, when evaluating potential toxicity of a particular chemical that is present in a product, testing should be performed with the product itself, with application methods approximating the likely in use conditions. On the other hand, when using *in vitro* permeation studies to determine intrinsic diffusion characteristics it is important to ensure that potential interfering factors such as the presence of excipients are avoided.

In many instances the ultimate purpose of conducting *in vitro* permeation studies is to predict in use or real practical behavior. It is likely that different *in vitro* methods will better predict this behavior for different chemicals or even different presentations of these chemicals. Thus, where possible the design of *in vitro* permeation studies should be guided by correlations with measurement of actual performance or toxicity in the real situation. As these data become available it should be possible to tailor individual studies for particular purposes.

REFERENCES

1. Organisation for Economic Cooperation and Development. OECD Guideline for Testing of Chemicals No. 428: Skin Absorption: In Vitro Methods. OECD, Paris, France, 2004; 1–8.
2. Organisation for Economic Cooperation and Development. OECD Series on Testing and Assessment No. 28: Guidance Document for the Conduct of Skin Absorption Studies. OECD. 2004:1–31.
3. CHILCOTT RP, BARAI N, BEEZER AE, BRAIN SI, BROWN MB, BUNGE AL, BURGESS SE, CROSS S, DALTON CH, DIAS M, FARINHA A, FINNIN BC, GALLAGHER SJ, GREEN DM, GUNT H, GWYTHER RL, HEARD CM, JARVIS CA, KAMIYAMA F, KASTING GB, LEY EE, LIM ST, McNAUGHTON GS, MORRIS A, NAZEMI MH, PELLETT MA, DU PLESSIS J, QUAN YS, RAGHAVAN SL, ROBERTS M, ROMONCHUK W, ROPER CS, SCHENK D, SIMONSEN L, SIMPSON A, TRAVERSA BD, TROTTET L, WATKINSON A, WILKINSON SC, WILLIAMS FM, YAMAMOTO A, HADGRAFT J. Inter- and intralaboratory variation of *in vitro* diffusion cell measurements: An international multicenter study using quasi-standardized methods and materials. *Journal of Pharmaceutical Sciences* 2005; 94: 632–638.
4. VAN DE SANDT JJ, van BURGSTEDEN JA, CAGE S, CARMICHAEL PL, DICK I, KENYON S, KORINTH G, LARESE F, LIMASSET JC, MAAS WJ, MONTOMOLI L, NIELSEN JB, PAYAN JP, ROBINSON E, SARTORELLI P, SCHALLER KH, WILKINSON SC, WILLIAMS FM. *In vitro* predictions of skin absorption of caffeine, testosterone, and benzoic acid: A multi-centre comparison study. *Regulatory and Toxicological Pharmacology* 2004; 39: 271–281.
5. SCHEUPLEIN RJ, BLANK IH. Permeability of the skin. *Physiological Reviews* 1971; 51: 702–747.
6. FRANZ TJ. Percutaneous absorption: On the relevance of *in vitro* data. *Journal of Investigative Dermatology* 1975; 64: 190–195.
7. FRANZ TJ. The finite dose technique as a valid *in vitro* model for the study of percutaneous absorption in man. In: Simon GA, Paster A, Klingberg M, Kaye M, eds. *Skin: Drug Application and Evaluation of Environmental Hazards. Current Problems in Dermatology.* Karger, Basel, Switzerland, 1978; 58–68.
8. BRONAUGH RL, STEWART RF. Methods for *in vitro* percutaneous absorption studies. IV. The flow-through diffusion cell. *Journal of Pharmaceutical Sciences* 1985; 74: 64–67.
9. HOLLAND JM, KAO JY, WHITAKER MJ. A multisample apparatus for kinetic evaluation of skin penetration *in vitro:* The influence of viability and metabolic status of the skin. *Toxicology and Applied Pharmacology* 1984; 72: 272–280.
10. COLLIER SW, SHEIKH NM, SAKR A, LICHTIN JL, STEWART RF, BRONAUGH RL. Maintenance of skin viability during *in vitro* percutaneous absorption/metabolism studies. *Journal of Toxicology and Applied Pharmacology* 1989; 99: 522–533.

11. BRONAUGH RL, STEWART RF. Methods for *in vitro* percutaneous absorption studies. III. Hydrophobic compounds. *Journal of Pharmaceutical Sciences* 1984; 73: 1255–1258.
12. BRONAUGH RL, STEWART RF. Methods for *in vitro* percutaneous absorption studies: VI. Preparation of the barrier layer. *Journal of Pharmaceutical Sciences* 1986; 75: 1094–1097.
13. SCOTT RC, RAMSEY JD. Comparison of the *in vivo* and *in vitro* percutaneous absorption of a lipophilic molecule (cypermethrin, a pyrethroid insecticide). *Journal of Investigative Dermatology* 1987; 89: 142–146.
14. RAMSEY JD, WOOLLEN BH, AUTON TR, SCOTT RC. The predictive accuracy of *in vitro* measurements for the dermal absorption of a lipophilic penetrant (fluazifop-butyl) through rat and human skin. *Fundamental and Applied Toxicology* 1994; 23: 230–236.
15. RAMSEY JD, WOOLLEN BH, AUTON TR, BATTEN TR, LEESER PL. Pharmacokinetics of fluazifop-butyl in human volunteers. II. Dermal dosing. *Human and Experimental Toxicology* 1992; 11: 247–254.
16. BRONAUGH RL, FRANZ TJ. Vehicle effect on percutaneous absorption: *In vivo* and *in vitro* comparisons. *British Journal of Dermatology* 1986; 115: 1–11.
17. BRONAUGH RL, STEWART RF, CONGDON ER. Methods for *in vitro* percutaneous absorption studies. II: Animal models for human skin. *Toxicology Applied Pharmacology* 1982; 62: 481–488.
18. BARBERO AM, FRASCH HF. Pig and guinea pig skin as surrogates for human *in vitro* penetration studies: A quantitative review. *Toxicology in Vitro* 2009; 23: 1–13.
19. EPPLER AR, KRAELING ME, WICKETT RR, BRONAUGH RL. Assessment of skin absorption and irritation potential of arachidonic acid and glyceryl arachidonate using *in vitro* diffusion cell techniques. *Food and Chemical Toxicology* 2007; 45: 2109–2117.
20. SOUTHWELL JD, BARRY BW, WOODFORD R. Variations in permeability of human skin within and between specimens. *International Journal of Pharmaceutics* 1984; 18: 299–309.
21. BENFELDT E, HANSEN SH, VOLUND A, MENNE T, SHAH VP. Bioequivalence of topical formulations in humans: Evaluation by dermal microdialysis sampling and the dermatopharmacokinetics method. *Journal of Investigative Dermatology* 2007; 127: 170–178.
22. TETTEY-AMLALO RN, KANFER I, SKINNER MF, BENFELDT E, VERBEECK RK. Application of dermal microdialysis for the evaluation of bioequivalence of a ketoprofen topical gel. *European Journal of Pharmaceutical Sciences* 2009; 36: 219–225.
23. WILLIAMS AC, CORNWELL PA, BARRY BW. On the non-Gaussian distribution of human skin permeabilities. *International Journal of Pharmaceutics* 1992; 86: 69–77.
24. CHIOU YB, BLUME-PEYTAVI U. Stratum corneum maturation: A review of neonatal skin function. *Skin Pharmacology and Physiology* 2004; 17: 57–66.
25. NICOLOVSKI J, STAMATAS GN, KOLLIAS N, WIEGAND BC. Barrier function and water-holding and transport properties of infant stratum corneum are different from adult and continue to develop through the first year of life. *Journal of Investigative Dermatology* 2008; 128: 1728–1736.
26. TAKAHASHI M, WATANABE H, KUMAGAI H, NAKAYAMA Y. Physiological and morphological changes in facial skin with aging. *Journal of the Society of Cosmetic Chemists Japan* 1989; 23: 22–30.
27. MARRAKCHI S, MAIBACH HI. Sodium lauryl sulfate-induced irritation in the human face: Regional and age-related differences. *Skin Pharmacology and Physiology* 2006; 19: 177–180.
28. ROSKOS KV, MAIBACH HI, GUY RH. The effect of ageing on percutaneous absorption in man. *Journal of Pharmacy and Biopharmaceutics* 1989; 17: 617–630.
29. SOLASSOL I, CAUMETTE L, BRESSOLLE F, GARCIA F, THEZENAS S, ASTRE C, CULINE S, COULOUMA R, PINGUET F. Inter- and intra-individual variability in transdermal fentanyl absorption in cancer pain patients. *Oncology Reports* 2005; 14: 1029–1036.
30. GROVE GL. Physiologic changes in older skin. *Clinical Geriatric Medicine* 1989; 5: 115–125.
31. ROSKOS KV, BIRCHER AJ, MAIBACH HI, GUY RH. Pharmacodynamic measurements of methyl nicotinate percutaneous absorption: The effect of aging on microcirculation. *British Journal of Dermatology* 1990; 122: 165–171.
32. FARAGE MA, MILLER KW, ELSNER P, MAIBACH HI. Intrinsic and extrinsic factors in skin ageing: A review. *International Journal of Cosmetic Science* 2008; 30: 87–95.
33. ELIAS PM, GHADIALLY R. The aged epidermal permeability barrier: Basis for functional abnormalities. *Clinical Geriatric Medicine* 2002; 18: 103–120.

34. JENSEN JM, FORI M, WINOTO-MORBACH S, SEITE S, SCHUNCK M, PROKSCH E, SCHUTZE S. Acid and neutral sphingomyelinase, ceramide synthase, and acid ceramidase activities in cutaneous aging. *Experimental Dermatology* 2005; 14: 609–618.

35. CHOI EH, MAN MO, XU P, XIN S, LIU Z, CRUMRINE DA, JIANG YJ, FLUHR JW, FEINGOLD KR, ELIAS PM, MAURO TM. Stratum corneum acidification is impaired in moderately aged human and murine skin. *Journal of Investigative Dermatology* 2007; 127: 2847–2856.

36. SRIDEVI S, DIWAN PV. Optimized transdermal delivery of ketoprofen using pH and hydroxypropyl-b-cyclodextrin as co-enhancers. *European Journal of Pharmacy and Biopharmaceutics* 2002; 54: 151–154.

37. HUANG ZR, HUNG CF, LIN YK, FANG JY. *In vitro* and *in vivo* evaluation of topical delivery and potential dermal use of soy isoflavones genistein and daidzein. *International Journal of Pharmaceutics* 2008; 364: 36–44.

38. SAUERMANN K, CLEMANN S, JASPERS S, GAMBICHLER T, ALTMEYER P, HOFFMANN K, ENNEN J. Age related changes of human skin investigated with histometric measurements by confocal laser scanning microscopy *in vivo*. *Skin Research Technology* 2002; 8: 52–56.

39. HOLOWATZ LA, THOMPSON-TORGERSON CS, KENNEY WL. Altered mechanisms of vasodilation in aged human skin. *Exercise and Sport Science Review* 2007; 35: 119–125.

40. CROSS SE, ROBERTS MS. Use of *in vitro* human skin membranes to model and predict the effect of changing blood flow on the flux and retention of topically applied solutes. *Journal of Pharmaceutical Sciences* 2008; 97: 3442–3450.

41. MARZULLI FN, MAIBACH HI. Permeability and reactivity of skin as related to age. *Journal of the Society of Cosmetic Chemists* 1984; 35: 95–102.

42. ROSKOS KV, MAIBACH HI. Percutaneous absorption and age: Implications for therapy. *Drugs Aging* 1992; 2: 432–449.

43. WEDIG JH, MAIBACH HI. Percutaneous penetration of dipyrithione in man: Effect of skin color (race). *Journal of the American Academy of Dermatology* 1981; 5: 433–438.

44. KOMPAORE F, MARTY J-P, DUPONT C. *In vivo* evaluation of the stratum corneum barrier function in Blacks, Caucasians and Asians with two noninvasive methods. *Skin Pharmacology* 1993; 6: 200–207.

45. WEIGAND DA, HAYGOOD C, GAYLOR JR. Cell layers and density of negro and Caucasian SC. *Journal of Investigative Dermatology* 1974; 62: 563–568.

46. RIENERTSON RP, WHEATLEY VR. Studies on the chemical composition of human epidermal lipids. *Journal of Investigative Dermatology* 1959; 32: 49–59.

47. MANGELSDORF S, OTBERG N, MAIBACH HI, SINKGRAVEN R, STERRY W, LADEMANN J. Ethnic variation in vellus hair follicle size and distribution. *Skin Pharmacology and Physiology* 2006; 19: 159–167.

48. LEOPOLD CS, MAIBACH HI. Effect of lipophilic vehicles on *in vivo* skin penetration of methyl nicotinate in different races. *International Journal of Pharmaceutics* 1996; 139: 161–167.

49. WICKREMA SINHA AJ, SHAW SR, WEBER DJ. Percutaneous absorption and excretion of tritium-labeled diflorasone diacetate, a new topical corticosteroid in the rat, monkey and man. *Journal of Investigative Dermatology* 1978; 71: 372–377.

50. LOTTE C, WESTER RC, ROUGIER A, MAIBACH HI. Racial differences in the *in vivo* percutaneous absorption of some organic compounds: A comparison between black, Caucasian and Asian subjects. *Archives of Dermatological Research* 1993; 284: 456–459.

51. RAWLINGS AV. Ethnic skin types: Are there differences in skin structure and function? *International Journal of Cosmetic Science* 2006; 28: 79–93.

52. HARRISON SM, BARRY BW, DUGARD PH. Effects of freezing on human skin permeability. *Journal of Pharmacy and Pharmacology* 1984; 36: 261–262.

53. KASTING GB, BOWMAN LA. Electrical analysis of fresh excised human skin: A comparison with frozen skin. *Pharmaceutical Research* 1990; 7: 1141–1146.

54. WESTER RC, CHRISTOFFEL J, HARTWAY T, POBLETE N, MAIBACH HI, FORSELL J. Human cadaver skin viability for *in vitro* percutaneous absorption: Storage and detrimental effects of heat-separation and freezing. *Pharmaceutical Research* 1998; 15: 82–84.

55. SINTOV AC, BOTNER S. Transdermal drug delivery using microemulsion and aqueous systems: Influence of skin storage conditions on the *in vitro* permeability of diclofenac from aqueous vehicle systems. *International Journal of Pharmaceutics* 2006; 311: 55–62.

56. AHLSTROM LA, CROSS SE, MILLS PC. The effects of freezing skin on transdermal drug penetration kinetics. *Journal of Veterinary Pharmacology and Therapeutics* 2007; 30: 456–463.

57. BRAIN KR, WALTERS KA, WATKINSON AC. Methods for studying percutaneous absorption. In: Walters KA, ed. *Dermatological and Transdermal Formulations*. Marcel Dekker, New York, 2002; 197–269.

58. WALTERS KA, BRAIN KR, HOWES D, JAMES VJ, KRAUS AL, TEETSEL NM, TOULON M, WATKINSON AC, GETTINGS SD. Percutaneous penetration of octyl salicylate from representative sunscreen formulations through human skin *in vitro*. *Food and Chemical Toxicology* 1997; 35: 1219–1225.

59. OKAMOTO H, KOMATSU H, HASHIDA M, SEZAKI H. Effects of β-cyclodextrin and di-O-methyl-β-cyclodextrin on the percutaneous absorption of butylparaben, indomethacin and sulfanilic acid. *International Journal of Pharmaceutics* 1986; 30: 35–45.

60. DÍEZ-SALES O, WATKINSON AC, HERRÁEZ-DOMINGUEZ M, JAVALOYES C, HADGRAFT J. A mechanistic investigation of the *in vitro* human skin permeation enhancing effect of Azone®. *International Journal of Pharmaceutics* 1996; 129: 33–40.

61. PANNATIER A, JENNER P, TESTA B, ETTER JC. The skin as a drug-metabolizing organ. *Drug Metabolism Reviews* 1978; 8: 319–343.

62. BICKERS DR, DUTTA-CHOUDHURY T, MUKHTAR H. Epidermis: Site of drug metabolism in neonatal rat skin. Studies on cytochrome P-450 content and mixed function oxidase and epoxide hydrolase activity. *Molecular Pharmacology* 1982; 21: 239–247.

63. MARTIN RJ, DENYER SP, HADGRAFT J. Skin metabolism of topically applied compounds. *International Journal of Pharmaceutics* 1987; 39: 23–32.

64. ZHANG Q, GRICE JE, WANG G, ROBERTS MS. Cutaneous metabolism in transdermal drug delivery. *Current Drug Metabolism* 2009; 10: 227–235.

65. STEINSTRÄSSER I, MERKLE HP. Dermal metabolism of topically applied drugs: Pathways and models reconsidered. *Pharmaceutica Acta Helvetiae* 1995; 70: 3–24.

66. KAO J, CARVER MP. Cutaneous metabolism of xenobiotics. *Drug Metabolism Reviews* 1990; 22: 363–410.

67. BARON JM, WIEDERHOLT T, HEISE R, MERK HF, BICKERS DR. Expression and function of cytochrome P450-dependent enzymes in human skin cells. *Current Medicinal Chemistry* 2008; 15: 2258–2264.

68. FINNEN MJ, SHUSTER S. Phase I and phase 2 drug metabolism in isolated epidermal cells from adult hairless mice and in whole human hair follicles. *Biochemical Pharmacology* 1985; 34: 3571–3575.

69. TÄUBER U. Metabolism of drugs on and in the skin. In: Brandau R, Lippold BH, eds. *Dermal and Transdermal Absorption*. Wissenschaftliche Verlagsgesellschaft, Stuttgart, Germany, 1982; 133–151.

70. FRUTON JS. On the proteolytic enzymes of animal tissues. *Journal of Biological Chemistry* 1946; 166: 721–738.

71. OESCH F, FABIAN E, OESCH-BARTLOMOWICZ B, WERNER C, LANDSIEDEL R. Drug-metabolizing enzymes in the skin of man, rat, and pig. *Drug Metabolism Reviews* 2007; 39: 659–698.

72. NOHYNEK GJ, ANTIGNAC E, RE T, TOUTAIN H. Safety assessment of personal care products/cosmetics and their ingredients. *Toxicology and Applied Pharmacology* 2010; 243: 239–259.

73. KAO J, HALL J. Skin absorption and cutaneous first pass metabolism of topical steroids: *In vitro* studies with mouse skin in organ culture. *The Journal of Pharmacology and Experimental Therapeutics* 1987; 241: 482–487.

74. BUCKS DAW. Skin structure and metabolism: Relevance to the design of cutaneous therapies. *Pharmaceutical Research* 1984; 1: 148–153.

75. FANG JY, LEU YL. Prodrug strategy for enhancing drug delivery via skin. *Current Drug Discovery Technology* 2006; 3: 211–224.

76. GUSEK DB, KENNEDY AH, MCNEILL SC, WAKSHULL E, POTTS RO. Transdermal drug transport and metabolism. I. Comparison if *in vitro* and *in vivo* results. *Pharmaceutical Research* 1989; 6: 33–39.

77. POTTS RO, MCNEILL SC, DESBONNET CR, WAKSHULL E. Transdermal drug transport and metabolism. II The role of competing kinetic events. *Pharmaceutical Research* 1989; 6: 119–124.

78. CHOI H-K, FLYNN GL, AMIDON GL. Transdermal delivery of bioactive peptides: The effect of n-decylmethyl sulfoxide, pH, and inhibitors on enkephalin metabolism and transport. *Pharmaceutical Research* 1990; 7: 1099–1106.

79. BROOKES FL, HUGO WB, DENYER SP. Transformation of betamethasone 17-valerate by skin microflora. Proceedings of the British Pharmaceutical Conference, Edinburgh, 1982.

80. DENYER SP, HUGO WB, O'BRIEN M. Metabolism of glyceryl trinitrate by skin staphylococci. *Journal of Pharmacy and Pharmacology* 1984; 36: 61P.

81. DENYER SP, GUY RH, HADGRAFT J, HUGO WB. The microbial degradation of topically applied drugs. *International Journal of Pharmaceutics* 1985; 26: 89–97.

82. LIU P, HIGUCHI WI, GHANEM A-H, KURIHARA-BERGSTROM T, GOOD WR. Quantitation of simultaneous diffusion and metabolism of β=estradiol in hairless mouse skin: Enzyme distribution and intrinsic diffusion/metabolism parameters. *International Journal of Pharmaceutics* 1990; 64: 7–25.

83. WILTON COOMES M, NORLING AH, POHL RJ, MÜLLER D, FOUTS JR. Foreign compound metabolism by isolated skin cells from the hairless mouse. *The Journal of Pharmacology and Experimental Therapeutics* 1983; 225: 770–777.

84. MERK HF, MUKHTAR H, SCHUTTE B, KAUFMANN I, DAS M, BICKERS DR. 7-ethoxyresorufin-o-deethylase activity in human hair roots: A potential marker for toxifying species of cytochrome P-450 isozymes. *Biochemical Biophysical Research Communications* 1987; 148: 755–761.

85. HSIA SL, MUSSALLEM AJ, WITTEN VH. Further metabolic studies of hydrocortisone-4-14C in human skin. *The Journal of Investigative Dermatology* 1965; 45: 384–388.

86. LODÉN M. The *in vitro* hydrolysis of diisopropyl fluoro-phosphate during penetration through human full-thickness skin and isolated epidermis. *The Journal of Investigative Dermatology* 1985; 85: 335–339.

87. THOMPSON S, SLAGA TJ. Mouse epidermal aryl hydrocarbon hydroxlase. *The Journal of Investigative Dermatology* 1976; 66: 108–111.

88. HSIA SL, HAO Y-L. Metabolic transformations of cortisol-4[14C] in human skin. *Biochemistry* 1966; 5: 1469–1464.

89. WEINSTEIN GD, FROST P, HSIA SL. *In vitro* interconversion of estrone and 17β-estradiol in human skin and vaginal mucosa. *The Journal of Investigative Dermatology* 1968; 51: 4–10.

90. HEWITT PG, PERKINS J, HOTCHKISS SAM. Metabolism of fluroxypyr, fluroxypyr methyl ester, and the herbicide fluroxypyr methylheptyl ester I: During percutaneous absorption through fresh rat and human skin *in vitro*. *Drug Metabolism and Disposition* 2000; 28: 748–754.

91. STORM JE, BRONOUGH RL, AS C, SIMMONS JE. Cutaneous metabolism of nitroglycerin in viable rat skin *in vitro*. *International Journal of Pharmaceutics* 1990; 65: 265–268.

92. FOX JL, YU C-D, HIGUCHI WI, HO NFH. General physical model for simultaneous diffusion and metabolism in biological membranes. The computational approach for the steady-state case. *International Journal of Pharmaceutics* 1979; 2: 41–57.

93. HADGRAFT J. Theoretical aspects of metabolism in the epidermis. *International Journal of Pharmaceutics* 1980; 4: 229–239.

94. SUGIBAYASHI K, HAYASHI T, HTANAKA T, OGIHARA M, MORIMOTO Y. Analysis of simultaneous transport and metabolism of ethyl nicotinate in hairless rat skin. *Pharmaceutical Research* 1996; 13: 855–860.

95. BODERKE P, SCHITTKOWSKI K, WOLFF M, MERKLE HP. Modelling of diffusion and concurrent metabolism in cutaneous tissue. *Journal of Theoretical Biology* 2000; 204: 393–407.

Chapter 6

Skin Permeation Assessment: Tape Stripping

Sandra Wiedersberg and Sara Nicoli

INTRODUCTION

The stratum corneum (SC)—the outermost layer of the epidermis—is a stratified layer, 10–20 µm thick, composed of flattened keratinized cells embedded in a multilamellar lipid matrix. The peculiar composition and organization of intercellular lipids determines SC barrier properties, preventing excessive water loss to the external environment, and representing the rate-limiting barrier for transport of xenobiotics across the skin.

Tape stripping is a minimally invasive procedure for SC removal and sampling. It consists of the sequential application and removal of an adhesive tape strip onto the skin surface in order to collect microscopic layers (0.2–1 µm) of SC (Fig. 6.1). The procedure is relatively painless and not particularly invasive, because only dead cells embedded in the lipid matrix are removed. Moreover, even if the skin stripping results in barrier disruption, a homeostatic repair response in the epidermis takes place rapidly, which results in rapid restoration of the original barrier function.[1]

Tape stripping is used to evaluate skin barrier function,[2] to investigate pathologies of the skin,[3] and to monitor gene expression.[4] It can also be used to evaluate the exposure to toxic substances like pesticides[5] or metals.[6] The main application of the tape-stripping technique, however, is to assess the local bioavailability (BA) of drugs whose target is the SC, such as antifungals,[7–11] ultraviolet (UV) filters,[12–15] keratolytics,[16–18] and antiseptics.[19]

Since the SC is in most cases the main barrier to the penetration of topically applied drugs, it has been argued that drug level therein should be correlated with those attained in the viable epidermis and dermis, where many dermatological diseases are located. This hypothesis was tested (even if not fully validated) by Rougier et al.,[20] who found a linear correlation between the amount of chemical (sodium

Transdermal and Topical Drug Delivery: Principles and Practice, First Edition. Edited by Heather A.E. Benson, Adam C. Watkinson.
© 2012 John Wiley & Sons, Inc. Published 2012 by John Wiley & Sons, Inc.

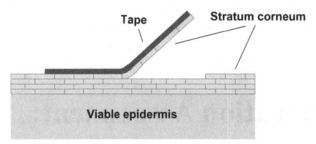

Figure 6.1   Schematic representation of the tape-stripping technique.

benzoate, caffeine, benzoic acid, acetyl salicylic acid) absorbed across the skin following a 30-minute application and the quantity recovered in the SC by tape stripping after an identical, but independent, administration procedure. So, if there is a
correlation between drug levels in the SC and drug levels in the underlying tissues,
then the tape-stripping technique can be theoretically used to determine the BA of
all topical drugs.

APPLICATIONS OF TAPE STRIPPING

Bioavailability and Bioequivalence (BA/BE) of Topical Products: The Dermatopharmacokinetic (DPK) Approach

BA is defined as the "rate and extent to which the drug is absorbed from the formulation and becomes available at the site of action" (as stated in 21 CFR 320.1[21]).
The efficiency of topical drug delivery is notoriously poor, with typical BAs of only
a few percent of the applied dose, and a major reason for this disappointing situation
is the absence of a quantitative and validated methodology with which to quantify
the rate and extent of drug delivery to a target into the skin.

Several *in vivo* and *in vitro* methods have been evaluated to assess skin permeation in terms of BA, and are summarized in Figure 6.2.

For the moment, the only acceptable methods to assess the BA/BE of topically
applied drug formulations are clinical trials between generic and original products
and pharmacodynamic response studies. Comparative clinical trials are considered
to be the "gold standard," but these studies are relatively insensitive, costly, time-
consuming, and require large numbers of subjects.[22] In contrast, pharmacodynamic
response studies are relatively easy to perform, expose the subjects to only a small
amount of the formulation for a short period of time, are fairly reproducible,
and require a relatively small number of subjects.[23] The vasoconstrictor assay for
topical corticosteroids, for instance, quantifies the ability of steroids to produce
vasoconstriction of the skin microvasculature, leading to blanching (whitening)
at the site of application. The intensity of skin blanching has been correlated with
drug potency and the degree of drug delivery through the SC.[24] The vasoconstrictor

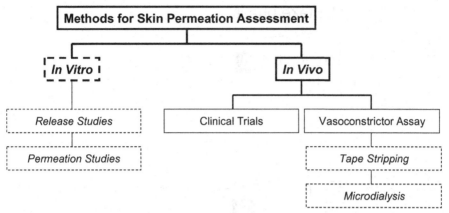

Figure 6.2   Authority-accepted methods for skin permeation assessment in terms of BA/BE; italicized legends signify those methods that are still under evaluation.

assay was adopted in 1995 for BE determination by the U.S. Food and Drug Administration (FDA).[23]

For all other topically applied drugs, however, there are currently no noninvasive or minimally invasive techniques that are acceptable to the regulatory bodies and comparative clinical trials are compulsory. In an effort to address this situation and to provide viable alternatives for BE determination, significant efforts are being directed to the DPK approach, microdialysis, and the use of *in vitro* experiments.[25]

The DPK method uses tape stripping to measure drug concentration in the SC. The SC is collected by successive application and removal of adhesive tapes that are subsequently extracted and analyzed for the drug. In theory, the DPK approach may be applied to all topical drugs. The principal assumption is that the amount of drug recovered from the SC, the usual barrier to percutaneous absorption, is directly correlated with the amount reaching the target cells. In other words, it is hypothesized that the rate and extent of drug disposition in the SC will reflect that achieved at target sites, which are further into the skin.

The FDA Draft Guidance

The DPK concept, which evolved from a series of earlier studies reported by Rougier et al.,[20] was introduced in a Draft Guidance from the FDA in 1998.[26] The Draft Guidance allows the assessment of both drug uptake into and drug elimination (clearance) from the SC as a function of time after application and after removal of the formulation, respectively. At specific times (four time points for the uptake phase and four time points for the clearance phase) (Fig. 6.3), layers of the SC are sequentially removed from the treated site with 12 adhesive tapes; the first two tapes are discarded and tape strips 3–12 are combined and quantified for the drug. The amount of drug in the first two tape-strips is not included in the assessment due to

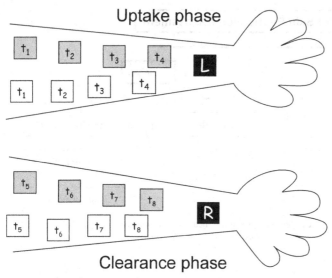

Figure 6.3 Scheme of FDA Draft Protocol for the comparison between a reference formulation (gray sites) and a generic one (white sites) at four uptake times (t_1–t_4; left arm) and four clearance times (t_5–t_8; right arm). After drug application (t_1–t_4) and clearance (t_5–t_8) the skin is stripped 12 times; the first two strips are discarded and the drug is quantified in the remaining 10 to build an amount-time curve as illustrated in Figure 6.4.

the possibility of incomplete removal of the product from the skin surface. The time points for drug uptake and clearance are not specified, except for the longest uptake time, which is supposed to be long enough that drug uptake is at steady state.

From the DPK profile of drug mass in the SC as a function of time, pharmacokinetic parameters such as the area under the curve (AUC), the maximum amount drug in the tape strips (A_{max}), and the time (T_{max}) at which A_{max} is attained are deduced and used to characterize the local BA (Fig. 6.4), in a manner analogous to that using plasma concentrations after oral administration.

In 2002, a comparative study using tretinoin gels was performed in two laboratories and produced conflicting results.[27–29] This, in addition to doubts regarding reproducibility, flaws resulting from the similar design of the approach to oral bioequivalence (BE) assessment, and criticism that quantification of the amount of SC removed should be better controlled,[30] led to the withdrawal of the Draft Guidance.

Furthermore, the large number of subjects (49) and application sites (1176) needed to set up and validate the BE study (one reference and two generics), minimized the advantages of the DPK approach compared to the clinical study it is meant to replace. Due to the abovementioned concerns, a critical reevaluation of the DPK method is in progress, with a clear objective being to validate a refined approach. The priorities of the refinement are to improve the efficiency and accuracy of a new DPK approach.

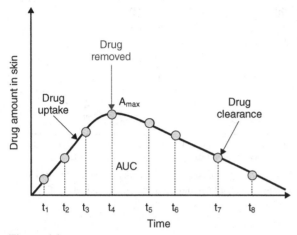

Figure 6.4   Schematic representation of the DPK approach as proposed by the FDA. The total amount of drug in the SC after four uptake times and four clearance times, obtained as illustrated in Figure 6.3, are plotted as a function of time. The area under the curve (AUC) and the maximum drug amount found in the SC (A_{max}) are mainly used to compare formulations.

Opportunities to Improve the DPK Approach

Drug Distribution Profiles Across the SC   As mentioned above, one weakness of the draft FDA protocol is represented by the uncertainty in the amount of the SC collected. In fact, 10 strips do not necessarily remove the same amount of SC since several factors such as skin hydration, vehicle composition, and cohesion between corneocytes, can influence the amount of SC that is removed by a single strip. Additionally, even if the same amount of SC is removed in all volunteers, SC thickness shows significant intersubject variability (approximately from 7 to 19 μm^{31}), so for subjects with a thicker SC, an important amount of drug remains in the barrier after tape stripping is completed. Thus, normalization of SC thickness is a prerequisite to facilitate comparison between subjects and between formulations. Briefly, the important parameter to consider during tape stripping is neither the number of strips collected nor the thickness of SC removed, but the fraction of the barrier removed (x/L); that is, the thickness removed (x) divided by the total SC thickness (L). This parameter represents the relative depth within the SC and varies between 0, at the skin surface and 1 at the interface with the viable epidermis.

To emphasize the importance of this point, transepidermal water loss (TEWL)—a measure of the integrity of the SC—has been determined after each tape strip (Fig. 6.5) and then plotted as a function of either tape-strip number (panel a), or microns of SC removed (panel b), or fraction of SC removed (panel c). While great variability is apparent in panels a and b, the data collapse onto a much more uniform curve in panel c, supporting the idea that it is the relative position within the SC (x/L) that is of prime importance. Detailed information concerning the experimental assessment of this parameter is in the section "Experimental Procedure and Validation."

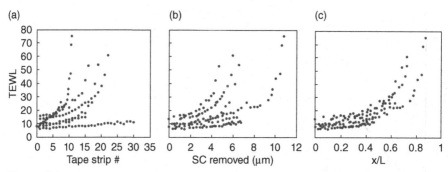

Figure 6.5   Transepidermal water loss (TEWL)—a measure of the integrity of the SC—plotted as a function of tape-strip number (panel a), micrometer of SC removed (panel b), or fraction of SC removed x/L (panel c) for different subjects.

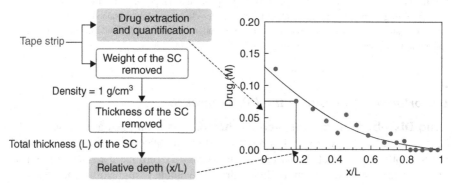

Figure 6.6   Schematic representation of the procedure used to construct a drug distribution profile inside the SC. From each strip the drug is extracted and quantified and the weight of SC removed is determined. By knowing the total SC thickness L (determined as described in the section "Determination of the total SC thickness"), the x/L value can be calculated.

With knowledge of x/L and quantification of the drug on each separate strip (including the first two strips that are suggested to be discarded in the FDA approach), it is possible to construct the drug distribution profile across the SC. The procedure and the obtained profile are schematically illustrated in Figure 6.6.

This approach has two important advantages compared to the FDA Draft Guidance: First, reduced data variability: despite the relatively small number of subjects involved in these kind of studies (four to six per experiment), the results reported have always been reasonably reproducible.[32–34] Second, the tape-stripping approach can be integrated with predictive mathematical models to further reduce the number of experiments necessary to undertake a BE study, as explained below.

THE UPTAKE PHASE   The concentration profile as a function of relative position within the SC can be fitted to the appropriate solution to Fick's second law of diffusion (Eq. 6.1), assuming that an infinite dose is applied, that the SC is a homogeneous barrier and contains no drug at $t = 0$, and that drug diffusivity in the SC is slow compared to uptake by the cutaneous microcirculation, that is, "sink" conditions apply for the drug at the SC–viable epidermis interface:

$$C_x = KC_v \left[1 - \frac{x}{L} - \frac{2}{\pi} \sum_{n=1}^{\infty} \frac{1}{n} \sin\left(n\pi \frac{x}{L} \right) \exp\left(-\frac{D}{L^2} n^2 \pi^2 t \right) \right],$$ (6.1)

where C_x is the drug concentration at position x in the SC at exposure time t and C_v is the drug concentration in the vehicle. The fitting (an example is shown in Fig. 6.6) yields values for the drug's SC–vehicle partition coefficient (K) and for D/L^2, a first-order rate constant comprising the ratio of the drug diffusivity (D) in the SC to the thickness (L) squared of the barrier. Subsequently, using the derived parameters, K and D/L^2, Equation 6.1 can be integrated across the SC thickness (i.e., from $x/L = 0$ to $x/L = 1$) to yield the amount of drug per area unit of SC thickness (Q) (milligrams per cubic centimeter or M):

$$Q = \int_0^1 C_x d\left(\frac{x}{L} \right) = KC_v \left[\frac{1}{2} - \frac{4}{\pi^2} \sum_{n=0}^{\infty} \frac{1}{(2n+1)^2} \exp\left(-\frac{D}{L^2}(2n+1)^2 \pi^2 t \right) \right].$$ (6.2)

The derived values of Q can be used to compare the relative BA of a drug delivered from different vehicles.

The DPK parameters derived from one experiment, characterizing drug partitioning (K) and diffusivity (D/L^2) into and through the SC, can be substituted in Equation 6.2 to predict the evolution of Q as a function of time. Herkenne et al.,[32] using the K and D/L^2 values obtained from a 30-minute exposure, satisfactorily predicted ibuprofen uptake for longer application times (Fig. 6.7), suggesting that reliable and quantitative information can be obtained with this approach. A similarly good prediction was obtained for terbinafine[9] and betamethasone 17-valerate (BMV) delivery.[34]

This approach can significantly simplify a DPK protocol for the comparison of formulations due to the lower variability observed (because x/L is measured), the need for fewer volunteers, and, thanks to the predictive power of the method, fewer time points (i.e., application sites) are necessary.

An important issue, when using this approach, is the choice of the exposure period used for the determination of K and D/L^2. This period should be long enough to allow the achievement of a measurable profile inside the SC, but not so long that the steady state has been reached. In the latter case, the profile inside the membrane becomes linear (see Fig. 6.8), information on the diffusive parameter D/L^2 is lost and Equations 6.1 and 6.2 simplify respectively to:

$$C_x = KC_v \left[1 - \frac{x}{L} \right]$$ (6.3a)

and

$$Q = \frac{KC_v}{2}.$$ (6.3b)

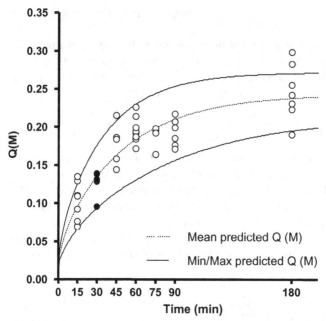

Figure 6.7 Comparison of experimental and predicted Q values. The individual ($n = 4$–7) experimentally determined amounts (Q) as a function of time are plotted together with the mean prediction (central curve) and the limits of the predictions based on the 30-minute K and D/L^2 values. Used with permission.[32]

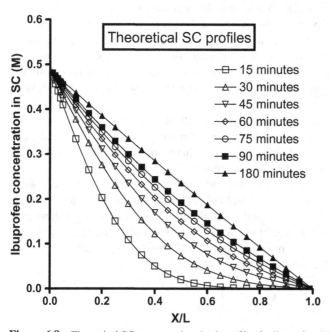

Figure 6.8 Theoretical SC concentration-depth profiles for ibuprofen delivered from a saturated solution 75:25 v/v PG:water as a function of different uptake periods. The profile becomes more linear with increasing uptake periods. Used with permission.[32]

116

Reddy et al. suggested therefore that the exposure period should be greater that $0.06 \cdot t_{lag}$ and less than $0.6 \cdot t_{lag}$,[35] where t_{lag} represents the lag time for a chemical to penetrate the SC (and correspond to $L^2/[6 \cdot D]$). It is worth mentioning that in order to get to steady state, exposure times should be greater than about $2.4 \cdot t_{lag}$.[36]

A potential problem for the tape-stripping approach is that drug in the SC will continue to diffuse during the time that it takes to apply and remove all the single tape strips. Unless the tape-stripping procedure is fast, the concentration measured in each tape will be different from the concentration when the exposure period ended, which would affect estimated values for diffusion and partition coefficients. In most cases, however, the time it takes to tape-strip a site is relatively short compared to the lag time of the drug, so diffusion during the tape-stripping procedure will be insignificant and the concentration profile represented by the tape strips should fairly represent the concentration profile in the SC at the end of exposure. Just for some small molecules—for example, chloroform—the diffusion is so fast that the total amount of chemical in the SC changes during the course of tape stripping.

As recommended by Reddy et al.,[35] if the time to tape-strip is less than $0.2 \cdot t_{lag}$ for an exposure period longer than $0.3 \cdot t_{lag}$, then diffusion during the tape-stripping procedure should not significantly affect tape-stripping concentrations. If the exposure time is less than $0.3 \cdot t_{lag}$, then the tape-stripping procedure of a site needs to be completed within $0.02 \cdot t_{lag}$.

THE CLEARANCE PHASE   The majority of investigations undertaken to date have focused upon the uptake phase of DPK. Less attention, though, has been given to the elimination, or clearance, phase of the DPK profile, which may have a significant impact on the key metrics classically derived from BA/BE studies.

The physicochemical factors controlling drug concentration in the SC are different during the uptake and clearance phases. In principle, the uptake phase is affected by both partitioning from the formulation to the SC as well as diffusion through the SC, at least until the steady state is established. By contrast, the clearance phase (permeation/diffusion of the drug from the SC into deeper skin layers) should be less dependent on the vehicle and is a function primarily of the properties of the drug itself (lipophilicity, receptor affinity, etc.). Theoretically, it should be possible to anticipate the clearance behavior of a drug from the SC, considering its diffusivity (D/L^2) and the drug level inside the SC when the clearance starts.

Reddy et al.[35] provide recommendations on the timing of such experiments: unless clearance can be studied without reaching the steady state, this makes interpretation of the data more complicated and more assumptions are needed. For this reason, exposure time should be chosen so as to get the steady state (i.e., greater than $2.4 \cdot t_{lag}$). Recommendations on the choice of the delay time (t_{delay}) after the exposure has ended suggest that this should be long enough for the concentration profile to change appreciably (t_{delay} greater than about $0.3 \cdot t_{lag}$), but not so long that the analytical errors become significant relative to the average concentration of the drug in the tape strips. In this condition, the clearance is described by a first-order elimination rate constant equal to D/L^2.

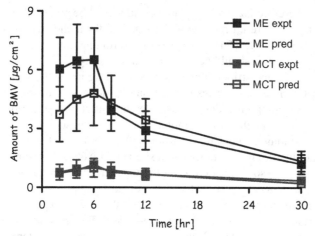

Figure 6.9   Experimental (expt) and predicted (pred) values of betamethasone 17-valerate (BMV) in the SC versus time following delivery from medium-chain triglycerides (MCT) and microemulsion (ME) vehicles (mean ± standard deviation $n = 6$). The predicted clearance phase from 6 to 30 hours is based upon a first-order elimination rate . Used with permission.[37]

For BMV, for example, after 6 hours of exposure, it was possible to predict the amounts of drug in the SC during the clearance phase (i.e., up to 24 hours after removing the formulation) when considering D/L^2 as a first-order elimination rate constant, as illustrated in Figure 6.9.[37] This approach is not feasible if the exposure time is too short (and in particular shorter than $1.2 \cdot t_{lag}$) because in this case much of the drug is still in the outermost layers of the SC when the clearance starts and so much of the drug has to diffuse across the entire SC to clear, thus delaying the decay.[11]

Despite the good results obtained in predicting drug clearance, as a matter of fact, the fate of a topically applied drug after removal of the formulation may not be dependent solely upon its physicochemical properties, but also upon the manner in which the active species is presented to the skin, that is, the formulation.

It has been demonstrated that, even with a simple cosolvent vehicle (water : propylene glycol [PG] 25:75), the behavior of one constituent (PG) is very complex, having a direct influence on the drug's (ibuprofen) DPK, not only during the uptake phase, but also during the clearance phase. It appears that, once the formulation is removed, the faster elimination of PG causes ibuprofen to precipitate within the SC and, hence, delays significantly its diffusion out of the membrane.[38]

Because topical formulations are typically complex, involving excipients which are volatile, or which can solubilize the drug within the outer SC but penetrate at different rates, or which act as enhancers that increase the permeability of the skin, there are manifold ways in which the constituents of a vehicle may influence DPK. It follows that comparison between putatively bioequivalent topical drug products must involve careful examination of the potential effects of different excipients and the manner in which their behavior may impact on the rate and extent at which the active attains its site of action.

The "Two-Time" Approach   As previously stated, one of the perceived problems of the FDA Draft Guidance was that the DPK method proposed was so complex that the time and cost involved to set up and validate the technique would undermine the advantages of the approach. In the so-called two-time method,[11,39,40] a substantial reduction in both method complexity and data variability is achieved by taking into account the uncertainties in the amount of SC collected and the effectiveness of drug removal at the end of the application period.

The key features of this approach are: (1) analysis of just one uptake time and one elimination time (instead of four of each, as suggested in the FDA Draft Guidance) per formulation; (2) an improved cleaning procedure before the tape stripping starts (so that the drug is reliably removed from the skin surface); (3) removal of nearly all the SC during tape stripping (and therefore most, if not all, of the drug); and (4) including information from all tape strips (i.e., the first tape strips are not discarded) in calculating drug uptake.

In this method, the parameter used to verify BE between a generic and a reference formulation is simply the total amount of drug measured in the SC (nanogram per square centimeter) after a specified uptake time and a specified clearance time. If the ratio of the total drug amounts in the SC satisfies the "80–125 rule" for both uptake and clearance, then the two formulations are bioequivalent (Fig. 6.10).

The "two-time" procedure is much simpler than the original FDA Draft Guidance and should therefore be considerably less sensitive to interlaboratory differences. The reduced number of treated sites means that replicate measurements can be made

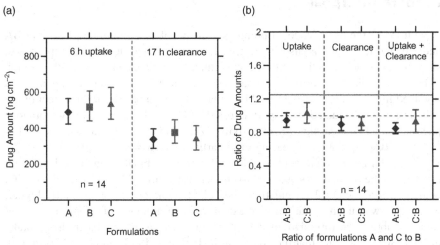

Figure 6.10   BE assessment of the generic 1% econazole creams (products A and C) compared with the reference listed drug (product B). Panel (a) shows the drug amounts per area (mean ± 90% confidence interval) for the three econazole nitrate products after 6 hours uptake and 17 hours clearance measured in 14 volunteers determined in duplicate. Panel (b) shows the ratio of the log-transformed amount of drug in the SC (mean ± 90% confidence interval) after 6 hours uptake, 17 hours clearance, and uptake and clearance combined. Traditionally, to be considered bioequivalent, the 90% confidence interval of the ratio must fall entirely within the indicated 0.8–1.25 interval. Used with permission.[11,41]

and greater statistical power can be achieved with fewer volunteers. Quantification of the SC is not necessary in this case, since the entire SC is removed. Further, the change in the metrics used—from AUC and A_{max} of the FDA protocol to drug amount in the SC at one uptake time and one clearance time—allows differences in BE for clearance and uptake to be discriminated in a manner which the AUC, as a time-weighted average, might miss. Indeed, the relative contributions of the absorption and clearance phases to the AUC can be altered significantly by the duration of the application time. As a result, it is possible that, using the FDA Draft protocol, two testing laboratories could reach contradictory conclusions simply because different drug application and sampling times were chosen.

Reanalysis of a previously reported tretinoin DPK study using the "two-time" method[39] led to conclusions identical to those obtained originally (based on analysis of the entire 8-time-point DPK experiment). Moreover, a BE study on econazole nitrate creams (a reference product and two generics) supported the robustness of the method obtaining conclusive results from a cohort of only 14 volunteers.[11]

The positive results obtained, however, are for now limited to only two drugs (tretinoin and econazole). Further investigations, using other compounds, are essential. Another important point is that, because drug levels are determined at as few as one uptake and one clearance time, guidelines for the correct selection of these times need to be developed.

In Vitro and *In Vivo* Tape Stripping for Research Purposes

In addition to the use of tape stripping as a means of determining topical drug BA and BE, the technique is also interesting for research and development purposes, since the approach, together with the abovementioned data analysis (see the section "The Uptake Phase"), allows mechanistic understanding of various phenomena involved in SC drug penetration and its enhancement. In particular, the effect of the vehicle can be elucidated. Transport across the SC can be enhanced by two obvious phenomena: (1) increasing drug diffusivity (D/L^2) and (2) increasing drug solubility in the SC ($C_{S,SC}$), that is, increasing drug partitioning ($K = C_{S,SC}/C_{S,V}$).

The addition of oleic acid to a formulation of terbinafine increased the drug uptake into the SC that was ascribed to an increase in drug diffusivity inside the SC; compared to the control formulation, the D/L^2 parameter was significantly higher, whereas K was unchanged.[7] In contrast, increasing amounts of PG in a series of saturated ibuprofen formulations caused a significant enhancement in drug uptake into the SC, suggesting that the cosolvent had increased the compound's solubility in the barrier.[42] An effect on the drug solubility in the SC was also found for BMV when delivered at equal thermodynamic activity from a microemulsion (ME) as compared to a reference vehicle comprising medium-chain triglycerides (MCT).[33] Interestingly, the values of K and D/L^2 deduced from the concentration profiles were not significantly different between the two vehicles. However, the deduced solubility of BMV in the SC was highly vehicle dependent, implying that components of the

ME had also been taken up into the SC in sufficient quantities to alter the drug's solubility in the barrier.

The tape-stripping technique can also be used to study the fate of excipients in the vehicle after formulation application. For example, the concentration profile of PG across the SC under different experimental conditions has been determined to understand the cosolvent clearance kinetics.[38] The SC profiles obtained after a 30-minute application and a 30-minute clearance time under both occluded and nonoccluded conditions suggested that PG is eliminated from the SC by both diffusion deeper into the skin and by evaporation from the skin surface. The tape-stripping technique, associated with attenuated total reflectance–Fourier transform infrared (ATR-FTIR) analysis of the tapes, has also been used to study the effect of different vehicles on human SC.[43,44]

In vitro tape stripping has become a valid research tool and useful and relevant measurements have been made on *ex vivo* porcine skin, a reasonable model for human skin due to its similar histology, lipid composition, and SC barrier function[45]; moreover, porcine SC thickness (8.5 ± 3.0 μm) is similar to that measured on the human forearm (11.7 ± 3.2 μm)[31]). Ibuprofen uptake from four different vehicles (PG : water mixtures 25 : 75, 50 : 50, 75 : 25, and 100 : 0) *in vivo* into human SC and *ex vivo* into SC on the porcine ear was very similar and the calculated K and D/L^2 parameters from the respective concentration-depth profiles were in good agreement.[31]

It is also worth noting that a modification of the tape-stripping technique has been used to study transfollicular drug penetration.[46] The technique, called "differential stripping," combines conventional tape stripping with cyanoacrylate skin surface biopsy[47] to obtain the follicular contents. This method has been evaluated both *in vitro* and *in vivo* and permits the drug accumulated in the SC to be differentiated from that accumulated in hair follicles.[48]

PERSPECTIVE AND LIMITATION OF TAPE STRIPPING AND DPK APPROACH

DPK, using tape stripping, appears to offer a reliable means with which to quantify the effective amount of drug penetrating into the major barrier to percutaneous absorption, the SC. The technique is simple and relatively noninvasive. While the proposed FDA Draft Guidance in 1998 showed some clear weaknesses, important progress has already been made with regard to (1) quantification and standardization of the amount of SC removed, (2) a new cleaning procedure to reduce variability by improving removal of residual drug before tape stripping, and (3) including drug present on all tape strips when comparing the amounts taken up into the SC from different products. Equally, DPK parameters, characterizing drug partitioning and diffusivity into and through the SC, can be deduced and used to quantify, respectively, the extent and rate of drug delivery.

The value of improved DPK procedures has been demonstrated for the assessment of the BA of drugs whose site of action is the SC itself, such as antifungal drugs,[7-10] keratolytics,[16-18] UVA/UVB filters,[12-15] and antiseptics.[19] Despite significant progress, however, the DPK method is not presently approved by the FDA, and some valid concerns remain.

First, is the method adequate to assess the BE of drugs which treat target sites other than the SC? In the case of corticosteroids, for example, the target receptors are within the viable epidermis and dermis, not in the SC. Despite some recent data[33] which support the idea that formulations which change drug uptake into the SC will also elicit a concomitant impact on delivery to the underlying viable tissue, there remains a need for further investigation.

Second, if the drug penetration occurs predominantly through another pathway, such as hair follicles, will the DPK method accurately reflect therapeutic effectiveness?

Third, as skin barrier function might be perturbed in dermatological disease, are BA/BE studies conducted on healthy skin relevant to the clinical situation?

Although thorough validation of the DPK measures against clinical outcomes has not yet been demonstrated, it must be remembered that, apart from the vasoconstrictor assay (which is clearly restricted to topical glucocorticoids), there are currently no alternative techniques that can replace clinical studies and that are acceptable to regulatory bodies. For this reason, and considering the striking improvements made after the withdrawal of the FDA Draft Guidance, the DPK method remains the most promising, minimally invasive approach for assessing the BA/BE of topically applied drugs.

EXPERIMENTAL PROCEDURE AND VALIDATION

Formulation Application

The formulations are applied on a defined skin area, mostly on the volar forearm, at least 4 cm from either the wrist or the bend of the elbow. The area of formulation application is typically between 3 and 10 cm^2 and depends upon the ability of the drug to penetrate the SC: for a poorly penetrating drug, it may be necessary to increase the application area (and then the stripped area) to have enough drug in the tape strips for reliable quantification.

Semisolid formulations can be applied using Hill Top Chambers® (Hill Top Research, Cincinnati, OH) affixed to the skin with adhesive tape. Ungelled, liquid formulation may be applied via a foam tape, into which a hole had been cut. The foam tape needs to be applied to the forearm, a piece of tissue to soak the liquid is inserted, and the liquid formulation is added; finally, the foam tape system is covered by an occlusive or nonocclusive tape to prevent any loss of the formulation (Fig. 6.11).

Skin Surface Cleaning

After the desired application time, the formulation is removed and the treated skin site is cleaned. Depending on the viscosity of the formulation, a simple cleaning

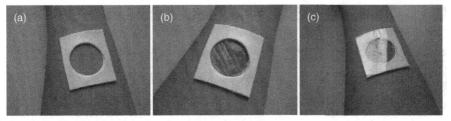

Figure 6.11 Formulation application. (a) Application of foam tape to limit the application area, (b) insertion of tissue to soak in the applied liquid formulation and (c) occlusive covering of the application area with tape.

procedure with a dry paper towel may not be sufficient. Especially for semisolid products, a more aggressive cleaning approach is warranted: excess formulation may be trapped in the skin "furrows," distorting the drug accumulation results and the calculation of "pure" SC/vehicle partitioning coefficient deduced from the analysis of the tape strips (see the section "The Uptake Phase") It has been shown[11,34] that cleaning more aggressively with isopropyl alcohol (IPA) resulted in a lower apparent uptake of drug into the SC. A quick cleaning with IPA wipes is safe; IPA residue left after cleaning evaporates rapidly and IPA contact with skin is too short (relative to time for diffusion in SC) to perturb the amount of absorbed drug. The careful evaluation and validation of an efficient skin cleaning procedure at the end of the application period is a prerequisite.

Tape-Stripping Procedure

The tapes are cut and allowed to equilibrate for at least 12 hours in the laboratory.

The SC sampling site is delimited by a template to leave an exposed skin area which is less than the skin site treated with the formulation. The template is centered over the drug application site immediately before tape stripping begins. This template ensures that all tape strips are removed from the same site (and eliminates any potential problems created by the formulation spreading over the skin). The size of the piece of tape used for stripping is bigger than the opening in the template but smaller than the external dimensions of the template to ensure removing skin layers on the desired skin area only.

The tape is applied to the template, pressed down, and then removed in one quick movement (Fig. 6.12). The first tape strips remove a substantial amount of SC, which tends to progressively reduce as the stripping proceeds to the deeper layers.

The number of strips to collect varies from about 12 to 30,[11] the actual number depending upon the individual's SC thickness, formulation applied, the adhesiveness of the tape used, and whether or not it is necessary to completely remove the SC (see in this regard the two approaches in the sections "Drug Distribution Profiles Across the SC" and "The 'Two-Time' Approach"). To monitor the procedure, the

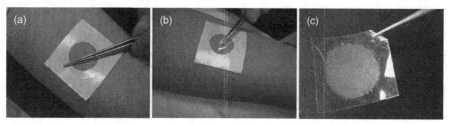

Figure 6.12   Tape-stripping procedure. (a) Application of a template over the drug application site and placing the tape strip on the template. (b) Removing of the tape strip with one quick movement. (c) Resulting tape strip with SC removed.

TEWL is measured before the stripping and then every five strips: the tape stripping is continued until the TEWL reaches fourfold (for removing at least 75 % of the SC) or eightfold (total removal of the SC) the initial (basal) value.

The tape stripping should be performed as quickly as possible, in order to minimize the effect of drug diffusion during the procedure (see specific comments at the end of the section "The Uptake Phase").

Quantification of the SC Removed

Several factors, such as skin hydration, vehicle composition, cohesion between corneocytes, and inter-individual differences in total SC thickness[49–52] can influence the amount of SC that is removed by a single tape strip. For this reason, the quantification of the amount stripped, depending on the data processing chosen, might be very important. Quantification can be done gravimetrically, using a spectophotometric method, by chemical quantification (i.e., protein assay) of the SC on the tape strips or using imaging methods.

In the gravimetric approach, the SC is measured by the difference between the pre- and poststripping weight of the tape. From this mass, and knowing the active area of the tape (i.e., the area in contact with the skin), it is possible to calculate the SC thickness removed (using an SC density of 1 g/cm^3) as a function of stripping, and hence the corresponding position (or depth, x) within the barrier. Although this approach is the simplest and most frequently used one, it is not without problems: the procedure is laborious and precision can be low due to static electricity on the tapes and small amounts of SC removed relative to the mass of the tape. When using this method, it is compulsory to have a balance with a sensitivity of at least 10 μg.

The spectrophotometric method is based on the determination of the absorbance (scattering, reflection, and diffraction) of the corneocyte aggregates, attached to the tape, in the visible spectral range. This technique also has the potential to quantify the drug directly on the tape strips if it has an absorbance clearly separated from those of the SC. Indeed, there have already been some promising correlations observed between the weight of the SC removed and the absorbance at 430 nm of SC stripped off with Tesa tape (No. 5529, Beiersdorf AG, Hamburg, Germany).[53,54] However, using a more adhesive tape like Scotch book tape (3M, St. Paul, MN), the correlation between this measurement and the mass of SC is unsatisfactory unless those tapes with an inhomogeneous layer of SC are ignored.[55] To-date, however, this approach has not been fully optimized or characterized.

The extraction and quantification of proteins from tapes using the protein assay[51,56–58] should ultimately be amenable to high-throughput screening, a clear advantage if the DPK method is used routinely. However, the protein assay is a destructive test, often incompatible with drug extraction and quantification.

Most recently, a novel imaging method to quantify SC on tapes has been investigated. High-resolution images are taken of each tape under carefully controlled optical conditions. Statistical analysis on the distribution of the pixels provides a mean grayscale value that offers a relative measure of SC content of the tapes. The approach has been shown to be rapid, simple, sensitive, and precise. Further, the grayscale values have been shown to be a useful relative measure of SC amount per tape for the determination of SC total thickness in drug permeation experiments, and for full DPK studies of acyclovir creams.[55]

Quantification of the Drug in the Tape Strips

Quantification of the drug in the tape strips is generally made by high-performance liquid chromatography (HPLC) after a suitable extraction procedure. The detection method can be UV, fluorescence, or mass spectrometry depending on the characteristic of the drug, the required detection limit, and the available equipment.

The extraction process should guarantee stability of the drug and good recovery percentages. The analytical method should be specific (the SC, the adhesive, or possible formulation components shall not interfere with the analysis) and sensitive.

Validation of the procedure can be done by spiking tape-stripped samples of untreated SC with a known amount of drug solution (chosen to meet the expected range of concentration to be found in the *in vivo* samples) and proceeding to extraction and analysis. A substantial analytical effort is necessary in order to set up a validated procedure that allows the achievement of reproducible and reliable tape-stripping data.

Since the amount of drug accumulated in the SC is generally low, the sensitivity of the method is one of the key issues of the tape-stripping protocol, mainly when it is necessary to determine the drug content in the individual tapes. If this is not necessary, in order to increase the sensitivity, different tapes can be combined before the extraction procedure.

Besides the HPLC, other analytical methods avoiding the extraction step are possible: ATR-FTIR has been used for the quantification of terbinafine[8] and cyanophenol as a model compound,[59] while a direct spectrophotometric method on the tape itself has been used for UV filter quantification.[60]

Determination of the Total SC Thickness

In some cases, the determination of the total SC thickness of each subject involved in the study is necessary (see the section "Drug Distribution Profiles across the SC").

If it is the case, the total SC thickness has to be determined on an untreated skin site. Approximately 30 tapes are cut into pieces of for example, 2.5 × 2.5 cm and allowed to equilibrate for at least 12 hours in the laboratory. The weight of each tape is determined using a balance with a sensitivity of at least 10 μg.

A template (e.g., piece of polypropylene foil), into which a hole has been cut (e.g., 2.0 cm diameter), is affixed onto an untreated skin site to ensure a constant skin area that must be smaller than the pieces of tape. The initial TEWL is measured.

Baseline TEWL ($TEWL_0$) across unstripped SC of thickness L is given by Fick's first law of diffusion:

$$TEWL_0 = \frac{D \cdot K}{L} \Delta C, \qquad (6.4)$$

where D and K are the diffusion coefficient of water in the SC and the SC-viable tissue partition coefficient of water, respectively, and ΔC is the water concentration gradient across the SC.

Subsequently, the SC is progressively removed by repeated adhesive tape stripping and the TEWL is measured after each tape strip removed. Each tape is reweighed after stripping to assess the mass of SC removed. From this mass, and knowing the stripping area and the density of the SC (1 g/cm^3), it is possible to calculate the thickness of SC removed with each tape. After tape stripping has removed a depth x of SC, the TEWL will have increased to a new value given by:

$$TEWL_x = \frac{D \cdot K}{(L - x)} \Delta C. \qquad (6.5)$$

Tape stripping is continued until the TEWL reaches at least fourfold the initial value. This is to ensure that at least 75 % of the SC is removed.

The total thickness of the SC is then calculated from the x-axis intercept of a graph of 1/TEWL versus the cumulative thickness of SC removed (Fig. 6.13) by linear regression:

$$\frac{1}{TEWL_x} = \frac{L}{D \cdot K \cdot \Delta C} - \frac{x}{D \cdot K \cdot \Delta C}. \qquad (6.6)$$

Most recently, two alternative nonlinear models were proposed, which suggest that the linear model may overestimate the SC thickness. This is explained by the removal of loose outer layers of SC, which do not contribute significantly to barrier function but are included into the linear regression.[61]

Data Processing

The data processing depends upon the approach chosen: if a drug distribution profile inside the SC has to be built, the drug concentration in each tape strip (milligrams per cubic centimeter, M) is plotted as a function of its position within the normalized SC thickness (x/L) (Fig. 6.6). These profiles are then fitted to the appropriate solution

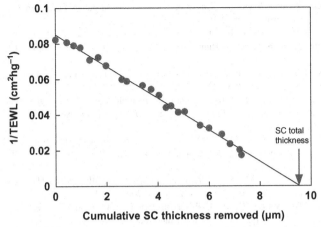

Figure 6.13   Plot of 1/TEWL versus cumulative SC thickness removed from one volunteer. Total thickness of the SC equals 9.55 μm.

of Fick's second law of diffusion to calculate the relevant parameters (see the section "Drug Distribution Profiles across the SC").

If the "two-time" method is used, the total amount of drug per square centimeter is calculated and compared to the value obtained using the reference formulation (Fig. 6.10).

ACKNOWLEDGMENTS

We thank Prof. Annette Bunge and Prof. Richard H. Guy for encouraging us in the fascinating field of skin research, for numerous stimulating discussions, and for critically reading this manuscript.

REFERENCES

1. MENON GK, FEINGOLD KR, ELIAS PM. Lamellar body secretory response to barrier disruption. *J Invest Dermatol* 1992; 98: 279–289.
2. VAN DER VALK PG, MAIBACH HI. A functional study of the skin barrier to evaporative water loss by means of repeated cellophane-tape stripping. *Clin Exp Dermatol* 1990; 15: 180–182.
3. PIÉRARD-FRANCHIMONT C, PIÉRARD GE. Assessment of aging and actinic damages by cyanoacrylate skin surface strippings. *Am J Dermatopathol* 1987; 9: 500–509.
4. MARIONNET C, BERNERD F, DUMAS A, et al. Modulation of gene expression induced in human epidermis by environmental stress *in vivo*. *J Invest Dermatol* 2003; 121: 1447–1458.
5. WU C-F, CHIU H-H. Rapid method for determining dermal exposures to pesticides by use of tape stripping and FTIR spectroscopy: A pilot study. *J Occup Environ Hyg* 2007; 4: 952–958.
6. CULLANDER C, GRANT PG, BENCH G. Development of a low-metal adhesive tape to detect and localize metals in or on the stratum corneum at parts per million levels. *Skin Pharmacol Physiol* 2001; 14: 46–51.

7. ALBERTI I, KALIA YN, NAIK A, et al. *In vivo* assessment of enhanced topical delivery of terbinafine to human stratum corneum. *J Control Release* 2001; 71: 319–327.

8. ALBERTI I, KALIA YN, NAIK A, et al. Effect of ethanol and isopropyl myristate on the availability of topical terbinafine in human stratum corneum, *in vivo*. *Int J Pharm* 2001; 219: 11–19.

9. ALBERTI I, KALIA YN, NAIK A, et al. Assessment and prediction of the cutaneous bioavailability of topical terbinafine, *in vivo*, in man. *Pharm Res* 2001; 18: 1472–1475.

10. PERSHING LK, NELSON JL, CORLETT JL, et al. Assessment of dermatopharmacokinetic approach in the bioequivalence determination of topical tretinoin gel products. *J Am Acad Dermatol* 2003; 48: 740–751.

11. N'DRI-STEMPFER B, NAVIDI WC, GUY RH, et al. Improved bioequivalence assessment of topical dermatological drug products using dermatopharmacokinetics. *Pharm Res* 2009; 26: 316–328.

12. JACOBI U, WEIGMANN H-J, BAUMANN M, et al. Lateral spreading of topically applied UV filter substances investigated by tape stripping. *Skin Pharmacol Physiol* 2004; 17: 17–22.

13. TEICHMANN A, JACOBI U, WEIGMANN HJ, et al. Reservoir function of the stratum corneum: Development of an *in vivo* method to quantitatively determine the stratum corneum reservoir for topically applied substances. *Skin Pharmacol Physiol* 2005; 18: 75–80.

14. GAMER AO, LEIBOLD E, VAN RAVENZWAAY B. The *in vitro* absorption of microfine zinc oxide and titanium dioxide through porcine skin. *Toxicol in Vitro* 2005; 20: 301–307.

15. WISSING SA, MÜLLER RH. Solid lipid nanoparticles as carrier for sunscreens: *In vitro* release and *in vivo* skin penetration. *J Control Release* 2002; 81: 225–233.

16. BASHIR SJ, DREHER F, CHEW AL, et al. Cutaneous bioassay of salicylic acid as a keratolytic. *Int J Pharm* 2005; 292: 187–194.

17. SCHWARB FP, GABARD B, RUFLI T, et al. Percutaneous absorption of salicylic acid in man after topical administration of three different formulations. *Dermatology* 1999; 198: 44–51.

18. TSAI J-C, CHUANG S-A, HSU M-Y, et al. Distribution of salicylic acid in human stratum corneum following topical application *in vivo*: A comparison of six different formulations. *Int J Pharm* 1999; 188: 145–153.

19. LBOUTOUNNE H, CHAULET J-F, PLOTON C, et al. Sustained ex vivo skin antiseptic activity of chlorhexidine in poly([epsilon]-caprolactone) nanocapsule encapsulated form and as a digluconate. *J Control Release* 2002; 82: 319–334.

20. ROUGIER A, DUPUIS D, LOTTE C, et al. *In vivo* correlation between stratum corneum reservoir function and percutaneous absorption. *J Invest Dermatol* 1983; 81: 275–278.

21. National Archives and Records Administration. Code of Federal Regulations (Title 21) Food and Drugs. Available at: http://www.access.gpo.gov/cgi-bin/cfrassemble.cgi?title=200121 (accessed August 1, 2011).

22. SHAH VP, FLYNN GL, YACOBI A, et al. Bioequivalence of topical dermatological dosage forms-methods of evaluation of bioequivalence. *Pharm Res* 1998; 15: 167–171.

23. Food and Drug Administration. Guidance for Industry. Topical Dermatologic Corticosteroids: *In vivo* Bioequivalence. Rockville, MD: Food and Drug Administration, 1995.

24. HAIGH JM, KANFER I. Assessment of topical corticosteroid preparations: The human skin blanching assay. *Int J Pharm* 1984; 19: 245–262.

25. SHAH VP. Topical drug products—Microdialysis: Regulatory perspectives. *Int J Clin Pharmacol Ther* 2004; 42: 379–381.

26. Food and Drug Administration. Guidance for Industry. Topical Dermatologic Drug Product NDAs and ANDAs—*In Vivo* Bioavailability, Bioequivalence, *In Vitro* Release, and Associated Studies. Draft Guidance. Rockville, MD: Food and Drug Administration, June 1998.

27. CONNER DP. Differences in DPK Methods. Advisory Committee for Pharmaceutical Sciences Meeting. Rockville, MD: Food and Drug Administration, November 29, 2001. Available at: http://www.fda.gov/ohrms/dockets/ac/01/slides/3804s2_05_conner/index.htm (accessed August 1, 2011).

28. FRANZ TJ. Study #1, Avita Gel 0.025% vs Retin-A Gel 0.025%. Advisory Committee for Pharmaceutical Sciences Meeting. Rockville, MD: Food and Drug Administration, November 29, 2001.

29. PERSHING LK. Bioequivalence Assessment of Three 0.025% Tretinoin Gel Products: Dermatopharmacokinetic vs. Clinical Trial Methods. Advisory Committee for Pharmaceutical Sciences Meeting. Rockville, MD: Food and Drug Administration, November 29, 2001.

30. Food and Drug Administration. Guidance for industry on special protocol assessment; Rockville, MD: Food and Drug Administration, availability. *Fed Reg* 2002; 67: 35122.

31. HERKENNE C, NAIK A, KALIA YN, et al. Pig ear skin ex vivo as a model for *in vivo* dermatopharmacokinetic studies in man. *Pharm Res* 2006; 23: 1850–1856.

32. HERKENNE C, NAIK A, KALIA YN, et al. Dermatopharmacokinetic prediction of topical drug bioavailability *in vivo*. *J Invest Dermatol* 2007; 127: 887–894.

33. WIEDERSBERG S, LEOPOLD CS, GUY RH. Pharmacodynamics and dermatopharmacokinetics of betamethasone 17-valerate: Assessment of topical bioavailability. *Br J Dermatol* 2009; 160: 676–686.

34. WIEDERSBERG S, LEOPOLD CS, GUY RH. Dermatopharmacokinetics of betamethasone 17-valerate: Influence of formulation viscosity and skin surface cleaning procedure. *Eur J Pharm Biopharm* 2009; 71: 362–366.

35. REDDY MB, STINCHCOMB AL, GUY RH, et al. Determining dermal absorption parameters *in vivo* from tape strip data. *Pharm Res* 2002; 19: 292–298.

36. BUNGE AL, CLEEK RL, VECCHIA BE. A new method for estimating dermal absorption from chemical exposure. 3. Compared with steady-state methods for prediction and data analysis. *Pharm Res* 1995; 12: 972–982.

37. WIEDERSBERG S, GUY RH. Dermatopharmacokinetics of betamethasone 17-valerate: Prediction of bioavailability. In: Brain KR, Walters KA, eds. *Perspectives in Percutaneous Penetration*, Vol. 11. STS Publishing, Cardiff, 2008; 101.

38. NICOLI S, BUNGE AL, DELGADO-CHARRO MB, et al. Dermatopharmacokinetics: Factors influencing drug clearance from the stratum corneum. *Pharm Res* 2009; 26: 865–871.

39. N'DRI-STEMPFER B, NAVIDI WC, GUY RH, et al. Optimizing metrics for the assessment of bioequivalence between topical drug products. *Pharm Res* 2008; 25: 1621–1630.

40. NAVIDI W, HUTCHINSON A, N'DRI-STEMPFER B, et al. Determining bioequivalence of topical dermatological drug products by tape-stripping. *J Pharmacokinet Pharmacodyn* 2008; 35: 337–348.

41. BUNGE AL, GUY RH. Therapeutic Equivalence of Topical Products: Revised Final report. Submitted to Department of Health and Human Services, Food and Drug Administration, 2008.

42. HERKENNE C, NAIK A, KALIA YN, et al. Effect of propylene glycol on ibuprofen absorption into human skin *in vivo*. *J Pharm Sci* 2008; 97: 185–197.

43. DIAS M, NAIK A, GUY RH, et al. *In vivo* infrared spectroscopy studies of alkanol effects on human skin. *Eur J Pharm Biopharm* 2008; 69: 1171–1175.

44. CURDY C, NAIK A, KALIA YN, et al. Non-invasive assessment of the effect of formulation excipients on stratum corneum barrier function *in vivo*. *Int J Pharm* 2004; 271: 251–256.

45. SEKKAT N, KALIA YN, GUY RH. Biophysical study of porcine ear skin *in vitro* and its comparison to human skin *in vivo*. *J Pharm Sci* 2002; 91: 2376–2381.

46. KNORR F, LADEMANN J, PATZELT A, et al. Follicular transport route—Research progress and future perspectives. *Eur J Pharm Biopharm* 2009; 71: 173–180.

47. TEICHMANN A, JACOBI U, OSSADNIK M, et al. Differential stripping: Determination of the amount of topically applied substances penetrated into the hair follicles. *J Invest Dermatol* 2005; 125: 264–269.

48. PATZELT A, RICHTER H, BUETTEMEYER R, et al. Differential stripping demonstrates a significant reduction of the hair follicle reservoir *in vitro* compared to *in vivo*. *Eur J Pharm Biopharm* 2008; 70: 234–238.

49. KALIA YN, ALBERTI I, SEKKAT N, et al. Normalization of stratum corneum barrier function and transepidermal water loss *in vivo*. *Pharm Res* 2000; 17: 1148–1150.

50. VAN DER MOLEN RG, SPIES F, VAN'T NOORDENDE JM, et al. Tape stripping of human stratum corneum yields cell layers that originate from various depths because of furrows in the skin. *Arch Dermatol Res* 1997; 289: 514–518.

51. BASHIR SJ, CHEW A-L, ANIGBOGU A, et al. Physical and physiological effects of stratum corneum tape stripping. *Skin Res Technol* 2001; 7: 40–48.

52. JACOBI U, MEYKADEH N, STERRY W, et al. Effect of the vehicle on the amount of stratum corneum removed by tape stripping. *J Dtsch Dermatol Ges* 2003; 1: 884–889.
53. WEIGMANN H-J, LADEMANN J, MEFFERT H, et al. Determination of the horny layer profile by tape stripping in combination with optical spectroscopy in the visible range as a prerequisite to quantify percutaneous absorption. *Skin Pharmacol Appl Skin Physiol* 1999; 12: 34–45.
54. WEIGMANN H-J, LINDEMANN U, ANTONIOU C, et al. UV/VIS absorbance allows rapid, accurate, and reproducible mass determination of corneocytes removed by tape stripping. *Skin Pharmacol Appl Skin Physiol* 2003; 16: 217–227.
55. RUSSELL LM, GUY RH. Dermato-pharmacokinetics: An approach to evaluate topical drug bioavailability. PhD thesis. University of Bath, 2008.
56. LINDEMANN U, WEIGMANN H-J, SCHAEFER H, et al. Evaluation of the pseudo-absorption method to quantify human stratum corneum removed by tape stripping using protein absorption. *Skin Pharmacol Appl Skin Physiol* 2003; 16: 228–236.
57. DREHER F, ARENS A, HOSTYNEK JJ, et al. Colorimetric method for quantifying human stratum corneum removed by adhesive-tape-stripping. *Acta Derm Venereol* 1998; 78: 186–189.
58. DREHER F, MODJTAHEDI BS, MODJTAHEDI SP, et al. Quantification of stratum corneum removal by adhesive tape stripping by total protein assay in 96-well microplates. *Skin Res Technol* 2005; 11: 97–101.
59. STINCHCOMB AL, PIROT F, TOURAILLE GD, et al. Chemical uptake into human stratum corneum *in vivo* from volatile and non-volatile solvents. *Pharm Res* 1999; 16: 1288–1293.
60. WEIGMANN H-J, JACOBI U, ANTONIOU C, et al. Determination of penetration profiles of topically applied substances by means of tape stripping and optical spectroscopy: UV filter substance in sunscreens. *J Biomed Opt* 2005; 10: 014009-1-7.
61. RUSSELL LM, WIEDERSBERG S, DELGADO-CHARRO MB. The determination of stratum corneum thickness: An alternative approach. *Eur J Pharm Biopharm* 2008; 69: 861–870.

Chapter 7

Skin Permeation Assessment: Microdialysis

Rikke Holmgaard, Jesper B. Nielsen, and Eva Benfeldt

INTRODUCTION

The most dependable data for drug penetration through the skin are obtained from human studies. However, in the initial development of a new drug, human studies are generally not feasible. As a result, *in vitro*, *ex vivo*, or animal models are often used as screening models to assess transdermal drug absorption profiles. Establishing the correlation between these models and human *in vivo* cutaneous absorption is eventually the challenge.

The pharmacokinetics of systemically administered drugs has, as a golden standard, always been studied using blood sampling. Blood samples are, however, not appropriate or feasible when it comes to studies of pharmacokinetics of topically applied drugs with the pharmacological target in the skin, since only a fraction of the drug present in the formulation/cream applied to the skin surface will reach the systemic blood circulation. This fraction does not necessarily reflect the concentration in the target organ, the skin.

Through the latest decades the microdialysis (MD) sampling methodology has gained ground. The approval of MD probes for use in humans by the U.S. Food and Drug Administration (FDA) and the European Union Conformité Européenne[1] has made clinical studies based on MD feasible and increased the use of the method; progress has also been made in dermal microdialysis (DMD) methodology for advanced studies of transdermal and topical drug penetration.

This chapter will give an update on theory and practice and a detailed description of experimental procedures including the manufacturing of probes, calibration, study design, sample analysis, and interpretation of MD data. The study planning required for successful sampling, as well as the current status regarding regulatory authorities, will be described.

Transdermal and Topical Drug Delivery: Principles and Practice, First Edition. Edited by Heather A.E. Benson, Adam C. Watkinson.
© 2012 John Wiley & Sons, Inc. Published 2012 by John Wiley & Sons, Inc.

HISTORY

The MD technique was originally developed for neuropharmacological research in the 1960s.[2] The dialytrodes were then further developed and in 1974 Ungerstedt and Pycock reported on the use of "hollow fibers,"[3] a structure which has gradually improved and today is known as the concentric probe (see later). Subsequently, the technique was subspecialized and it is currently used in many different tissues in animal models as well as in human studies.[1] DMD was first described in a human study regarding percutaneous absorption of ethanol in 1991.[4]

MD methodology provides the opportunity of sampling free unbound local drug concentrations in a site-specific or tissue-specific fashion in pharmacokinetic studies. Considerable experience ranging from *in vitro* to *in vivo* studies in animals, patients, and healthy volunteers has accumulated over recent years and several thousand MD publications are published to date.

For reviews of MD we recommend: Groth et al.,[5] Plock and Kloft,[6] the FDA-AAPS White Paper,[1] Schmidt et al.,[7] and most recently Holmgaard et al.[8]

MD METHODOLOGY

MD is one of the few techniques that provide *in vivo* chronological, real-time information about the pharmacokinetics of drugs, obtained from the extracellular fluid phase at the site of action, that is, in the target tissue.

The MD principle can be compared with the function of an artificial blood vessel. MD sampling is achieved by placing a membrane (probe) in the tissue (Fig. 7.1).[5] This probe, which is permeable to water and small molecules, is continuously perfused with a physiological buffer (the perfusate) at a low flow rate. Unbound substances present in the extracellular fluid can cross the membrane and enter the flowing perfusate in the lumen of the probe by passive diffusion, driven by the concentration gradient. The rate of entry into the lumen of the probe is determined by the physicochemical properties of the substance such as the size and solubility properties, including charge of the molecule. Furthermore, active tissue processes such as blood flow, the membrane material, and wall thickness all influence the rate

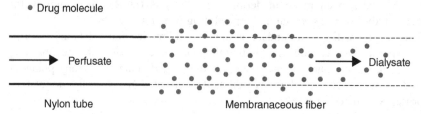

Figure 7.1 Principle of MD sampling by a linear probe. The perfusate is pumped through the probe at a preset low flow rate. During the passage through the membranaceous portion, which can be from 1 to 4 cm long, the diffusion of small molecules across the membrane takes place. The perfusate is now termed the dialysate.

Table 7.1   Factors Affecting RR

Substance-specific parameters
- Lipophilicity
- Molecular weight
- Protein binding
- Solubility
- Adherence to probe and tubes

Choice of instrumentation
- Probe membrane material and design
- Perfusate composition and flow rate

Experimental procedures
- Probe depth in the dermis (for topically applied substances)
- Application of heat or cooling
- Vasoconstriction or -dilatation

Endogenous parameters
- Tissue
- Blood flow in the tissue
- Metabolism in the skin
- Temperature

The concentration of substance around the probe does in theory *not* affect the RR.

Source: Modified from Holmgaard et al.[8]

at which a substance enters the perfusate (see Table 7.1). Larger molecules such as proteins and enzymes cannot cross the membrane. Molecules with moderate to high lipophilicities (logPow > 2.5–3) are a specific challenge in relation to finding a suitable perfusate. Details about this and the determination of recovery are given later in this chapter.

The MD system consists of a probe, a pump, and vials in which the perfusate is collected. The system can be connected to an automated sampler/collector or to online (or even online bedside) analysis.

In the following section the focus is on the use of MD in the skin—the dermis.

EXPERIMENTAL PROCEDURE AND CONSIDERATIONS

The preparations and considerations required when planning a DMD study are summarized in Table 7.2.[5] Whether the study is performed *in vitro*, *in vivo*, with animals, or with humans, several of the considerations are identical.

Probe

The method is minimally invasive and is based on local sampling using thin dialysis catheters with a semipermeable membrane (Fig. 7.2).[9] The design of the probes

Table 7.2   Necessary steps in Preparation of Human MD Experiments

1. Preparations:
    - *In vitro* recovery and loss: linearity.
    - Ensure reproducible, stable recovery over a concentration range and time.
    - Establish that analysis is sensitive enough in the low concentration range.
2. Consider:
    - Choosing a calibrator.
    - The possible effect of probe modifications introduced at a later stage (guide wire in lumen, sterilization procedures).
    - That *in vivo* recovery is likely to be ≪ than *in vitro* recovery, due to skin metabolism and vascularization.
    - If studies of drug protein-binding effects or animal studies are needed.
3. Human protocol work:
    - Include pilot experiments and await analysis of pilot samples.
    - Amend setup (flow rate, probe type, perfusate composition) if necessary.

Source: Modified from Groth et al.[5]

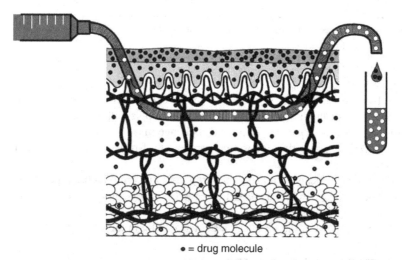

● = drug molecule

Figure 7.2   Illustration of the MD probe placed in the dermis, sampling increasing dermal drug concentrations following topical drug penetration. Source: Benfeldt et al. 1999.[9]

differs in size, shape, and material depending on the intended site of implantation. The probes can be divided into four categories: the linear probe, the loop probe, the side-by-side probe, and the concentric probe (Fig. 7.3).[10] For DMD, the linear probe type is typically used. Different types of linear probes are available and the majority of these probes are inserted in the skin through a small guide cannula (Fig. 7.4a) as the probes are made of fragile material. Probes for MD are commercially available, but can also be made on-site in the laboratory, for example, taken from a hemodialy-

A　　　B　　　　C　　　　D

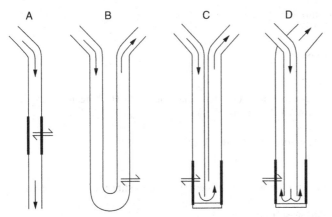

Figure 7.3　Illustration of the four types of probes. A. The linear probe. B. The loop probe. C. The side-by-side probe. D. The concentric probe. Source: Gunaratna et al.[10]

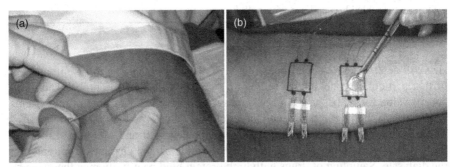

Figure 7.4　(a) The insertion of the guide cannula in the dermis. (b) The probes inserted in the dermis; perfusion has been started and the topical formulation is being applied.

sis cylinder, which contains many thousand fibers. Placing a guide wire inside the fiber and connecting a tube at the end of the fiber creates a functioning probe. The presence of the wire inside the probe will not affect recovery[11] but allows probe depth in the skin to be measured with ultrasound and will also stiffen the probe, which eases dermal insertion. For a manual of probe manufacturing, see Table 7.3. The linear probe has a unidirectional flow and a very small diameter compared to the other probe types—down to approximately 200 μm for some structures.[12] Linear probes will, however, need to penetrate the skin twice (Fig. 7.4), since they have both an inlet and an outlet puncture.

The exchange of molecules between the perfusate and the extracellular fluid will depend on the probe type. The probe has a membranaceous part characterized by a porous structure allowing the exchange of smaller molecules across the membrane. The pores are different in size for different types of probe designs. The pore

Table 7.3 Probe Manufacturing

Materials:
- Lamp with magnifying glass
- Stanley knife
- Tweezers
- Gambro GFS 16+ hemodialysis cylinder (Gambro Dialysaten AG, Hechingen, Germany)
- Guide wire (Sandvik steel 0.10 mm) (Sandvik Steel, Norway)
- Acetone
- Nylon tube (Portex flexible grade) (Portex, Berck-sur-Mer, France)
- Cyanoacrylate glue (Loctite) (Super Attak, Loctite, Denmark)

Procedure:
- Open the hemodialysis cylinder a few days before use. Keep the fibers in an air-sealed box when not in use.
- Degrease the guide wire using acetone.
- Insert the wire in the hemodialysis fiber under magnifying glass.
- Insert the fiber (2.5 cm) in the nylon tube.
- Close the connection with a drop of glue.
- Let the glue dry for 6 hours.
- Store in air-sealed box and use within 48 hours.

size will determine the upper molecular size of analytes that can diffuse in and out of that particular probe—described as the "cut-off value" of the probe. The usual cut-off value for probes used in low flux systems is <20 kDa, in high flux systems is 40–70 kDa, but membranes with larger cut-off values (up to 3000 kDa) exist.[13,14] The concentric probes are commercially available at 20 and 100 kDa. Low flux probe types exclude larger molecules such as proteins and enzymes from entering the dialysate. Sampling of drugs with high protein binding affinity may therefore be associated with very low drug concentration in the dialysate. The exclusion of enzymes will, however, secure that no enzymatic degradation of analyte occurs in the dialysate.

The probe can be used as a sampling tool ("recovery") as well as a tool for drug delivery ("loss"), since compounds in the perfusate can be delivered to the tissue at the same time as analytes in the extracellular fluid are gained from the tissue by diffusion in the opposite direction. An important methodological feature of the MD sampling process is that neither extraction nor delivery of fluid from/to the tissue occurs—a feature that makes the method very appropriate for use in, for example, small animals or in pediatric patients.

A new probe type, which has recently been introduced, is the open-coil probe known from open-flow microperfusion (OFM). The principle resembles MD but is essentially different since no dialysis occurs. The technique involves the placement of an open coil-like probe type in the tissue, followed by slow perfusion from a pump. This promising sampling technique may in the future solve some of the difficulties that have been experienced using DMD since the technique is not affected by the size, shape, and lipophilicity of the drugs to the same extent as DMD.

These challenges will be described later. For further information about OFM, see References 15–17.

Perfusate

The perfusate is a tissue-compatible fluid, which is pumped through the probe at a low flow rate (typically 0.9–1.5 μL/min.), higher if periprobe drug concentrations and recovery are both high. In DMD the perfusate is most often an isotonic saline solution or a Ringer solution, thus a hydrophilic environment. Most often the flow rate has to be kept low to assure an acceptable relative recovery (RR) of the drug/ test substance across the membrane (for RR, see below). When the perfusate flows through the membranaceous area of the probe, dialysis takes place and the perfusate becomes the dialysate, which is collected in the sampling vial or injected directly into the analytical system. The hydrophilic environment inside the probe determines that a very lipophilic drug will usually have a low RR. Modifying the perfusate by adding substances such as albumin, Intralipid® (Baxter Healthcare, Deerfield, IL), or Encapsin® (Cerestar USA, Hammond, IN) will make the perfusate more attractive to lipophilic substances.[12,18] Other binding agents such as cyclodextrins have been shown to increase MD RR,[19,20] as has the addition of small organic molecules such as ethanol, propylene glycol, and dimethyl sulfoxide when sampling hydrophilic analytes *in vitro*.[21]

Application Site

The volar forearm is the standard area for investigations of skin penetration and barrier function by noninvasive measurements in DMD.[22–29] It is easily accessible, usually not hairy, and not very convex (Fig. 7.4).

To avoid discomfort only one arm is used for MD at a time, which allows the test person to use the other arm during the experiment. Blood drawn from this arm can provide measurements of plasma drug concentrations and thus the systemic drug delivery, if relevant.

Insertion of Probes

The probes are inserted under clean procedures after gentle soap wash of the skin area. To minimize the discomfort during insertion, local anesthesia can be used[30–32] or the skin can be anaesthetized by application of ice packs onto the skin, which has been shown to provide sufficient reduction in pain/discomfort.[29,33] The probes are inserted using a 19–23 G cannula as a guide, placed horizontally in the dermis (Fig. 7.4). The probe, which has been submerged in a 70% ethanol bath for 20 minutes before insertion, is then inserted in the opposite direction through the open tip of the hollow cannula and tested by a short flush of perfusate to secure the functionality. Subsequently the guide cannula is withdrawn with the probe still in place. The accuracy of placing the probe at the intended depth in the skin depends on the training and experience of the laboratory personnel.[9]

Measuring Probe Depth by Ultrasound Scanning

To verify the probe depth and the dermis location, an ultrasound scan (normally by 20 MHz ultrasound scanning) can be used. The laboratory-made linear probes used in DMD contain a stainless steel wire in the lumen, which makes it easy to visualize the probe position in the skin by ultrasound scanning.[11] Theoretically, probe depth would be expected to affect the amount of drug sampled following topical application. However, several studies have not been able to demonstrate a correlation between the depth of the probe and the drug concentration in the dialysate.[27,29,34–36] The only study demonstrating a correlation between depth and drug concentration included different skin layers (both dermal and subcutaneous probe placement).[37] The recommendation is to measure the probe depth in three separate scans along the length of the probe *in situ*. With experience, probes can be inserted with great accuracy and low variability,[29,34] for example, 0.7 ± 0.15 mm mean $\pm$ standard deviation (SD).[27] The preferable insertion depth is 0.6–1.0 mm (in the dermis).

The overall conclusion is that since the inter-individual variability in skin penetration is around 40%–60%[34,38] and thereby a major contributor to the variability in cutaneous drug delivery, the small variability in probe depth probably has no significant influence on the drug concentration in the sample.

Tissue Trauma

Even though MD is known as a minimally invasive technique, the tissue trauma and histamine release induced by probe insertion cause a reversible response in the skin (Table 7.4). The tissue response diminishes after a period of 40–135 minutes in human skin.[30,39–41] A proper equilibration period of a minimum of 90 minutes is therefore advisable before sampling can begin.[31] Local anesthesia can be used during insertion[30–32] and has shown to reduce trauma reaction[31] as well as minimizing pain/discomfort. A pharmacokinetic interaction between the anesthesia and the test substance must here be considered.

Table 7.4   Skin Reaction

Early response (transient):
• Histamine release
• Increase in the local blood flow
• Increased skin thickness
• Hyperemia
Late response (>24 hours):
• Lymphocyte infiltration
• Fibrin deposits
If volunteer predisposed:
• Keloid formation

The presence of a DMD probe elicits an inflammatory response after some time. No signs of tissue inflammation are described within the initial 6–10 hours after probe insertion; but infiltration of lymphocytes will arise later, and after 32 hours scar tissue may appear.[40,42] Following insertion of concentric probes, more extensive tissue disruption compared to a linear probe has been reported,[42,43] which is properly caused by the larger diameter of the guide cannula used for implantation of concentric probes (e.g., ~500 μm).[42] In our experience the development of skin changes, visible at clinical examination after, for example, 3 months, is very rare. One exception is if the volunteer or patient is prone to keloid formation, and for this reason we recommend screening for this as an exclusion criterion of the study protocol, thus avoiding DMD in keloid-prone individuals.

Pump

The MD pumps controlling the flow are very exact precision pumps with very limited intra- and interexperimental variation in flow rate. Portable pumps are available, an advantage in experiments that run over several hours and where a volunteer may have to change position now and then. The pumps are for continuous use but the flow rate has to be tested frequently in basic experiments by gravimetric control of volume delivery conducted at different flow settings.

CALIBRATION

Calibration is important when studying a new drug or analyte. Since the MD probe is continuously perfused with fresh perfusate, full equilibrium across the membrane cannot be established. A steady-state rate of molecule exchange across the MD membrane is, however, reached and the dialysate concentration is therefore a fraction of the actual concentration in the tissue. Calibration and an estimate of the RR are therefore necessary if the intention is quantitative MD.

$$RR = C_{dialysate} / C_{periprobe\ fluid}.$$

RR is the ratio between the drug concentration in the dialysate and the drug concentration in the periprobe fluid.[44]

In vitro calibration does not substitute the *in vivo* calibration but will give an indication of the RR and subsequently the feasibility of *in vivo* MD sampling of the particular test substance (Table 7.1). Thus, using *in vitro* calibration it is possible to predict and minimize some of the recovery challenges in the *in vivo* study. Both dialysis and retrodialysis can be used for *in vitro* calibration (see below).[45] The *in vitro* settings for perfusate flow rate, temperature, and sampling intervals should be the same as for the planned *in vivo* experiment.[46] In general, the RR is much higher *in vitro* than *in vivo* due to, for example, the tortuosity of the path of the molecule in the tissue, the effects of temperature, blood flow, and tissue metabolism.[47] *In vivo* calibration can be made using different methods. The dialysis membrane allows for both uptake (recovery) and delivery (loss) of an analyte, depending on whether the substance is initially present in the medium/tissue or has been added to the perfusate. The transport (loss/recovery) across the membrane is in theory symmetrical, although in practice this is not always so due to, for example, the (predominantly lipophilic) test substance binding to the probe material, or other artifactual situations.[5]

The actual amount of analyte collected by the probe during a finite period of time is called the "absolute recovery." A higher flow rate leads to a greater absolute recovery of molecules—and a dilution of the dialysis sample due to the higher flow. The flow rate of the perfusate influences the RR, which decreases as the flow rate increases.[48] The RR is also determined by the physicochemical properties of the analyte and proteins binding in the tissue, the tissue temperature, probe type, and probe length as well as the membrane material. Consequently, the RR will vary with changes in the experimental set-up (Table 7.1) but is not affected by the peri-probe concentration of the analyte—for further information, see the review by Holmgaard et al.[8]

No-Net-Flux Method

This method is also known as the zero-net-flux method. Different concentrations of the analyte flows through the probe and, depending on the direction of the concentration gradient between perfusate and periprobe fluid, the analyte will diffuse in or out of the probe. If the concentration in the periprobe fluid is equal to the concentration in the dialysate, no-net-flux of analyte will occur. By plotting the perfusate versus dialysate concentrations, the extracellular concentration outside the probe can be identified. No assumptions about the analyte and its behavior in the periprobe fluid have to be made as the RR is interpolated and not extrapolated.[6]

Stop-Flow/Flow-Rate Method

Calibration is achieved by varying the perfusate flow rate. The theoretical total equilibrium between probe and periprobe fluid is achieved at a zero flow rate, where the C_d is identical to the actual concentration, C_p, in the extracellular fluid surrounding the probe (periprobe fluid). Through measurement of RR at decreasing perfusate flow rates, an estimate of the zero flow RR can be made by extrapolation.[49]

Retrodialysis

Retrodialysis is also known as the delivery method.[50] The method is defined as the loss/diffusion of molecules from the perfusate to the surroundings under sink conditions. The idea is that the *in vivo* loss mirrors the *in vivo* recovery. Again, this method relies on the symmetry of the dialysis process across the membrane.

The calibration is made by spiking the perfusate with the analyte of interest (*retrodialysis by drug*) or by adding a calibrator (*retrodialysis by calibrator*). Retrodialysis by drug requires a prolongation of an *in vivo* experimental protocol since the drug must be cleared from the extracellular fluid before experiments with dermal application can be initiated. If retrodialysis by calibrator is used, the calibrator chosen needs to be similar to the analyte regarding parameters such as diffusion, transportation, and metabolism in the tissue (some examples: lidocaine and prilocaine[51] or caffeine and theophylline[52]). The ultimate situation is when the loss of the calibrator is symmetrical to the recovery of the analyte during MD. The loss and recovery of the analyte and its calibrator are functions of their effective permeabilities—a reciprocal relation to their resistance to diffusion.[48] Whenever sampling of an analyte is performed during retrodialysis by calibrator, both compounds will have to be analyzed in the same sample.

PHARMACOKINETICS

Since the use of MD in human drug studies has become more and more accepted[1] the sampling of drugs by the use of different probes has become possible in almost all living tissues (muscle, skin, lung, myocardium, brain, and even malignant tumors). Real-time pharmacokinetic profiles of absorption, half-life, maximum concentration, area under the time versus concentration curve, metabolism, and elimination of drugs and other chemicals can be obtained from the site of action. Some of the pharmacokinetic studies using DMD sampling include the pre-clinical investigation of several new or approved antineoplastic drugs, employing the utility of sampling the drug simultaneously in both tumor and unaffected tissue. Estimating the $AUC_{tumor/tissue}$ ratio for a series of antineoplastic drugs in pre-clinical investigations supports the selection of the best candidate for further drug development. Thus, in a study of two antineoplastic drugs, sampled in cutaneous metastases of human malignant melanoma, it was possible to evaluate whether a lack of response to either drug was related to reduced target site concentration or to drug resistance in the malignant cells.[53,54] DMD has also been used to evaluate topical drug penetration into basal cell carcinoma prior to photodynamic therapy.[55,56]

Studies of drug penetration and drug metabolism in the skin was previously evaluated following suction blister[9] and skin biopsy techniques.[57] These techniques are more invasive than DMD and produce samples containing the entire drug concentration, that is, both bound and unbound drug. Since it is the level of unbound drug that determines the pharmacodynamic activity,[58-60] a measurement of the total drug concentration can be a misleading indicator of the active drug concentration at the target site. An advantage of MD is therefore that only the unbound fraction of the drug of interest is sampled.

The first human DMD studies examined the cutaneous penetration of ethanol and were followed by studies on the release of histamine in response to skin manipulation and the vascular changes in the skin after insertion of DMD probes.[4,30,39] Numerous studies have subsequently demonstrated the versatility of DMD sampling in pharmacokinetic studies. DMD allows not only sampling of the drug of interest in the dermis but also its metabolites.[9] DMD sampling of drugs that exercise their action in the skin or that can be followed by a biomarker gives the opportunity for pharmacokinetic–pharmacodynamic studies.[61] Transdermal drug studies have explored the kinetics of different drugs released from patches—for example, nicotine and estradiol—by the use of DMD.[35,37] Also, topical drugs for treatment of muscle inflammation—felbinac (transdermal therapeutic system [TTS]) and diclofenac (spray gel)—have been examined.[62,63] Both administration modalities proved to be possible alternatives to orally administered nonsteroidal anti-inflammatory drug (NSAID) for superficial muscle inflammation since high drug concentrations were found in the skin and subcutaneous tissues, respectively. Ketoprofen penetration kinetics following application as a TTS (with the target being intra-articular inflammation) has been sampled in the skin as well as in the knee joint. Sufficient drug concentration for inhibition of prostaglandin E2 production was found in the joint following topical application.[64] Bioavailability (BA) and the possibility of the DMD technique as a tool for the determination of bioequivalence (BE) (see later) has been studied in human *in vivo* studies of topical formulations of lidocaine,[25,34] ketoprofen,[29] and metronidazol.[65] For a thorough review of DMD studies of *in vivo* topical drug penetration see Holmgaard et al.[8]

BIOAVAILABLITY

The definition of BA is "the rate and extent to which the active ingredient or active moiety is absorbed from a drug product and becomes available at the site of action. For drug products that are not intended to be absorbed into the bloodstream, bioavailability may be assessed by measurements intended to reflect the rate and extent to which the active ingredient or active moiety becomes available at the site of action," as per the FDA "Guidance for Industry" 2002.[66]

A comparative BA study of orally administered ibuprofen versus topically administered ibuprofen has been undertaken by placing MD probes in the subcutaneous tissue as well as in the muscular tissue (the target sites), showing that the relative BA in both muscle and subcutaneous tissue after topical application was significantly higher than after oral administration and that the plasma levels measured were much lower.[67] This example illustrates the advantage of MD sampling in cases where target sites are accessible to MD.

MONITORING CHANGES IN BA BY DMD

Alterations in the BA of a topically applied drug may be caused by a damaged skin barrier, may be enhanced by iontophoresis, or can be caused by changes in cutaneous vascular tone.

Damaged Skin Barrier

A damaged skin barrier increases transepidermal water loss (TEWL)[68] and is expected to be associated with increased penetration of exogenous compounds. The increased penetration of a model compound, salicylic acid, has been studied by Benfeldt et al. following different barrier disruption methods employed in human volunteers as well as in hairless rats.[69,70] The studies demonstrated highly increased drug penetration where the barrier had been perturbed by either tape stripping or irritant dermatitis in both human and in rat skin (157- and 170-fold increased penetration, respectively). Recent studies have evaluated the penetration of acyclovir and salicylic acid on the disrupted skin barrier using DMD and tape stripping[71] and the penetration of a metronidazole cream formulation (1%) applied to the forearm skin in areas of both irritant dermatitis[27] and eczematous skin in patients suffering from atopic dermatitis.[72] The studies all demonstrated increased drug penetration in barrier-disrupted skin/diseased skin as well as demonstrated the usefulness of MD methodology for *in vivo* studies of commercially available formulations in healthy and diseased human skin.

Effect of Iontophoresis

Studies using DMD have assessed the effect of iontophoresis on topical drug delivery (Fig. 7.5) of several different drugs such as acyclovir,[73] propranolol,[28] methotrexate,[74] and flurbiprofen[75] to/through the skin and the subsequent systemic delivery.[73] The systemic exposure is limited while the drug quickly reaches a high concentration in the dermis and underlying tissue.

Blood Circulation

The BA of topically applied drugs depends on the local blood flow in the skin. Vasodilatation as well as vasoconstriction can be achieved in many ways and can

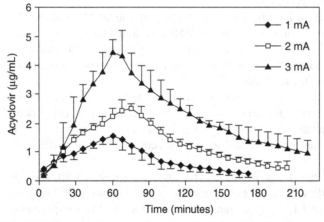

Figure 7.5 Dermal concentrations of acyclovir in rabbit skin after iontophoretic administration for 1 hour at 1, 2, or 3 mA, respectively. Source: Stagni et al.[73]

arise intentionally or unintentionally. It can be physiologically or pharmacologically induced and will affect the local blood flow significantly. The skin concentration of a topically applied drug will increase if the blood flow is diminished, whereas an increased blood flow enhances the uptake and subsequent systemic distribution and elimination of the drug from the skin.[42] Experimental DMD studies where vasoconstriction or vasodilatation has been induced have demonstrated that the BA of topically as well as systemically applied test substances is highly influenced by changes in the microcirculation of the skin[76-79]—an influence apparently much more significant than the influence of variations in probe depth.

BE OF TOPICALLY ADMINISTERED DRUGS

FDA describes BE as a comparative test between two products using specified criteria. BE is defined as "the absence of a significant difference in the rate and extent to which the active ingredient or active moiety in pharmaceutical equivalents or pharmaceutical alternatives becomes available *at the site of action* when administered at the same molar dose under similar conditions in an appropriately designed study."[66]

Present FDA requirements for BE determination of topical drug products depend on the pharmacological class of the dosage form. The blanching assay using a chromameter has been recommended for glucocorticoid dosage forms. All other topical drug products were first suggested to be determined using the dermatopharmacokinetic (DPK) methodology.[80] DPK, also known as tape stripping, is a well-known and validated method, which comprises successive application and removal of tape from the skin surface to remove the epidermis (see Chapter 6). FDA subsequently withdrew the draft guidance and the current determination of BE relies on comparative clinical trials between the generic drug and the innovator drug.[81] As clinical trials often require several hundreds of participants, this is therefore a very time-consuming and expensive procedure.[82]

In 2007, Benfeldt et al. investigated two commercially available topical lidocaine products (ointment 5% and cream 5%) by DMD and found these two products to be bioinequivalent (Fig. 7.6).[34] Statistic evaluations indicated that BE studies of topical formulations could be conclusive in as few as 18 subjects (when three probes are used per application site; see Table 7.5).

Using a set-up where only one formulation was investigated in four similar penetration areas on the volar forearm (Fig. 7.7), Tettey-Amlalo et al. could demonstrate a very low intraindividual variability of 10%, and a 68 % between-subjects variability and thus also an overall feasibility of conducting a conclusive BE study in 18 subjects.[29]

In comparison, it has been estimated that approximately 40–50 subjects are required for BE studies using the tape-stripping method and up to 300 subjects using the current clinical BE study design.[83] Thus, the present FDA requirement for BE determination, which relies on comparative clinical trials between the generic drug and the innovator drug, is a more time-consuming and expensive procedure.

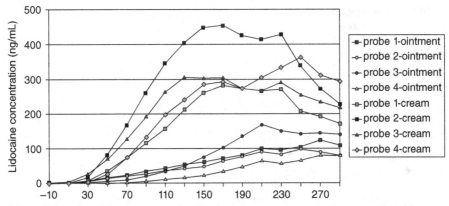

Figure 7.6 Microdialysate concentration data from the two separate experiments conducted in one volunteer. In the upper four graphs, the lidocaine concentration in dialysates from the four probes following topical application of the 5% cream formulation. In the lower four graphs, the lidocaine concentration in the dialysates from the four probes sampling topical penetration forms the 5% ointment formulation. The sample concentration is plotted at midinterval by convention. Source: Benfeldt et al.[34]

Table 7.5 BE Study Size Estimates

Probability (%)	Limits of variation (%)	Two probes per area	Three probes per area
BE study with two formulations in each subject			
80	<25 (80–125)	20	114
90	**<25**	**27**	**18**
90	<33	17	12
90	<50	10	7
BE study with one formulation in each subject			
80	<25 (80–125)	711	695
90	**<25**	**985**	**962**
90	<33	591	577
90	<50	922	292

Based on a DMD study of topical formulations in healthy human volunteers, where the inter-individual variability was found to account for 60% of the overall variability, the following numbers of volunteers could be calculated.

The criteria for limits of variation are those currently employed by the FDA, where the limit of variation described as "<25%" means less than factor 1.25 above and below the mean, thus between 125% and 100/1.25 = 80%. The study designs shown in bold, with 90% probability and limitation of variability to between 80% and 125%, corresponds to the current FDA criteria for BE determination.
Source: Modified from Benfeldt et al.[34]

Other studies have also proven that the DMD method is a valuable tool in the evaluation of the BE between two or more topical drug products.[25,34,65,84] The technique can be an appropriate method for studying drug penetration into the deeper skin layers and can obtain detailed pharmacokinetic information with real-time chronology. Another advantage is that DMD allows testing of both test and reference products at the same time in the same individuals.

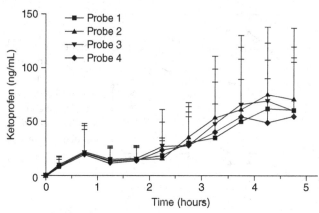

Figure 7.7   In a study of topical ketoprofen gel, applied to the skin surface on the volar aspect of the forearm, four probes inserted 3 cm apart were used ($n = 18$). Mean dialysate concentration versus time profiles ($\pm$SD) demonstrate a very small variability. Source: Tettey-Amlalo et al.[29]

ANALYTICAL ASPECTS

When planning a DMD study a close collaboration with the analyst is important, since some of the limitations of this method are related to two factors: extremely small dialysate volumes (1–30 µL) and very low drug concentration in these small samples. Very sensitive analytical methods or methods that can handle ultra-low volumes are therefore essential; for example, gas chromatography–mass spectrometry (GC-MS), capillary electrophoresis, liquid chromatography–mass spectrometry (LC-MS), or gas chromatography–flame photometric detector (GC-FPD).[85-88] It is important to realize that increasing sample volume by increasing the perfusate flow rate will result in sample dilution; slowing down perfusion rate will increase RR but result in small sample volumes. In the case of small sample volumes, pooling the dialysates from two or more probes should be considered; alternatively, prolongation of the sampling interval.

Online injection for analysis is possible and was first used in 1987 on freely moving rats[89] but is now also used in some cutaneous drug distribution studies.[90,91]

Review articles on analytical aspects related to MD can be recommended[23,92,93]

ADVANTAGES AND CHALLENGES

DMD allows the study of topically applied drugs by continuous real-time drug sampling in the living dermis and thereby pharmacokinetic investigations at the target site. Most methodological challenges can typically be identified and considered through well-planned *in vitro* experiments as part of the planning phase. Founded on pre-experimental troubleshooting and validation of the analytical method chosen, reproducible results with acceptable variability can be achieved for most drugs. The advantages and limitations of the DMD method raise questions that need to be addressed prior to choosing DMD for studies of topical formulations.

Advantages

- MD captures the pharmacological events where they take place in the tissues, providing high-resolution real-time details.
- There is no fluid extraction from the tissue.
- For topical drugs and formulations, DMD allows testing of both test and reference products at the same time in the same individuals.
- The drug of interest as well as its metabolites will be present in the dialysate.
- The probes allow sampling as well as delivery of substances.
- The method provides protein-free samples, which is often an analytical advantage.
- Immediate cessation of enzyme degradation once the drug has been sampled.
- DMD is an inexpensive method to use once the MD pumps have been purchased, since the probes can be manufactured in the laboratory at minimal cost (see Table 7.2).
- Multiple application or sampling sites can be planned.
- Good reproducibility.
- DMD sampling of topical drug formulation in the BA/BE setting does *not* depend on the drug concentrations in the formulations tested being the same.

Challenges

- Moderately or highly lipophilic drug molecules are often excellent for topical penetration but less favorable for sampling by DMD (for highly lipophilic drugs, the DPK method can be more suitable).
- An *in vitro* RR of less than 5% will most often characterize a compound as not suitable for MD studies due to an expected further reduction in *in vivo* recovery.
- Some topical formulations (e.g., topical corticosteroids) contain low drug concentrations and the analysis of the dialysate will predictably be challenging.
- For protein-bound substances it can be necessary to add protein content to the perfusate to increase recovery, which may result in more complex analytical procedures.

- Achieving low variability in probe insertion and probe manufacturing depends on experienced personnel.

- The dialysate concentration will decrease with increasing flow rate and vice versa since the RR of substances is flow dependent. However, if very low flow rates are used, the time resolution can be compromised.

- Extensive modifications of analytical procedures may be required prior to *in vivo* experiments.

- The duration of a DMD experiment is in many instances limited to 8–10 hours (this may be overcome if portable pumps are available).

REGULATORY AUTHORITIES

A challenge in biopharmaceutical research is finding a correlation between *ex vivo* and *in vivo* studies, and between animal and human studies for prediction of percutaneous absorption in humans.

In the "Critical Path Initiative" from 2004, the FDA puts focus on the challenges involved in the development of new drugs—from laboratory concept to commercial product.[94] They raise concern of the declining and languishing innovation of biomedical products due to the continuing increase in expenses of medical product development, process prolongation, and inefficiency. A call for new knowledge and methodologies for improving predictability and efficiency along the critical path was made, specifically for the assessment of BE of locally acting drugs such as topical and inhalation products. MD was mentioned as an *in vivo* sampling method and a possible research direction to address these problems.[95] The FDA has been receptive to MD data and has used MD data in both pre- and postauthorization situations, and as part of both pre-clinical and clinical pharmacological investigations, as an addition to *in vivo* BA experiments.[34] Additionally, MD has been recommended to pharmaceutical companies as a way to investigate specific safety topics related to systemic drug delivery of drugs intended for topical application and action.[1] In 2008, attention was drawn to DMD as a method offering opportunities for topical BE studies and to the method being in keeping with optimization of the critical path.[82]

Current determination of BE relies on comparative clinical trials between the generic drug and the innovator drug. As clinical trials often require several hundreds of participants, this is therefore a very time-consuming and expensive procedure.[82,83] The MD methodology has the potential of becoming central in the development of new drugs, and a valuable tool in the evaluation of BE between topical drug products since the technique enables sampling in the skin of pharmacokinetic information with real-time chronology. The technique may also be an appropriate method for studying drugs in the deeper layers of the skin.

REFERENCES

1. CHAURASIA CS, MULLER M, BASHAW ED, et al. AAPS-FDA workshop white paper: Microdialysis principles, application and regulatory perspectives. *Pharm Res* 2007; 24(5): 1014–1025.

2. BITO L, DAVSON H, LEVIN E, et al. The concentrations of free amino acids and other electrolytes in cerebrospinal fluid, *in vivo* dialysate of brain, and blood plasma of the dog. *J Neurochem* 1966; 13(11): 1057–1067.

3. UNGERSTEDT U, PYCOCK C. Functional correlates of dopamine neurotransmission. *Bull Schweiz Akad Med Wiss* 1974; 30(1–3): 44–55.

4. ANDERSON C, ANDERSSON T, MOLANDER M. Ethanol absorption across human skin measured by *in vivo* microdialysis technique. *Acta Derm Venereol* 1991; 71(5): 389–393.

5. GROTH L, GARCÍA ORTIZ P, BENFELDT E. Microdialysis methodology for sampling in the skin. In: Serup J, Jemec GBE, Grove G, eds. *Handbook of Non-Invasive Methods and the Skin*, 2nd ed. CRC Press, Boca Raton, FL, 2006; 443–454.

6. PLOCK N, KLOFT C. Microdialysis—Theoretical background and recent implementation in applied life-sciences. *Eur J Pharm Sci* 2005; 25(1): 1–24.

7. SCHMIDT S, BANKS R, KUMAR V, et al. Clinical microdialysis in skin and soft tissues: An update. *J Clin Pharmacol* 2008; 48(3): 351–364.

8. HOLMGAARD R, NIELSEN JB, BENFELDT E. Microdialysis sampling for investigations of bioavailability and bioequivalence of topically administered drugs: Current state and future perspectives. *Skin Pharmacol Physiol* 2010; 23(5): 225–243.

9. BENFELDT E, SERUP J, MENNE T. Microdialysis vs. suction blister technique for *in vivo* sampling of pharmacokinetics in the human dermis. *Acta Derm Venereol* 1999; 79(5): 338–342.

10. GUNARATNA C, LUNTE SM, ZUO H. Shunt probe: A new microdialysis probe design for *in vivo* drug metabolism studies. *Curr Sep* 1994; 13: 80–83.

11. KLIMOWICZ A, BIELECKA-GRZELA S, GROTH L, et al. Use of an intraluminal guide wire in linear microdialysis probes: Effect on recovery? *Skin Res Technol* 2004; 10(2): 104–108.

12. CARNEHEIM C, STAHLE L. Microdialysis of lipophilic compounds: A methodological study. *Pharmacol Toxicol* 1991; 69(5): 378–380.

13. SCHMELZ M, LUZ O, AVERBECK B, et al. Plasma extravasation and neuropeptide release in human skin as measured by intradermal microdialysis. *Neurosci Lett* 1997; 230(2): 117–120.

14. WINTER CD, IANNOTTI F, PRINGLE AK, et al. A microdialysis method for the recovery of IL-1 beta, IL-6 and nerve growth factor from human brain *in vivo*. *J Neurosci Methods* 2002; 119(1): 45–50.

15. BODENLENZ M, SCHAUPP LA, DRUML T, et al. Measurement of interstitial insulin in human adipose and muscle tissue under moderate hyperinsulinemia by means of direct interstitial access. *Am J Physiol Endocrinol Metab* 2005; 289(2): E296–E300.

16. ELLMERER M, WACH P, TRAJANOSKI Z, et al. Open flow microperfusion—Interstitial sampling of large molecules. *Proc Ann Int Conf IEEE EMBS* 1997; 19: 2381–2383.

17. ELLMERER M, SCHAUPP L, BRUNNER GA, et al. Measurement of interstitial albumin in human skeletal muscle and adipose tissue by open-flow microperfusion. *Amer J Physiol-Endocrinol Met* 2000; 278(2): E352–E356.

18. WARD KW, MEDINA SJ, PORTELLI ST, et al. Enhancement of *in vitro* and *in vivo* microdialysis recovery of SB-265123 using Intralipid (R) and Encapsin (R) as perfusates. *Biopharm Drug Dispos* 2003; 24(1): 17–25.

19. KHRAMOV AN, STENKEN JA. Enhanced microdialysis extraction efficiency of ibuprofen *in vitro* by facilitated transport with beta-cyclodextrin. *Anal Chem* 1999; 71(7): 1257–1264.

20. KHRAMOV AN, STENKEN JA. Enhanced microdialysis recovery of some tricyclic antidepressants and structurally related drugs by cyclodextrin-mediated transport. *Analyst* 1999; 124(7): 1027–1033.

21. SUN L, STENKEN JA. Improving microdialysis extraction efficiency of lipophilic eicosanoids. *J Pharmaceut Biomed Anal* 2003; 33(5): 1059–1071.

22. BENFELDT E. *In vivo* microdialysis for the investigation of drug levels in the dermis and the effect of barrier perturbation on cutaneous drug penetration. Studies in hairless rats and human subjects. *Acta Derm Venereol Suppl (Stockh)* 1999; 206: 1–59.

23. DAVIES MI, COOPER JD, DESMOND SS, et al. Analytical considerations for microdialysis sampling. *Adv Drug Deliv Rev* 2000; 45(2–3): 169–188.

24. KORINTH G, JAKASA I, WELLNER T, et al. Percutaneous absorption and metabolism of 2-butoxyethanol in human volunteers: A microdialysis study. *Toxicol Lett* 2007; 170(2): 97–103.

25. KREILGAARD M, KEMME MJ, BURGGRAAF J, et al. Influence of a microemulsion vehicle on cutaneous bioequivalence of a lipophilic model drug assessed by microdialysis and pharmacodynamics. *Pharm Res* 2001; 18(5): 593–599.

26. MORGAN CJ, RENWICK AG, FRIEDMANN PS. The role of stratum corneum and dermal microvascular perfusion in penetration and tissue levels of water-soluble drugs investigated by microdialysis. *Br J Dermatol* 2003; 148(3): 434–443.

27. ORTIZ PG, HANSEN SH, SHAH VP, et al. The effect of irritant dermatitis on cutaneous bioavailability of a metronidazole formulation, investigated by microdialysis and dermatopharmacokinetic method. *Contact Dermatitis* 2008; 59(1): 23–30.

28. STAGNI G, O'DONNELL D, LIU YJ, et al. Intradermal microdialysis: Kinetics of iontophoretically delivered propranolol in forearm dermis. *J Control Release* 2000; 63(3): 331–339.

29. TETTEY-AMLALO RN, KANFER I, SKINNER MF, et al. Application of dermal microdialysis for the evaluation of bioequivalence of a ketoprofen topical gel. *Eur J Pharm Sci* 2009; 36(2–3): 219–225.

30. ANDERSON C, ANDERSSON T, WARDELL K. Changes in skin circulation after insertion of a microdialysis probe visualized by laser Doppler perfusion imaging. *J Invest Dermatol* 1994; 102(5): 807–811.

31. GROTH L, SERUP J. Cutaneous microdialysis in man: Effects of needle insertion trauma and anaesthesia on skin perfusion, erythema and skin thickness. *Acta Derm Venereol* 1998; 78(1): 5–9.

32. PETERSEN LJ. Measurement of histamine release in intact human skin by microdialysis technique. Clinical and experimental findings. *Dan Med Bull* 1998; 45(4): 383–401.

33. KELLOGG DL, ZHAO JL, WU Y. Neuronal nitric oxide synthase control mechanisms in the cutaneous vasculature of humans *in vivo. J Physiol (London)* 2008; 586(3): 847–857.

34. BENFELDT E, HANSEN SH, VOLUND A, et al. Bioequivalence of topical formulations in humans: Evaluation by dermal microdialysis sampling and the dermatopharmacokinetic method. *J Invest Dermatol* 2007; 127(1): 170–178.

35. HEGEMANN L, FORSTINGER C, PARTSCH B, et al. Microdialysis in cutaneous pharmacology: Kinetic analysis of transdermally delivered nicotine. *J Invest Dermatol* 1995; 104(5): 839–843.

36. MULLER M, MASCHER H, KIKUTA C, et al. Diclofenac concentrations in defined tissue layers after topical administration. *Clin Pharmacol Ther* 1997; 62(3): 293–299.

37. MULLER M, SCHMID R, WAGNER O, et al. In-vivo characterization of transdermal drug transport by microdialysis. *J Control Release* 1995; 37(1–2): 49–57.

38. LARSEN RH, NIELSEN F, SORENSEN JA, et al. Dermal penetration of fentanyl: Inter- and intraindividual variations. *Pharmacol Toxicol* 2003; 93(5): 244–248.

39. ANDERSON C, ANDERSSON T, ANDERSSON RG. *In vivo* microdialysis estimation of histamine in human skin. *Skin Pharmacol* 1992; 5(3): 177–183.

40. KROGSTAD AL, JANSSON PA, GISSLEN P, et al. Microdialysis methodology for the measurement of dermal interstitial fluid in humans. *Br J Dermatol* 1996; 134(6): 1005–1012.

41. PETERSEN LJ, SKOV PS, BINDSLEV-JENSEN C, et al. Histamine release in immediate-type hypersensitivity reactions in intact human skin measured by microdialysis. A preliminary study. *Allergy* 1992; 47(6): 635–637.

42. AULT JM, RILEY CM, MELTZER NM, et al. Dermal microdialysis sampling *in vivo. Pharm Res* 1994; 11(11): 1631–1639.

43. AULT JM, LUNTE CE, MELTZER NM, et al. Microdialysis sampling for the investigation of dermal drug transport. *Pharm Res* 1992; 9(10): 1256–1261.

44. BENVENISTE H, HUTTEMEIER PC. Microdialysis—Theory and application. *Prog Neurobiol* 1990; 35(3): 195–215.

45. SCHELLER D, KOLB J. The internal reference technique in microdialysis: A practical approach to monitoring dialysis efficiency and to calculating tissue concentration from dialysate samples. *J Neurosci Methods* 1991; 40(1): 31–38.

46. GROTH L. Cutaneous microdialysis. Methodology and validation. *Acta Derm Venereol Suppl (Stockh)* 1996; 197: 1–61.

47. LAFONTAN M, ARNER P. Application of in situ microdialysis to measure metabolic and vascular responses in adipose tissue. *Trends Pharmacol Sci* 1996; 17(9): 309–313.

48. WANG Y, WONG SL, SAWCHUK RJ. Microdialysis calibration using retrodialysis and zero-net flux: Application to a study of the distribution of zidovudine to rabbit cerebrospinal fluid and thalamus. *Pharm Res* 1993; 10(10): 1411–1419.
49. JACOBSON I, SANDBERG M, HAMBERGER A. Mass transfer in brain dialysis devices—A new method for the estimation of extracellular amino acids concentration. *J Neurosci Methods* 1985; 15(3): 263–268.
50. STAHLE L, ARNER P, UNGERSTEDT U. Drug distribution studies with microdialysis. III: Extracellular concentration of caffeine in adipose tissue in man. *Life Sci* 1991; 49(24): 1853–1858.
51. KREILGAARD M. Dermal pharmacokinetics of microemulsion formulations determined by *in vivo* microdialysis. *Pharm Res* 2001; 18(3): 367–373.
52. STAHLE L, SEGERSVARD S, UNGERSTEDT U. Drug distribution studies with microdialysis. 2. Caffeine and theophylline in blood, brain and other tissues in rats. *Life Sci* 1991; 49(24): 1843–1852.
53. BLOCHL-DAUM B, MULLER M, MEISINGER V, et al. Measurement of extracellular fluid carboplatin kinetics in melanoma metastases with microdialysis. *Br J Cancer* 1996; 73(7): 920–924.
54. JOUKHADAR C, KLEIN N, MADER RM, et al. Penetration of dacarbazine and its active metabolite 5-aminoimidazole-4-carboxamide into cutaneous metastases of human malignant melanoma. *Cancer* 2001; 92(8): 2190–2196.
55. SANDBERG C, HALLDIN CB, ERICSON MB, et al. Bioavailability of aminolaevulinic acid and methyl-aminolaevulinate in basal cell carcinomas: A perfusion study using microdialysis *in vivo*. *Br J Dermatol* 2008; 159(5): 1170–1176.
56. WENNBERG AM, LARKO O, LONNROTH P, et al. Delta-aminolevulinic acid in superficial basal cell carcinomas and normal skin—A microdialysis and perfusion study. *Clin Exp Dermatol* 2000; 25(4): 317–322.
57. ROLSTED K, BENFELDT E, KISSMEYER AM, et al. Cutaneous *in vivo* metabolism of topical lidocaine formulation in human skin. *Skin Pharmacol Physiol* 2009; 22(3): 124–127.
58. HERKENNE C, ALBERTI I, NAIK A, et al. *In vivo* methods for the assessment of topical drug bioavailability. *Pharm Res* 2008; 25(1): 87–103.
59. KUNIN CM, CRAIG WA, KORNGUTH M, et al. Influence of binding on the pharmacologic activity of antibiotics. *Ann N Y Acad Sci* 1973; 226: 214–224.
60. MERRIKIN DJ, BRIANT J, ROLINSON GN. Effect of protein binding on antibiotic activity *in vivo*. *J Antimicrob Chemother* 1983; 11(3): 233–238.
61. KREILGAARD M. Influence of microemulsions on cutaneous drug delivery. *Adv Drug Deliv Rev* 2002; 54(Suppl 1): S77–S98.
62. BRUNNER M, DEHGHANYAR P, SEIGFRIED B, et al. Favourable dermal penetration of diclofenac after administration to the skin using a novel spray gel formulation. *Br J Clin Pharmacol* 2005; 60(5): 573–577.
63. SHINKAI N, KORENAGA K, TAKIZAWA H, et al. Percutaneous penetration of felbinac after application of transdermal patches: Relationship with pharmacological effects in rats. *J Pharm Pharmacol* 2008; 60(1): 71–76.
64. SHINKAI N, KORENAGA K, MIZU H, et al. Intra-articular penetration of ketoprofen and analgesic effects after topical patch application in rats. *J Control Release* 2008; 131: 107–112.
65. ORTIZ PG, HANSEN SH, SHAH VP, et al. Are marketed topical metronidazole creams bioequivalent? Evaluation by *in vivo* microdialysis sampling and tape-stripping methodology. *Skin Pharmacol Physiol* 2011; 24(1): 44–53.
66. FDA. Guidance for Industry Bioavailability and Bioequivalence Studies for Orally Administered Drug Products—General Considerations. Available at: www.fda.gov/OHRMS/DOCKETS/98fr/3657gd2.pdf.
67. TEGEDER I, MUTH-SELBACH U, LOTSCH J, et al. Application of microdialysis for the determination of muscle and subcutaneous tissue concentrations after oral and topical ibuprofen administration. *Clin Pharmacol Ther* 1999; 65(4): 357–368.
68. VAN DER VALK PGM, NATER JP, BLEUMINK E. Skin irritancy of surfactants as assessed by water vapor loss measurements. *J Invest Dermatol* 1984; 82(3): 291–293.

69. BENFELDT E, SERUP J. Effect of barrier perturbation on cutaneous penetration of salicylic acid in hairless rats: *In vivo* pharmacokinetics using microdialysis and non-invasive quantification of barrier function. *Arch Dermatol Res* 1999; 291(9): 517–526.

70. BENFELDT E, SERUP J, MENNE T. Effect of barrier perturbation on cutaneous salicylic acid penetration in human skin: *In vivo* pharmacokinetics using microdialysis and non-invasive quantification of barrier function. *Br J Dermatol* 1999; 140(4): 739–748.

71. KLIMOWICZ A, FARFAL S, BIELECKA-GRZELA S. Evaluation of skin penetration of topically applied drugs in humans by cutaneous microdialysis: Acyclovir vs. salicylic acid. *J Clin Pharm Ther* 2007; 32(2): 143–148.

72. ORTIZ PG, HANSEN SH, SHAH VP, et al. Impact of adult atopic dermatitis on topical drug penetration: Assessment by cutaneous microdialysis and tape stripping. *Acta Derm Venereol* 2009; 89(1): 33–38.

73. STAGNI G, ALI ME, WENG D. Pharmacokinetics of acyclovir in rabbit skin after IV-bolus, ointment, and iontophoretic administrations. *Int J Pharm* 2004; 274(1–2): 201–211.

74. STAGNI G, SHUKLA C. Pharmacokinetics of methotrexate in rabbit skin and plasma after iv-bolus and iontophoretic administrations. *J Control Release* 2003; 93(3): 283–292.

75. MATHY FX, LOMBRY C, VERBEECK RK, et al. Study of the percutaneous penetration of flurbiprofen by cutaneous and subcutaneous microdialysis after iontophoretic delivery in rat. *J Pharm Sci* 2005; 94(1): 144–152.

76. BORG N, GOTHARSON E, BENFELDT E, et al. Distribution to the skin of penciclovir after oral famciclovir administration in healthy volunteers: Comparison of the suction blister technique and cutaneous microdialysis. *Acta Derm Venereol* 1999; 79(4): 274–277.

77. BOUTSIOUKI P, THOMPSON JP, CLOUGH GF. Effects of local blood flow on the percutaneous absorption of the organophosphorus compound malathion: A microdialysis study in man. *Arch Toxicol* 2001; 75(6): 321–328.

78. JOUKHADAR C, DEHGHANYAR P, TRAUNMULLER F, et al. Increase of microcirculatory blood flow enhances penetration of ciprofloxacin into soft tissue. *Antimicrob Agents Chemother* 2005; 49(10): 4149–4153.

79. RIVIERE JE, WILLIAMS PL. Pharmacokinetic implications of changing blood-flow in skin. *J Pharm Sci* 1992; 81(6): 601–602.

80. US FDA. Guidance for Industry: Topical Dermatological Drug Product NDAs and ANDAs—*In Vivo* Bioavailability, Bioequivalence, *In Vitro* Release, and Associated Studies. Draft Guidance, June 1998, U.S. Department of Health and Human Services, Food and Drug Administration, Center for Drug Evaluation and Research (CDER). 1998. Available at: www.fda.gov/ohrms/dockets/ac/00/backgrd/3661b1c.pdf.

81. US FDA. Guidance for industry on special protocol assessment; availability. *Fed Reg* 2002; 67: 35122.

82. LIONBERGER RA. FDA critical path initiatives: Opportunities for generic drug development. *AAPS J* 2008; 10(1): 103–109.

83. SHAH VP, FLYNN GL, YACOBI A, et al. Bioequivalence of topical dermatological dosage forms— Methods of evaluation of bioequivalence. *Pharm Res* 1998; 15(2): 167–171.

84. MCCLEVERTY D, LYONS R, HENRY B. Microdialysis sampling and the clinical determination of topical dermal bioequivalence. *Int J Pharm* 2006; 308(1–2): 1–7.

85. JOUKHADAR C, KLEIN N, DITTRICH P, et al. Target site penetration of fosfomycin in critically ill patients. *J Antimicrob Chemother* 2003; 51(5): 1247–1252.

86. LEVEQUE N, MURET P, MARY S, et al. Validation of a microdialysis-gas chromatographic-mass spectrometric method to assess 8-methoxypsoralen in psoriatic patient dermis. *J Chromatogr B* 2002; 780(1): 119–127.

87. LINDBERGER M, TOMSON T, WALLSTEDT L, et al. Distribution of valproate to subdural cerebrospinal fluid, subcutaneous extracellular fluid, and plasma in humans: A microdialysis study. *Epilepsia* 2001; 42(2): 256–261.

88. OBERTHUR C, HEINEMANN C, ELSNER P, et al. A comparative study on the skin penetration of pure tryptanthrin and tryptanthrin in Isatis tinctoria extract by dermal microdialysis coupled with isotope dilution ESI-LC-MS. *Planta Med* 2003; 69(5): 385–389.

89. Damsma G, Westerink BHC, Devries JB, Horn AS. Analysis and microdialysis of acetylcholine in the brain of freely moving rats. *Pharm Weekbl Sci* 1987; 9(6): 338.

90. Mathy FX, Vroman B, Ntivunwa D, et al. On-line determination of fluconazole in blood and dermal rat microdialysates by microbore high-performance liquid chromatography. *J Chromatogr B Analyt Technol Biomed Life Sci* 2003; 787(2): 323–331.

91. Mathy FX, Ntivunwa D, Verbeeck RK, et al. Fluconazole distribution in rat dermis following intravenous and topical application: A microdialysis study. *J Pharm Sci* 2005; 94(4): 770–780.

92. Nandi P, Lunte SM. Recent trends in microdialysis sampling integrated with conventional and microanalytical systems for monitoring biological events: A review. *Anal Chim Acta* 2009; 651(1): 1–14.

93. Williams FM. Evaluations and predictions of dermal absorption of toxic chemicals. *Toxicology* 2004; 202(1–2): 38.

94. US FDA. Challenge and Opportunity on the Critical Path to New Medicinal Products. 2004. Available at: www.nipte.org/docs/Critical_Path.pdf.

95. US FDA. Critical Path Opportunities for Generic Drugs. 2007. Available at: www.fda.gov/ScienceResearch/SpecialTopics/CriticalPathInitiative/CriticalPathOpportunitiesReports/ucm077250.htm.

Chapter 8

Skin Permeation: Spectroscopic Methods

Jonathan Hadgraft and Majella E. Lane

INTRODUCTION

Structure

The skin is a very complex heterogeneous membrane that provides a unique barrier to the loss of water from the body and the ingress of xenobiotics. In very simple terms, the outer layer, the stratum corneum, provides the major barrier and has a structure that has been likened to a brick wall. The bricks are the corneocytes, which are predominantly comprised of keratin, and the mortar, which is a complex mixture of lipids, including ceramides, cholesterol, cholesterol sulfate, and free fatty acids. The lipids are structured into ordered bilayers, the packing of which is very tight. The major route of permeation across the stratum corneum is via the lipid-filled intercellular channels and therefore the total barrier function is a result of the tortuous path and the necessity of the diffusant to cross sequentially numerous bilayers. A molecule, therefore, has to pass from lipophilic to hydrophilic domains, and it is not surprising that only a few substances have optimum properties to cross the skin. These are small molecules with reasonably balanced partition characteristics and good solubility in both water and oils. Examples of such include nicotine and nitroglycerin but even these only pass slowly through the skin.

In order to understand the nature of the barrier, a number of spectroscopic techniques have been used. This chapter examines some of these and highlights the uses to which they have been put in order to progress our understanding of this complex membrane. In fact, the heterogeneity of the skin makes interpretation of the signals complex, and sometimes it is easier to understand the barrier better by using model membranes with the caveat that they may not truly represent the skin itself.

Transdermal and Topical Drug Delivery: Principles and Practice, First Edition. Edited by Heather A.E. Benson, Adam C. Watkinson.
© 2012 John Wiley & Sons, Inc. Published 2012 by John Wiley & Sons, Inc.

Electromagnetic Spectrum

Most regions of the electromagnetic spectrum have been used to probe the skin, ranging from X-rays through ultraviolet (UV) to infrared (IR), sound waves, and radio waves, in the form of nuclear magnetic resonance (NMR). The types of features probed, at a molecular level, are the bilayer packing, molecular interactions, diffusion rates, and the spatial location of actives and formulation components with the stratum corneum and below. Some techniques can also be used to examine the nature of skin and to determine any abnormalities, and hence research has been proposed in the diagnosis area.

The various spectroscopic techniques will now be summarized. Since most of the literature is concerned with vibrational spectroscopy, namely IR and Raman, these will be considered first. The subject has also been considered in depth in many publications and so representative cases will only be considered.

VIBRATIONAL SPECTROSCOPIC METHODS

A typical IR spectrum of skin is shown in Figure 8.1. The features that are most commonly examined are the CH symmetric and asymmetric stretch at around 2850 and 2920/cm. Of particular interest in the fingerprint region is information about the carbonyl stretch and the amide 1 and amide 2 bands.

Puttnam first suggested the use of attenuated total reflectance–Fourier transform infrared (ATR-FTIR) spectroscopy for studying skin[1] but the technique remained rather dormant for a decade. Work in the mid-1980s showed the use of IR in an understanding of the role of the skin lipids in the overall permeation

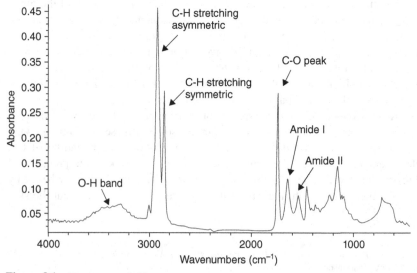

Figure 8.1 IR spectrum of skin.

process.[2,3] Polymorphism of the skin lipids has been demonstrated by considering the scissoring vibrations.[4] Lipid organization can also be inferred from spectroscopic data.[5,6]

The nature of the skin lipids could be altered by the ingress of formulation excipients such as octadecanoic acids[7] and oleic acid.[8] This clearly had implications in an understanding of the mechanisms of action of penetration enhancers. There is always a problem of separating the stretch frequency of the stratum corneum lipids from those of the enhancer; this can be resolved using perdeuterated material. Using this technique, it was possible to demonstrate that oleic acid forms phase-separated pools within the stratum corneum.[9] This contrasts with Azone® (Nelson Ltd., Irvine, CA), which appears to distribute homogeneously.[10]

The precise route of permeation has always been a matter of debate. The diffusion of water through porcine skin was followed as a function of temperature and, at the same time, the –CH stretch monitored.[11] Water permeability and the –CH stretch frequency appear highly correlated, implying that water transfer is related to its passage through the lipid-rich intercellular domains. The occlusive effects of hydrocolloids can be followed using Fourier transform infrared (FTIR) spectroscopy.[12]

Skin hydration improves permeability but IR data suggest that increased hydration does not affect lipid fluidity and therefore other mechanisms of action must be important.[13] Ethanol has also been used as a penetration enhancer, particularly in first-generation transdermal devices such as Duragesic® (Alza Corp., Vacaville, CA) for the delivery of fentanyl. The delivery of the active stops when the ethanol is depleted from the reservoir device. However, the enhancer effect must be solubility related, as there is no evidence that ethanol disorders the lipids in the skin.[14]

ATR-FTIR studies have been conducted *in vitro* to separate the effects of penetration enhancers, for example, Azone and Transcutol® (Gattefosse, Saint-Priest, France).[15] Combining *in vivo* skin stripping with ATR-FTIR also gives insight into the effects of enhancers on drug distribution.[16,17] Using perdeuterated solvents it is also possible to show that the degree of uptake of the enhancer is directly related to the disorder induced in the skin lipids.[18] Recently, this type of diffusion experiment has been used to follow permeation of commercial products through model membranes and skin; in order to achieve these, data deconvolution is necessary.[19] The experimental set-up for a typical ATR-FTIR diffusion experiment *in vitro* is illustrated in Figure 8.2.

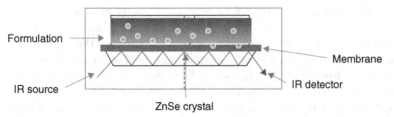

Figure 8.2   Typical ATR-FTIR experimental set-up for an *in vitro* membrane diffusion experiment.

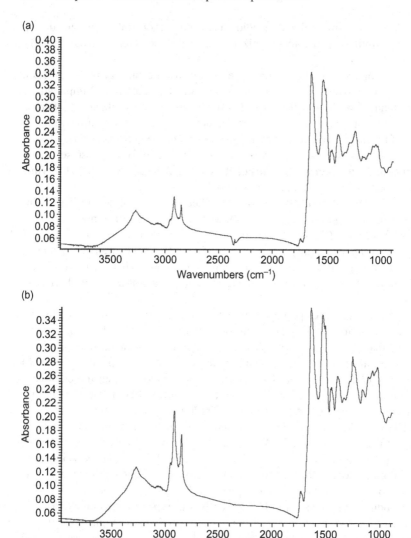

Figure 8.3   IR spectra from psoriatic skin (a) pre- and (b) post-treatment with UV radiation.

There is also evidence that IR can be used in diagnosis of skin disorders.[20] Unpublished data from our own laboratory shows a difference in the spectral signature from psoriatic skin pre- and post-treatment with UV radiation (Fig. 8.3).

Near infrared (NIR) has been used to monitor water profiles in atopy,[21] but the results were inconclusive; however, the study did indicate the uses of NIR in the study of skin. The technique was also used to follow the interactions of isopropyl myristate and polyethylene glycol on water distribution in normal and atopic skin

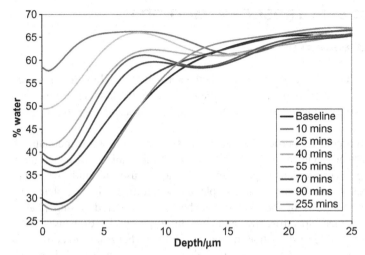

Figure 8.4 Hydration profiles of the volar forearm measured after 90 minutes occlusion and hydration. Source: Courtesy of Professor Paul J. Matts and Dr. Jonathan M. Crowther, Procter & Gamble, Egham, UK.

and differences were noted.[22] Water can also be examined *in vivo* within the stratum corneum using microwave dielectric analysis.[23]

Imaging using IR is also possible with a resolution down to about 2 μm. Using this with advanced chemometrics, it is possible to obtain spatial resolution of both active and excipients.[24–26] The conformation of the lipids can also be imaged.[27] It is also possible to determine the interaction of components of liposomes; for example, dimyristoylphosphatidylcholine with skin lipids.[28]

Raman spectroscopy is related to IR and has also been used beneficially to study skin. Similar spectral profiles are produced and intra- and intervariability from different skin samples are good.[29,30] It is interesting to note that the spectral signatures from skin that is over 5000 years old are similar to those found today.[31] It is possible to use confocal Raman *in vivo* and to depth profile the skin.[32–34] The hydration level of the skin can be followed[35] and Figure 8.4 illustrates the hydration profiles of the volar forearm measured before (baseline) and after 90 minutes occlusion with a wet towel and Parafilm®. A very recent study has demonstrated how it is possible to follow the permeation of both an active (retinol) and an excipient (propylene glycol).[36] It has also been used to monitor the penetration of dimethyl sulfoxide (DMSO).[37]

Depth profiling can also be conducted with photoacoustic FTIR spectroscopy and the diffusion of cyanodecane is 1.6 times higher in the inner regions of the stratum corneum than the outer.[38] There is an indication from our own *in vivo* studies on the −CH stretch frequency from confocal Raman that the fluidity of the lipids is higher the deeper into the stratum corneum.[39] This is consistent with the previous findings in the literature.

ELECTRONIC SPECTROSCOPIC METHODS

UV and Fluorescence

Diffuse reflectance UV can be used to examine the surface of the skin; at this wavelength of light, there is little penetration into the membrane. It can therefore be used to examine the disappearance of materials from the skin surface, for example, aminolevulinic acid.[40]

Skin has fluorescent properties and these can be used to monitor the state of the skin; this has been reviewed recently.[41] In terms of mechanisms of penetration and enhancer effects, fluorescence spectroscopy is largely used to study what has happened to probes within the skin. For example, the penetration enhancer oleic acid is known to create regions in the skin lipids that are disordered. Using phase-modulated fluorescence spectroscopy and the fluorophore 1,6-diphenyl-1,3,5-hexatriene, it was possible to show that the increased flux of benzoic acid across the skin, as a result of oleic acid, was directly related to fluorescence lifetime and anisotropy. There was a saturable effect with a limiting concentration of oleic acid.[42] It is also possible to monitor the fate of fluorescently tagged vesicles and particles.[43,44] *In vivo* fluorescence imaging has also been used in diagnosis and the study of skin lesions.[45]

Multiphoton femtosecond laser imaging systems have been used to study the skin and the localization of drugs and particulates within the skin. The technique uses a pulsed laser to excite endogenous fluorophores and actives or excipients if they are fluorescent. Deeper tissues such as collagen can also be visualized.[46,47]

NMR

NMR was used to study the hydration of stratum corneum and the mobility of water within guinea pig skin.[48,49] The presence of "free" and "bound" water has been observed.[50] More recently, the self-diffusion of water in the stratum corneum and viable epidermis has been measured.[51] Lipid constructs that mimic the structured lipids of the skin were examined using deuterium NMR and, like IR, thermally induced polymorphism has been detected together with lamellar structures.[52–54] NMR using stray field has also been successfully employed to follow water and also some cosmetic ingredients in the skin.[55,56] *In vivo* studies are also possible but the resolution prevents monitoring precise levels in the stratum corneum.[51]

^{19}F NMR has been used *in vivo* to follow the permeation of flurbiprofen through human and hairless rat skin. Not unexpectedly, the permeation through human skin was slower.[57] Water loss from samples of skin *in vitro* can be monitored together with the water distribution using stray-field NMR.[55,56] The major problem with the technique is the size of the equipment, although a relatively new NMR mouse may prove interesting.[58]

^{31}P NMR has been used to follow the metabolic processes in the skin and differences were noted between normal and psoriatic skin, the latter having elevated levels of phosphomonoester concentrations and higher phosphomonoester : phosphodiester ratios. These could be useful noninvasive markers to monitor treatment response in patients with psoriasis.[59]

MISCELLANEOUS SPECTROSCOPIC METHODS

Opto-Thermal Transient Emission Radiometry (OTTER)

OTTER uses pulsed laser excitation to induce temperature jumps of the order of a few degrees Celsius in the top few microns of the skin surface. These temperature jumps decay on a timescale of microseconds and do not materially increase the average substrate temperature or the rate of diffusion under study. They are observed with a high-speed IR detector sensitive to the heat radiation emitted by the surface. For biological tissue, this radiation is strongest in the mid-IR 6–13 μm band of wavelengths. The measurement captures the decay dynamics of this transient component of the heat radiation and relates it to the physical properties of the near-surface layers through mathematical models.[60] The technique has been used to measure skin water content *in vivo*,[61] the hydration profile within the stratum corneum *in vivo*, and how this profile changes in the presence of petroleum jelly and DMSO.[62] In a later study, the application of the technique to depth profile ethylene glycol after application to the volar forearm was also reported.[63]

Electron Spin Resonance (ESR)

ESR is also commonly described as electron paramagnetic resonance. Paramagnetic molecules have unpaired electrons and will absorb energy at particular values of an applied magnetic field. ESR is based on the same principles as NMR; however, microwave rather than radio wave frequencies are used and the spin transitions of the unpaired electrons rather than nuclei are recorded. The technique typically involves the incorporation of a paramagnetic probe molecule (usually a nitroxide free radical) into the system under investigation. Analysis of the probe's ESR spectrum provides information about the motional character of the probe in that particular environment. This in turn reflects the type and rate of molecular motion of the molecules comprising the membrane. Using 5-doxyl stearic acid as the probe, Gay and coworkers[64] showed that n-decylmethyl sulfoxide increased the degree of disorder in the lipid bilayer in the stratum corneum *in vitro*. Hatcher and Plachy[65] studied the diffusion of oxygen through human stratum corneum *in vitro*. Permeation of oxygen increased by 200% after application of DMSO and by 100% after application of decylmethyl sulfoxide (DEMSO), but was unaffected by oleic acid. Mukherjee et al. reported decreased mobility of the ESR probe 5-doxyl stearic acid in human stratum corneum after treatment with sodium lauryl sulfate or sodium dodecyl sulfate and suggested that this might reflect removal of fluid lipids from the stratum corneum.[66]

Impedance

The electrical impedance or resistance of the skin to an electric current has been used for many years to characterize skin permeability. The basis of impedance spectroscopy is the analysis of the impedance (resistance of alternating current) of an observed system subject to the applied frequency and exciting signal. The first reports of a correlation between impedance spectroscopy and water flux for *in vitro* skin treated with DMSO, detergents, and surfactants were noted by Allenby et al.[67] These workers also investigated the effects of pH and temperature on skin impedance. Clar et al. suggested that impedance could be used as a measure of skin hydration *in vivo*.[68] Yamamoto and Yamamoto showed that the electrical resistance of the skin was drastically reduced with progressive tape stripping.[69] Mize et al. demonstrated that skin impedance decreased during the first postnatal months of life and attributed this to an increase in skin hydration as a result of the greater functional maturity of eccrine sweat glands.[70] Gender and anatomic site were shown to affect skin impedance by Burstrom.[71] Ollmar and Emtestam used impedance to measure skin irritation induced by application of solutions of sodium lauryl sulfate,[72] and in a later study explored this technique to discriminate between atopic and normal skin.[73] Kalia and Guy characterized the effects of iontophoresis on human skin impedance *in vivo* and also showed that impedance spectroscopy and transepidermal water loss are complementary techniques for measuring skin permeability *in vivo*.[74] Impedance spectroscopy was used to investigate the residence time of local anesthetic formulations in skin *in vivo* by Woolfson et al.[75] Cancel and coworkers demonstrated reduced skin impedance and enhanced solute permeability *in vitro* after the application of low frequency ultrasound.[76] Formulation effects on, and uptake into, the SC were evaluated with impedance spectroscopy by Curdy et al. Lipophilic formulations increased impedance values consistent with the uptake of hydrocarbon ointment base components into the skin, which was also substantiated by transepidermal water loss (TEWL) and ATR-FTIR measurements.[77]

Laser-Induced Breakdown Spectroscopy (LIBS)

LIBS systems typically utilize a neodymium-doped yttrium aluminum garnet (Nd:YAG) solid-state laser and a spectrometer with a wide spectral range to generate energy in the NIR region of the electromagnetic spectrum, with a wavelength of 1064 nm. Excimer (Excited dimer)-type lasers have also been used, which generate energy in the visible and ultraviolet regions. Sun and coworkers demonstrated the feasibility of using LIBS to analyze trace elemental concentrations of zinc in the stratum corneum of human skin *in vivo* after application of zinc chloride solution and zinc oxide paste. In a related study,[78,79] LIBS was used to show the effectiveness of various commercial barrier creams to zinc absorption *in vivo*.

CONCLUSIONS AND FUTURE

There have been considerable developments in the instrumentation and data analysis associated with the major spectroscopic methods over the last 40 years. We believe that continued progress will advance our understanding of skin structure and function at the molecular level as well as the disposition of excipients in skin and their mechanisms of interaction with skin components. The major advances have been the transference of *in vitro* techniques to *in vivo* and it is anticipated that these will continue with enhanced resolution. This should allow the real-time monitoring of actives and excipients in the stratum corneum and perhaps into the deeper layers of the skin where topical activity is largely required.

REFERENCES

1. PUTTNAM NA. Attenuated total flectance studies of the skin. *J Soc Cosmet Chem* 1972; 23: 209–226.
2. KNUTSON K, POTTS RO, GUZEK DB, GOLDEN GM, McKIE JE, LAMBERT WJ, et al. Macro- and molecular physical-chemical considerations in understanding drug transport in the stratum corneum. *J Control Release* 1985; 2: 67–87.
3. POTTS RO, FRANCOEUR ML. Biophysics of stratum corneum barrier function. *Skin Pharmacol* 1989; 2(1): 51.
4. ONGPIPATTANAKUL B, FRANCOEUR ML, POTTS RO. Polymorphism in stratum corneum lipids. *Biochim Biophys Acta* 1994; 1190(1): 115–122.
5. MOORE DJ, REREK ME. Biophysics of skin barrier lipid organization. *J Dermatol Sci* 1998; 16(Suppl 1): S203–S20S.
6. MOORE DJ, REREK ME, MENDELSOHN R. Lipid domains and orthorhombic phases in model stratum corneum: Evidence from Fourier transform infrared spectroscopy studies. *Biochem Biophys Res Commun* 1997; 231(3): 797–801.
7. KNUTSON K, KRILL SL, ZHANG J. Solvent-mediated alterations of the stratum corneum. *J Control Release* 1990; 11(1–3): 93–103.
8. MAK VHW, POTTS RO, GUY RH. Oleic acid concentration and effect in human stratum corneum: Non-invasive determination by attenuated total reflectance infrared spectroscopy *in vivo*. *J Control Release* 1990; 12(1): 67–75.
9. ONGPIPATTANAKUL B, BURNETTE RR, POTTS RO, FRANCOEUR ML. Evidence that oleic acid exists in a separate phase within stratum corneum lipids. *Pharm Res* 1991; 8(3): 350–354.
10. HARRISON JE, GROUNDWATER PW, BRAIN KR, HADGRAFT J. Azone induced fluidity in human stratum corneum: A Fourier transform infrared spectroscopy investigation using the perdeuterated analogue. *J Control Release* 1996; 41(3): 283–290.
11. POTTS RO, FRANCOEUR ML. Lipid biophysics of water loss through the skin. *Proc Natl Acad Sci* 1990; 87: 3871–3873.
12. EDWARDSON PA, WALKER M, BREHENY C. Quantitative FT-IR determination of skin hydration following occlusion with hydrocolloid containing adhesive dressings. *Int J Pharm* 1993; 91(1): 51–57.
13. MAK VH, POTTS RO, GUY RH. Does hydration affect intercellular lipid organization in the stratum corneum? *Pharm Res* 1991; 8(8): 1064–1065.
14. BOMMANNAN D, POTTS RO, GUY RH. Examination of the effect of ethanol on human stratum corneum *in vivo* using infrared spectroscopy. *J Control Release* 1991; 16: 299–304.

15. HARRISON JE, WATKINSON AC, GREEN DM, HADGRAFT J, BRAIN K. The relative effect of Azone and Transcutol on permeant diffusivity and solubility in human stratum corneum. *Pharm Res* 1996; 13(4): 542–546.
16. ALBERTI I, KALIA YN, NAIK A, BONNY J, GUY RH. Effect of ethanol and isopropyl myristate on the availability of topical terbinafine in human stratum corneum, *in vivo*. *Int J Pharm* 2001; 219(1–2): 11–19.
17. ALBERTI I, KALIA YN, NAIK A, BONNY JD, GUY RH. *In vivo* assessment of enhanced topical delivery of terbinafine to human stratum corneum. *J Control Release* 2001; 71(3): 319–327.
18. DIAS M, NAIK A, GUY RH, HADGRAFT J, LANE ME. *In vivo* infrared spectroscopy studies of alkanol effects on human skin. *Eur J Pharm Biopharm* 2008; 69(3): 1171–1175.
19. RUSSEAU W, MITCHELL J, TETTEH J, LANE ME, HADGRAFT J. Investigation of the permeation of model formulations and a commercial ibuprofen formulation in Carbosil® and human skin using ATR-FTIR and multivariate spectral analysis. *Int J Pharm* 2009; 374(1–2): 17–25.
20. JACKSON M, KIM K, TETTEH J, MANSFIELD JR, DOLENKO B, SOMORJAI RL, et al. Cancer diagnosis by infrared spectroscopy: Methodological aspects. *SPIE Proc* 1998; 3257: 24–34.
21. DREASSI E, CERAMELLI G, FABBRI L, VOCIONI F, BARTALINI P, CORTI P. Application of near-infrared reflectance spectrometry in the study of atopy. Part 1. Investigation of skin spectra. *Analyst* 1997; 122(8): 767–770.
22. DREASSI E, CERAMELLI G, MURA P, PERRUCCIO PL, VOCIONI F, BARTALINI P, et al. Near-infrared reflectance spectrometry in the study of atopy. Part 2. Interactions between the skin and polyethylene glycol 400, isopropyl myristate and hydrogel. *Analyst* 1997; 122(8): 771–776.
23. NAITO S, HOSHI M, YAGIHARA S. Microwave dielectric analysis of human stratum corneum *in vivo*. *Biochim Biophys Acta* 1998; 1381(3): 293–304.
24. BONCHEVA M, TAY FH, KAZARIAN SG. Application of attenuated total reflection Fourier transform infrared imaging and tape-stripping to investigate the three-dimensional distribution of exogenous chemicals and the molecular organization in Stratum corneum. *J Biomed Opt* 2008; 13(6): 064009.
25. ANDANSON JM, HADGRAFT J, KAZARIAN SG. In situ permeation study of drug through the stratum corneum using attenuated total reflection Fourier transform infrared spectroscopic imaging. *J Biomed Opt* 2009; 14(3): 034011.
26. TETTEH J, MADER KT, ANDANSON JM, MCAULEY WJ, LANE ME, HADGRAFT J, et al. Local examination of skin diffusion using FTIR spectroscopic imaging and multivariate target factor analysis. *Anal Chim Acta* 2009; 642(1–2): 246–256.
27. MENDELSOHN R, FLACH CR, MOORE DJ. Determination of molecular conformation and permeation in skin via IR spectroscopy, microscopy, and imaging. *Biochim Biophys Acta Biomembr* 2006; 1758(7): 923–933.
28. XIAO C, MOORE DJ, FLACH CR, MENDELSOHN R. Permeation of dimyristoylphosphatidylcholine into skin—Structural and spatial information from IR and Raman microscopic imaging. *Vibrat Spectrosc* 2005; 38(1–2): 151–158.
29. BARRY BW, EDWARDS HGM, WILLIAMS AC. Fourier-transform Raman and infrared vibrational study of human skin—Assignment of spectral bands. *J Raman Spectrosc* 1992; 23(11): 641–645.
30. WILLIAMS AC, BARRY BW, EDWARDS HG, FARWELL DW. A critical comparison of some Raman spectroscopic techniques for studies of human stratum corneum. *Pharm Res* 1993; 10(11): 1642–1647.
31. WILLIAMS AC, EDWARDS HGM, BARRY BW. The [']Iceman': Molecular structure of 5200-year-old skin characterised by Raman spectroscopy and electron microscopy. *Biochim Biophys Acta* 1995; 1246(1): 98–105.
32. CASPERS PJ, LUCASSEN GW, BRUINING HA, PUPPELS GJ. Automated depth-scanning confocal Raman microspectrometer for rapid *in vivo* determination of water concentration profiles in human skin. *J Raman Spectrosc* 2000; 31(8–9): 813–818.
33. CASPERS PJ, LUCASSEN GW, CARTER EA, BRUINING HA, PUPPELS GJ. *In vivo* confocal Raman microspectroscopy of the skin: Noninvasive determination of molecular concentration profiles. *J Invest Dermatol* 2001; 116(3): 434–442.
34. EGAWA M, KAJIKAWA T. Changes in the depth profile of water in the stratum corneum treated with water. *Skin Res Technol* 2009; 15(2): 242–249.

35. Crowther JM, Sieg A, Blenkiron P, Marcott C, Matts PJ, Kaczvinsky R, et al. Measuring the effects of topical moisturizers on changes in stratum corneum thickness, water gradients and hydration *in vivo*. *Br J Dermatol* 2008; 159(3): 567–577.

36. Park K. Confocal Raman spectroscopy to study *in vivo* skin penetration of retinol. *J Control Release* 2009; 138(1): 1.

37. Caspers PJ, Williams AC, Carter EA, Edwards HGM, Barry BW, Bruining HA, et al. Monitoring the penetration enhancer dimethyl sulfoxide in human stratum corneum *in vivo* by confocal Raman spectroscopy. *Pharm Res* 2002; 19(10): 1577–1580.

38. Hanh BD, Neubert RHH, Wartewig S, Lasch J. Penetration of compounds through human stratum corneum as studied by Fourier transform infrared photoacoustic spectroscopy. *J Control Release* 2001; 70(3): 393–398.

39. Hadgraft J, Matts PJ, Lane ME, Crowther JM. *In vivo* depth profiling of the lipids of the skin using laser confocal Raman spectroscopy. Unpublished data. 2009.

40. Kim K-H, Jheon S, Kim J-K. *In vivo* skin absorption dynamics of topically applied pharmaceuticals monitored by fiber-optic diffuse reflectance spectroscopy. *Spectrochim Acta A Mol Biomol Spectrosc* 2007; 66(3): 768–772.

41. Kollias N, Zonios G, Stamatas GN. Fluorescence spectroscopy of skin. *Vibrat Spectrosc* 2002; 28(1): 17–23.

42. Garrison MD, Doh LM, Potts RO, Abraham W. Effect of oleic acid on human epidermis: Fluorescence spectroscopic investigation. *J Control Release* 1994; 31(3): 263–269.

43. Alvarez-Román R, Naik A, Kalia YN, Fessi H, Guy RH. Visualization of skin penetration using confocal laser scanning microscopy. *Eur J Pharm Biopharm* 2004; 58(2): 301–316.

44. Lombardi Borgia S, Regehly M, Sivaramakrishnan R, Mehnert W, Korting HC, Danker K, et al. Lipid nanoparticles for skin penetration enhancement—correlation to drug localization within the particle matrix as determined by fluorescence and parelectric spectroscopy. *J Control Release* 2005; 110(1): 151–163.

45. Fischer F, Gudgin Dickson EF, Pottier RH. *In vivo* fluorescence imaging using two excitation and/or emission wavelengths for image contrast enhancement. *Vibrat Spectrosc* 2002; 30(2): 131–137.

46. Konig K, Ehlers A, Stracke F, Riemann I. *In vivo* drug screening in human skin using femtosecond laser multiphoton tomography. *Skin Pharmacol Physiol* 2006; 19(2): 78–88.

47. Stracke F, Weiss B, Lehr CM, Koenig K, Schaefer UF, Schneider M. Multiphoton microscopy for the investigation of dermal penetration of nanoparticle-borne drugs. *J Invest Dermatol* 2006; 126(10): 2224–2233.

48. Packer KJ, Sellwood TC. Proton magnetic resonance studies of hydrated stratum corneum part 1. Spin-lattice and transverse relaxation. *J Chem Soc Faraday Trans II* 1978; 74: 1579–1591.

49. Packer KJ, Sellwood TC. Proton magnetic resonance studies of hydrated stratum corneum part 2. Self-diffusion. *J Chem Soc Faraday Trans II* 1978; 74: 1592–1606.

50. Foreman MI, Bladon P, Pelling P. Proton NMR studies of human stratum corneum. *Bioeng Skin* 1979; 2: 48–58.

51. McDonald PJ, Akhmerov A, Backhouse LJ, Pitts S. Magnetic resonance profiling of human skin *in vivo* using GARField magnets. *J Pharm Sci* 2005; 94(8): 1850–1860.

52. Abraham W, Downing DT. Deuterium NMR investigation of polymorphism in stratum corneum lipids. *Biochim Biophys Acta* 1991; 1068(2): 189–194.

53. Abraham W, Downing DT. Lamellar structures formed by stratum corneum lipids *in vitro*: A deuterium nuclear magnetic resonance (NMR) study. *Pharm Res* 1992; 9(11): 1415–1421.

54. Kitson N, Thewalt J, Lafleur M, Bloom M. A model membrane approach to the epidermal permeability barrier. *Biochemistry* 1994; 33(21): 6707–6715.

55. Dias M, Hadgraft J, Glover PM, McDonald PJ. Stray field magnetic resonance imaging: A preliminary study of skin hydration. *J Phys D Appl Phys* 2003; 36(4): 364–368.

56. Backhouse L, Dias M, Gorce JP, Hadgraft K, McDonald PJ, Wiechers JW. GARField magnetic resonance profiling of the ingress of model skin-care product ingredients into human skin *in vitro*. *J Pharm Sci* 2004; 93(9): 2274–2283.

57. KOCH RL, MICALI G, BURT CT, LEE DJ, WEST DP, SOLOMON LM. Measurement of flurbiprofen absorption *in vivo* through human skin using 19fluorine—Nuclear magnetic resonance. *J Invest Dermatol* 1993; 100(4): 594.

58. BLÜMICH B, BLÜMLER P, EIDMANN G, GUTHAUSEN A, HAKEN R, SCHMITZ U, et al. The NMR-mouse: Construction, excitation, and applications. *Magn Reson Imaging* 1998; 16: 479–484.

59. ZEMTSOV A, DIXON L, CAMERON G. Human *in vivo* phosphorus 31 magnetic resonance spectroscopy of psoriasis: A noninvasive tool to monitor response to treatment and to study pathophysiology of the disease. *J Am Acad Dermatol* 1994; 30(6): 959–965.

60. IMHOF RE, ZHANG B, BIRCH DJS. Photothermal radiometry for NDE. In: Mandelis A, ed. 2nd ed. *Progress in Photothermal and Photoacoustic Science and Technology,* 11. PTR Prentice Hall, Englewood Cliffs, NJ, 1994; 185–236.

61. BINDRA RMS, IMHOF RE, MOCHAN A, ECCLESTON GM. Optothermal technique for in-vivo stratum-corneum hydration measurement. *J Phys IV (France)* 1994; 4(C7): 465–468.

62. XIAO P, IMHOF RE. Opto-thermal skin water concentration gradient measurement. *SPIE Proc* 1996; 2681: 31–41.

63. XIAO P, COWEN JA, IMHOF RE. In-vivo transdermal drug diffusion depth profiling—A new approach to opto-thermal signal analysis. *Anal Sci* 2001; 17: S349–SS52.

64. GAY CL, MURPHY TM, HADGRAFT J, KELLAWAY IW, EVANS JC, ROWLANDS CC. An electron spin resonance study of skin penetration enhancers. *Int J Pharm* 1989; 49: 39–45.

65. HATCHER ME, PLACHY WZ. Dioxygen diffusion in the stratum corneum: An EPR spin label study. *Biochim Biophys Acta* 1993; 1149(1): 73–78.

66. MUKHERJEE S, MARGOSIAK M, PROWELL S, LEI X, ARONSON M. *In vitro* spectroscopic study of surfactant-stratum corneum interactions. *J Invest Dermatol* 1994; 102(4): 606.

67. ALLENBY AC, FLETCHER J, SCHOCK C, TEES TFS. The effect of heat, pH and organic solvents on the electrical impedance and permeability of excised human skin. *Br J Dermatol* 1969; 81(4): 31–39.

68. CLAR EJ, HER CP, STURELLE CG. Skin impedance and moisturization. *J Soc Cosmet Chem* 1975; 26: 337–353.

69. YAMAMOTO T, YAMAMOTO Y. Electrical properties of the epidermal stratum corneum. *Med Biol Eng Comput* 1976; 14(2): 151–158.

70. MIZE MM, VILA-CORO AA, PRAGER TC. The relationship between postnatal skin maturation and electrical skin impedance. *Arch Dermatol* 1989; 125: 647–650.

71. BURSTROM L. Measurements of the impedance of the hand and arm. *Int Arch Occup Env Health* 1990; 62(6): 431–439.

72. OLLMAR S, EMTESTAM L. Electrical impedance applied to non-invasive detection of irritation in skin. *Contact Derm* 1992; 27(1): 37–42.

73. NICANDER I, OLLMAR S. Clinically normal atopic skin vs. non-atopic skin as seen through electrical impedance. *Skin Res Technol* 2004; 10(3): 178–183.

74. KALIA YN, GUY RH. The electrical characteristics of human skin *in vivo*. *Pharm Res* 1995; 12(11): 1605–1613.

75. WOOLFSON AD, MOSS GP, MCCAFFERTY DF, LACKERMEIER A, MCADAMS ET. Changes in skin A.C. impedance parameters *in vivo* during the percutaneous absorption of local anesthetics. *Pharm Res* 1999; 16(3): 459–462.

76. CANCEL LM, TARBELL JM, BEN-JEBRIA A. Fluorescein permeability and electrical resistance of human skin during low frequency ultrasound application. *J Pharm Pharmacol* 2004; 56(9): 1109–1118.

77. CURDY C, NAIK A, KALIA YN, ALBERTI I, GUY RH. Non-invasive assessment of the effect of formulation excipients on stratum corneum barrier function *in vivo*. *Int J Pharm* 2004; 271(1–2): 251–256.

78. SUN Q, TRAN M, SMITH BW, WINEFORDNER JD. Zinc analysis in human skin by laser induced-breakdown spectroscopy. *Talanta* 2000; 52(2): 293–300.

79. SUN Q, TRAN M, SMITH B, WINEFORDNER JD. In-situ evaluation of barrier-cream performance on human skin using laser-induced breakdown spectroscopy. *Contact Derm* 2000; 43(5): 259–263.

Chapter 9

Skin Permeation Assessment in Man: *In Vitro–In Vivo* Correlation

Paul A. Lehman, Sam G. Raney, and Thomas J. Franz

INTRODUCTION

The demonstration that the water barrier of skin "lives on" in the *ex vivo* state is the historical cornerstone upon which the validity of *in vitro* studies of percutaneous absorption rests.[1–3] These early studies not only established that the stratum corneum is the rate-limiting barrier to water loss from the skin, but that: (1) it remains structurally and functionally intact for many days under *in vitro* conditions and (2) it is not damaged by freezing for long periods of time and subsequent thawing. Understandably, these attributes underscore why excised human skin is commonly used as a surrogate for *in vivo* studies in living man. Although a substantial body of literature has emerged utilizing this model system, the degree to which the *in vitro* model mimics the living state and, therefore, the extent to which the data can be reliably extrapolated, need to be critically examined. Is it a perfect model and, if not, how reliable are the data?

IN VITRO–IN VIVO CORRELATION: TOPICAL DELIVERY

Validating the Model

The earliest systematic attempt to validate the *in vitro* excised skin model was that of Franz,[4] in which the absorption of 12 organic compounds was measured *in vitro* and the data compared to those obtained years earlier in living man by Feldmann

Transdermal and Topical Drug Delivery: Principles and Practice, First Edition. Edited by Heather A.E. Benson, Adam C. Watkinson.

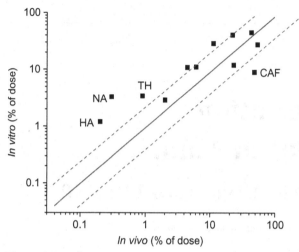

Figure 9.1   IVIV comparison (total absorption as percent of applied dose) for 12 organic compounds applied in an acetone vehicle. The solid line represents theoretical one-to-one correlation. The dashed lines represent ±threefold difference from perfect correlation. HA, hippuric acid; NA, nicotinic acid; TH, thiourea; CAF, caffeine. Source: Data taken from References 4 and 5.

and Maibach.[5] A comparison of both data sets found a clear, direct relationship between the two; however, the relationship was not 1 : 1 (Fig. 9.1). For four of the 12 compounds (caffeine, hippuric acid, nicotinic acid, thiourea), there were four- to 10-fold differences in total absorption between the *in vitro* and *in vivo* data.

A follow-up study explored the reason for the striking lack of *in vitro/in vivo* (IVIV) concordance for the four questionable compounds.[6] New *in vitro* and *in vivo* studies were conducted in which changes were made to both protocols in order to: (1) bring them into harmony and (2) correct potential flaws in the original *in vivo* study. Both sets of experiments were conducted on abdominal skin using radiolabeled compounds dissolved in acetone and applied at an identical compound dose. The application sites were protected nonocclusively to prevent rub off (*in vivo* only) and the skin surface was washed at 24 hours. Moreover, urine collection was extended until background levels of radioactivity were approached and not limited to 5 days as was the case in the first *in vivo* study. This was necessary since several compounds in the original study showed significant levels of radioactivity in the fifth day's collection, suggesting incomplete systemic clearance. Thus, although the *in vitro* study duration was only 2 days, it was recognized that longer periods of time might be required *in vivo* for some compounds to accommodate systemic distribution, metabolism, and excretion.

Excellent IVIV correlation was found in the new study and some of the reasons for the discrepancies in the original comparison were identified (Table 9.1). Longer urinary collection times were indeed needed for two compounds, thiourea and nicotinic acid, where it took 21 days before background levels of radioactivity were approached. It was also noted that an incorrect urinary correction factor had been

Table 9.1   Total Absorption from IVIV Study Conducted Under Harmonized Protocol

Compound	In vitro (% dose)	In vivo (% dose)
Caffeine	24.1 ± 3.90 (4)	22.1 ± 7.90 (4)
Hippuric acid	1.25 ± 0.25 (4)	1.0 ± 0.16 (6)
Nicotinic acid	2.3 ± 0.45 (4)	2.1 ± 0.40 (3)
Thiourea	4.6 ± 1.03 (5)	3.7 ± 0.65 (4)

Mean ± standard deviation (SD) (number of subjects or skin donors).
Source: Data adapted from Reference 6.

used for nicotinic acid in the original study. It had been assumed that nicotinic acid followed the same excretory pattern as nicotinamide, in which 90% of the radioactivity was excreted in the urine. In fact, it was found that only 15% of ^{14}C-nicotinic acid was excreted in the urine following intravenous administration in the rhesus monkey.[6] Regional variation (forearm vs. abdomen) may also have accounted for some of the differences noted earlier, but the new study was not designed to answer this question.

The second study makes it clear that absorption data obtained in living man should not automatically be assumed to be the "gold standard." The conduct of studies in living man is not always simple, particularly when dealing with compounds that are poorly absorbed, slowly absorbed and/or excreted (as seen above), or largely excreted in the feces. For example, assessment of dichloro-diphenyl-trichloroethane (DDT) percutaneous absorption in the rhesus monkey led to the finding that 375% of the applied dose was absorbed.[7] This irrational value was based upon the use of an erroneous correction factor—a result of only monitoring the urinary route of excretion and applying a correction factor (based on intravenous dosing) for excretion via other routes. As with all scientific experiments, inadequate protocol design or simple laboratory error can lead to flawed data.

Two additional IVIV correlation studies were subsequently conducted by Franz to further validate the use of excised human skin as a surrogate for living man: (1) a study to examine the effect of vehicle on absorption in collaboration with Bronaugh[8] and (2) a study of benzene absorption in man.[9] In both studies, IVIV correlation for total absorption was again found to be reasonably good, with *in vitro* differing from *in vivo* by no more than a factor of 2 (Table 9.2).

Other Validation Studies

Data from other laboratories also support the validity of the excised skin model, but often, due to various differences between the *in vitro* and *in vivo* protocols, the precise quantitative accuracy of the agreement is uncertain.[10–34] These include differences in: (a) anatomical skin site studied, (b) test compound dose, (c) vehicle dose, (d) composition of vehicle, (e) length of exposure/wash time, and (f) the temperature at which the *in vitro* study was run as well as the use of isothermal rather

Table 9.2   Total Absorption from IVIV Studies Conducted Under Harmonized Protocol

Compound	Vehicle	*In vitro* (% dose)	*In vivo* (% dose)
Benzoic acid	Petrolatum	46.5 ± 5.9 (6)	60.6 ± 10.7 (4)
Caffeine	Petrolatum	40.6 ± 2.2 (7)	40.6 ± 6.1 (5)
	EG Gel[b]	32.2 ± 7.3 (6)	55.6 ± 11.7 (4)
	Water Gel	5.1 ± 0.5 (7)	4.0 ± 0.5 (4)
Testosterone	Petrolatum	39.4 ± 1.2 (20)	49.5 ± 5.8 (3)
	EG Gel[b]	23.7 ± 2.0 (5)	36.3 ± 0.4 (4)
	Water Gel	41.4 ± 6.8 (8)	49.2 ± 4.7 (4)
Benzene[a]	Benzene	0.10 ± 0.004 (9)	0.05 ± 0.05 (4)

Mean ± standard error (# of subjects or skin donors).

[a] Not harmonized to body site, ventral forearm *in vivo* versus abdomen *in vitro*.

[b] Ethylene glycol.

Data adapted from references 8 and 9.

than anisothermal conditions. Lehman et al.[35] recently reviewed all of the previously cited work[4–6,8–34] and found 92 data sets could be extracted for IVIV comparison of 30 organic compounds (Table 9.3). Using total absorption as the metric for comparison, expressed as percent of applied dose, they found a clear tendency for the data to follow the line of perfect 1:1 correlation (Fig. 9.2). The average IVIV ratio across all values was 1.6; however, there were a few cases where the differences between the *in vitro* and *in vivo* values were quite large (range: 0.18–19.7).

Since most of the *in vitro* experiments from which the data of Figure 9.2 were derived utilized conditions that did not fully replicate those employed *in vivo*, they also analyzed a smaller group of 11 data sets from two studies[6,8] in which no differences between the *in vitro* and *in vivo* protocols existed. All test compounds were applied to abdominal skin at identical doses for the same defined exposure period. In addition, vehicle composition and vehicle dose were identical, and the temperature and water gradients normally existing across the skin *in vivo* were approximated *in vitro*. With these constraints they found an unmistakable improvement in IVIV correlation (Fig. 9.3). The average IVIV ratio for all 11 data sets closely approximated one (0.96) and, for any single compound, the difference between the *in vitro* and *in vivo* values was found to be less than two (range: 0.58–1.28).

This analysis makes it very clear that the data obtained in the excised human skin model closely replicate those obtained in living man when the two study protocols are well matched. Although the magnitude of the error introduced by small deviations between protocols in past studies is impossible to assess, the most common factor leading to exclusion of 81 of 92 data sets was found to be the use of skin from different body sites. Since the skin is not homogeneous over the whole body, and significant regional differences in absorption are well documented,[36] comparison of data from different body sites has unnecessarily distorted attempts to accurately quantify IVIV correlation. The second most common factor leading to exclusion of data was a disparity in the vehicle used: either a compositional

Table 9.3 Comparison of *In Vitro* and *In Vivo* Absorption Values (% of Applied Dose) for 92-Data Sets (Adapted from Reference 35)

Compound	Vehicle	% Absorbed			Reference	
	In vitro/In vivo	*In vitro*	*In vivo*	IVIV ratio	*In vitro*	*In vivo*
Acetylsalicylic acid	Acetone / same	40.5	21.8	1.86	4	5
Benezene	Benzene / same	0.1	0.05	2.00	9	9
Benzene	Benzene / same	0.1	0.07	1.43	9	34
Benzoic acid	Acetone / same	44.9	42.6	1.05	4	5
Benzoic acid	Ethanol / same	34.4	42.6	0.81	16	5
Benzoic acid	Petrolatum / same	46.5	60.6	0.77	8	8
Benzoic acid[a]	1:1 Aq Ethanol / Acetone	63.0	42.6	1.48	32	5
Benzoic acid[a]	1:1 Aq Ethanol / Acetone	51.5	42.6	1.21	32	5
Benzoic acid[a]	1:1 Aq Ethanol / Acetone	83.3	42.6	1.96	32	5
Benzoic acid[a]	1:1 Aq Ethanol / Acetone	86.8	42.6	2.04	32	5
Benzoic acid[a]	1:1 Aq Ethanol / Acetone	42.7	42.6	1.00	32	5
Benzoic acid[a]	1:1 Aq Ethanol / Acetone	68.8	42.6	1.62	32	5
Benzoic acid[a]	1:1 Aq Ethanol / Acetone	90.3	42.6	2.12	32	5
Benzoic acid[a]	1:1 Aq Ethanol / Acetone	77.8	42.6	1.83	32	5
Borax	Water / same	0.41	0.21	1.95	25	25
Boric acid	Water / same	1.75	0.23	7.61	25	25
Disodium octaborate	Aqueous ?? / same	0.19	0.12	1.58	25	25
Caffeine	Acetone / same	24.1	22.1	1.09	6	6
Caffeine	Eth. Glycol Gel / same	32.2	55.6	0.58	8	8
Caffeine	Petrolatum / same	40.6	40.6	1.00	8	8
Caffeine	Water gel / same	5.1	4.0	1.28	8	8
Caffeine[a]	1:1 Aq Ethanol / Acetone	19.1	22.1	0.86	32	6
Caffeine[a]	1:1 Aq Ethanol / Acetone	10.9	22.1	0.49	32	6
Caffeine[a]	1:1 Aq Ethanol / Acetone	11.3	22.1	0.51	32	6
Caffeine[a]	1:1 Aq Ethanol / Acetone	34.9	22.1	1.58	32	6

(*Continued*)

Table 9.3 (*Continued*)

Compound	Vehicle	% Absorbed			Reference	
	In vitro/In vivo	*In vitro*	*In vivo*	IVIV ratio	*In vitro*	*In vivo*
Caffeine[a]	1:1 Aq Ethanol / Acetone	21.7	22.1	0.98	32	6
Caffeine[a]	1:1 Aq Ethanol / Acetone	46.5	22.1	2.10	32	6
Caffeine[a]	1:1 Aq Ethanol / Acetone	23.5	22.1	1.06	32	6
Caffeine[a]	1:1 Aq Ethanol / Acetone	32.6	22.1	1.48	32	6
Caffeine[a]	1:1 Aq Ethanol / Acetone	20.1	22.1	0.91	32	6
Caffeine[a]	1:1 Aq Ethanol / Acetone	19.1	47.6	0.40	32	5
Caffeine[a]	1:1 Aq Ethanol / Acetone	10.9	47.6	0.23	32	5
Caffeine[a]	1:1 Aq Ethanol / Acetone	11.3	47.6	0.24	32	5
Caffeine[a]	1:1 Aq Ethanol / Acetone	34.9	47.6	0.73	32	5
Caffeine[a]	1:1 Aq Ethanol / Acetone	21.7	47.6	0.46	32	5
Caffeine[a]	1:1 Aq Ethanol / Acetone	46.5	47.6	0.98	32	5
Caffeine[a]	1:1 Aq Ethanol / Acetone	23.5	47.6	0.49	32	5
Caffeine[a]	1:1 Aq Ethanol / Acetone	32.6	47.6	0.68	32	5
Caffeine[a]	1:1 Aq Ethanol / Acetone	20.1	47.6	0.42	32	5
Chloramphenicol	Acetone / same	2.9	2.0	1.45	4	5
Chloroform[b]	Water / same	5.6	8.2	0.68	21	21
Chloroform[b]	Water / same	7.1	8.2	0.87	21	21
Chlorpyrifos	Dursban 4:water / same	19.7	1.0	19.70	27	26
Coumarin	Ethanol / 70% Aq ethanol	50.4	59.7	0.84	23	29
Diazinon	Acetone / Acetone	14.1	3.2	4.41	19	19
DNCB	Acetone / Acetone	27.5	53.1	0.52	4	5
DNCB	Acetone / Acetone	32.5	53.1	0.61	12	5
Fluazifop-butyl[c]	Aq Suspension / same	2.2	6.4	0.34	20	17

Table 9.3   (*Continued*)

Compound	Vehicle	% Absorbed			Reference	
	In vitro/In vivo	*In vitro*	*In vivo*	IVIV ratio	*In vitro*	*In vivo*
Fluazifop-butyl[c]	Aq Suspension / same	2.8	2.7	1.04	20	17
Fluazifop-butyl[c]	Aq Suspension / same	2.4	1.3	1.85	20	17
Hippuric acid	Acetone / same	1.25	1.0	1.25	6	6
Isophenos	Acetone / same	2.5	3.6	0.69	18	18
Lindane	Acetone / same	0.69	3.9[d]	0.18	24	11
Lindane	Emulsion / Acetone	3.2	8.3[d]	0.39	24	11
Lindane	93% white spirit / Acetone	15.3	8.3[d]	1.84	24	11
Lindane	White spirit / Acetone	25.7	8.3[d]	3.10	24	11
Lindane	Lotion (Kwell) / Acetone	71.7	8.3[d]	8.64	22	11
Mexoryl SX	o/w Emulsion / same	0.07	0.01	7.00	31	31
Nicotinamide	Acetone / same	28.8	11.1	2.59	4	5
Nicotinic acid	Acetone / same	2.3	2.1	1.10	6	6
Nicotinic acid	Ethanol / Acetone	0.6	2.1	0.29	16	6
Nitrobenzene	Acetone / same	7.8	1.5	5.20	12	5
o-Phenylphenol	60% Aq. ethanol / same	31.9	26.7	1.19	30	30
p-phenylenediamine	L'Oreal formulation / same	1.14	0.54	2.11	33	33
Phenol	Acetone / same	10.9	4.4	2.48	4	5
Phenol	Ethanol / 95% Ethanol	19.6	24.0	0.82	16	15
Propoxur	60% Aq. ethanol / same	9.7	3.7	2.62	28	28
Salicylic acid	Acetone / Acetone	12	22.8	0.53	4	5
Testosterone	Eth. glycol gel / same	23.7	36.3	0.65	8	8
Testosterone	Petrolatum / same	39.4	49.5	0.80	8	8
Testosterone	Water gel / same	41.4	49.2	0.84	8	8
Testosterone[a]	1:1 Aq ethanol / Acetone	8.4	13.2	0.64	32	10
Testosterone[a]	1:1 Aq ethanol / Acetone	6.3	13.2	0.48	32	10

(*Continued*)

Table 9.3   (*Continued*)

Compound	Vehicle	% Absorbed			Reference	
	In vitro/In vivo	*In vitro*	*In vivo*	IVIV ratio	*In vitro*	*In vivo*
Testosterone[a]	1:1 Aq ethanol / Acetone	3.9	13.2	0.30	32	10
Testosterone[a]	1:1 Aq ethanol / Acetone	13.5	13.2	1.02	32	10
Testosterone[a]	1:1 Aq ethanol / Acetone	8.5	13.2	0.64	32	10
Testosterone[a]	1:1 Aq ethanol / Acetone	38.9	13.2	2.95	32	10
Testosterone[a]	1:1 Aq Ethanol / Acetone	5.2	13.2	0.39	32	10
Testosterone[a]	1:1 Aq Ethanol / Acetone	5.3	13.2	0.40	32	10
Testosterone[a]	1:1 Aq Ethanol / Acetone	15.8	13.2	1.20	32	10
Testosterone[a]	1:1 Aq Ethanol / Acetone	8.4	18	0.47	32	13
Testosterone[a]	1:1 Aq Ethanol / Acetone	6.3	18	0.35	32	13
Testosterone[a]	1:1 Aq Ethanol / Acetone	3.9	18	0.22	32	13
Testosterone[a]	1:1 Aq Ethanol / Acetone	13.5	18	0.75	32	13
Testosterone[a]	1:1 Aq Ethanol / Acetone	8.5	18	0.47	32	13
Testosterone[a]	1:1 Aq Ethanol / Acetone	38.9	18	2.16	32	13
Testosterone[a]	1:1 Aq Ethanol / Acetone	5.2	18	0.29	32	13
Testosterone[a]	1:1 Aq Ethanol / Acetone	5.3	18	0.29	32	13
Testosterone[a]	1:1 Aq Ethanol / Acetone	15.8	18	0.88	32	13
Thiourea	Acetone / same	4.6	3.7	1.24	6	6
Triclopyr BEE	Neat / Garlon 4	0.7	1.7	0.41	16	14
Urea	Acetone / same	11.1	6.0	1.85	4	5

[a] *In vitro* data from individual laboratories of a multicenter study.

[b] Chloroform applied *in vitro* at two different doses.

[c] Fluazifop-butyl applied at three different doses in both studies.

[d] Value selected based on *in vivo* dose which best matched that used *in vitro*.

BEE, butoxyethyl ether; DNCB, dinitrochlorobenzene.

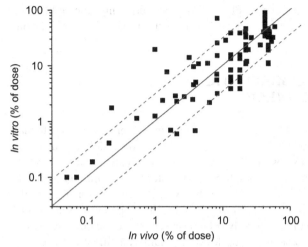

Figure 9.2 IVIV comparison (total absorption as percent of applied dose) for 92 data sets on 30 organic compounds, some in different vehicles or at different doses. The solid line represents theoretical one-to-one correlation. The dashed lines represent ±threefold difference from perfect correlation. Data from each individual laboratory of multicenter study[32] are plotted separately. Source: Data taken from References 4–6, 8–34.

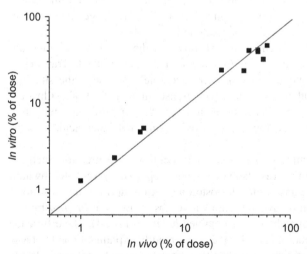

Figure 9.3 IVIV comparison (total absorption as percent of applied dose) for 11 data sets in which the *in vitro* and *in vivo* studies were performed on skin from the same anatomical site (abdomen) and where the two protocols were fully harmonized. The single exception (testosterone in ethylene glycol gel dosed *in vitro* at 2 $\mu g/cm^2$ vs. 3 $\mu g/cm^2$ *in vivo*) was considered inconsequential. The solid line represents theoretical one-to-one correlation. Source: Data taken from references 6 and 8.

difference or a difference in the dose applied. This is not surprising since it has long been known that the vehicle plays a critical rose in the process of percutaneous absorption.

IN VITRO–IN VIVO CORRELATION: TRANSDERMAL DELIVERY

Evidence that strongly supports the validity of data obtained from the excised human skin model can also be found in the field of transdermal drug delivery in which measurement of percutaneous absorption is a critical step in early product development. Its use is predicated on the assumption that the steady-state flux through skin *in vitro* is equivalent to the rate of input to the systemic circulation *in vivo*, the penultimate target for a transdermal product. Since the development of transdermal dosage forms for any given drug generally occurs subsequent to the development of other dosage forms, the therapeutic blood level (C_{ss}) and systemic clearance (Cl_s) are already known and allow calculation of the needed steady-state flux according to the following equation[37]:

$$J_{ss} \times A = C_{ss} \times Cl_s,$$

where

J_{ss} = steady-state flux through skin,

A = area of skin.

Thus, the tedious process of formulation development is greatly simplified since the target steady-state flux can be determined *in vitro* and the need to initially conduct trial-and-error clinical studies is precluded.

The effectiveness of this scheme was first shown by the Alza Corporation (Palo Alto, CA) during the development of the first transdermal product, Transderm-Scop®, and led them to conclude that "*in vitro* accurately predicted the situation which pertains *in vivo*."[38] Other studies involving transdermal products also illustrate the validity of the model. Excellent correlation between *in vitro* data with that obtained in living man has been found for nitroglycerin,[39] ketorolac acid,[40] selegiline,[41] and estradiol.[42]

There is no better example in the transdermal field of the degree to which the *in vitro* model replicates *in vivo* results than the work reported by Venkateschwaran on the development of transdermal testosterone (Androderm®) and estradiol (Alora®).[43] When expressed as average cumulative absorption, the *in vitro* rate of absorption profiles closely matched those obtained *in vivo* (Fig. 9.4). The difference in absorption noted for estradiol after 48 hours was readily explainable on the basis of the experimental conditions employed *in vitro* where, because the patch was larger than the chamber, only 67% of the total patch area was in contact with the skin. Thus, the rate of drug depletion from the patch *in vitro* was lower than that which would occur *in vivo* and the steady-state rate of absorption *in vitro* was extended for a longer period of time.

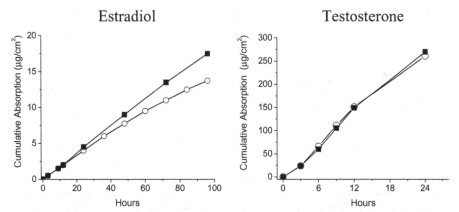

Figure 9.4   Comparison of the rate of absorption of estradiol and testosterone from separate transdermal systems as measured *in vitro* (■) in excised skin and *in vivo* (○) in human subjects. The *in vitro* rate was measured directly through excised skin; the *in vivo* rate was measured indirectly by determining drug loss from the patch. Source: Data taken from Reference 43.

IN VITRO–IN VIVO CORRELATION: BIOAVAILABILITY AND BIOEQUIVALENCE

Widespread use of the excised human skin model in the fields of toxicology and pharmacology generally fall into four areas: (1) to assess systemic risk associated with cutaneous exposure to various chemicals or drugs; (2) formulation development to achieve a target rate of absorption for transdermal drug products; (3) formulation optimization of topical drug and cosmetic products, to achieve either maximum bioavailability or some target bioavailability; and (4) screening drugs or a series of drug analogs to select the most bioavailable for further development. In the first two cases, it is crucial that the model properly reflects the *in vivo* state so that quantitatively accurate data are obtained, and the studies discussed in previous sections of this chapter have confirmed that the model achieves this goal.

Studies also exist confirming excellent IVIV correlation in the selection of vehicles for topical products such as creams, gels, and ointments that must achieve a target bioavailability (e.g., bioequivalence [BE] of generic topical drug products); here, the comparator *in vivo* data is a clinical end point rather than a numeric end point such as total absorption. An example of the utility of this approach is illustrated by the process used in the development of a generic ketoconazole cream.[44] A series of prototype formulations were prepared in which the concentration of two cosolvents were varied and ketoconazole absorption compared side by side to the reference listed drug (RLD) in the excised human skin model. The first attempt was unsuccessful in matching the bioavailability of the RLD, but the data obtained guided the preparation of additional formulations in which one was found that did demonstrate comparable bioavailability (Fig. 9.5). Subsequently, this formulation was shown by clinical trial to be bioequivalent to the RLD and approved by the

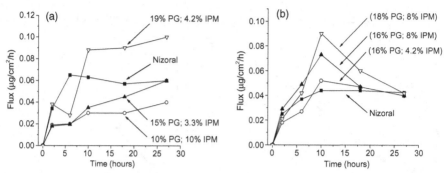

Figure 9.5   Comparison of *in vitro* rate of absorption profiles of test formulations of ketoconazole, with varying levels of propylene glycol (PG) and isopropylmyristate (IPM), to determine which best matches the original RLD (Nizoral Cream, Janssen Pharmaceutica, Titusville, NJ). (a) None of the first three formulations tested match the RLD. (b) One formulation from the second group of three formulations closely approximates the RLD.

U.S. Food and Drug Administration (FDA) with an AB rating (therapeutically equivalent).

In a similar manner, the excised human skin model has been used to determine "*in vitro* BE" of a number of prospective generic formulations to assure equivalence prior to conduct of the pivotal clinical trial. Franz et al.[45] evaluated absorption of the active pharmaceutical ingredient (API) from seven generic drug products during their pre-clinical development (two tretinoin gels, five glucocorticoid formulations) and compared it to that of the reference products in side-by-side studies. The test products were later evaluated by clinical trial or pharmacodynamic assay (vasoconstrictor [VC] test), where all were shown to be bioequivalent to the RLD and subsequently approved by the FDA.

The *in vitro* tretinoin product comparisons were designed as a simulated BE study with a sufficient number of replicate skin specimens run to calculate confidence intervals as required for BE clinical trials by the FDA. Both test products were found to be bioequivalent to the reference products (Table 9.4). The 90% confidence interval fell within the required interval (80%–125%) for all three primary end points with 0.01% tretinoin gel and for two of three primary end points with 0.025% tretinoin gel, with the third end point (maximum flux) barely missing (95.1%–127.9%).

The *in vitro* glucocorticoid data were also in agreement with the VC assay and found the test products to be equivalent to the reference products in four of five cases, with test:reference ratios ranging from 0.96 to 1.14 (Table 9.5). The glucocorticoid product, mometasone furoate ointment, was the sole exception, with a test:reference ratio of only 0.63. The explanation for this single discrepancy was found to be a result of the greater sensitivity of the *in vitro* method to detect differences between products, not a failure of the *in vitro* method.

The prior observation that the model may be more sensitive than the VC assay for the demonstration of BE is highly significant, but not totally unexpected. Other

Table 9.4   *In Vitro* Comparison of Primary End Points for Test and Reference Tretinoin Gels

	Test	Reference	Test/Reference	Confidence[a] interval
0.01% tretinoin				
AUC	3.00	2.97	1.02	97.06–107.46
J_{max}	0.55	0.57	1.04	92.53–115.05
T_{max}	3.60	3.57	1.04	92.23–116.37
0.025% tretinoin				
AUC	3.49	3.47	1.03	95.14–110.45
J_{max}	0.91	0.88	1.11	95.08–127.88
T_{max}	3.66	3.72	0.98	97.26–99.52

[a] The estimated error SD was used to compute the 90% confidence intervals for the ratio of the log-transformed Test and Reference means of each of the primary endpoints.

Source: Data taken from Reference 45.

AUC, area under absorption curve (total absorbed); J_{max}, maximum rate of absorption; T_{max}, time of maximum rate of absorption.

Table 9.5   Comparison of the BE of Five Generic Glucocorticoid Products (Test vs. Reference) as Determined by the *In Vivo* VC Assay and the *In Vitro* Excised Skin Model

	In vitro absorption (ng/cm^2/48 h)			VC assay ($-AUEC_{0-24h}$)		
	Test	Reference	Test/ Reference	Test	Reference	Test/ Reference
Alclometasone cream	4.52	4.39	1.03	18.7	16.8	1.10
Alclometasone ointment	66.95	70.00	0.96	16.0	17.4	0.92
Halobetasol cream	110.4	96.9	1.14	33.1	30.7	1.08
Halobetasol ointment	246.7	256.3	0.96	28.6	28.5	1.00
Mometasone ointment	213.4	338.7	0.63	13.7	12.3	1.11

All values represent the mean.

Source: Data taken from Reference 45.

striking examples exist. As part of a program to develop a more efficacious topical formulation of betamethasone valerate, a new and innovative thermolabile foam formulation of the drug was compared to the traditional lotion formulation by both VC assay and clinical trial. By clinical trial, the foam formulation was found to be 50% more efficacious in the treatment of scalp psoriasis than the lotion formulation. Although this was supported by *in vitro* permeation data that demonstrated a three-fold greater rate of absorption from the foam, VC assay failed to reveal the greater potency of the foam formulation.[46,47]

Similarly, it has been shown in the *in vitro* permeation model that the percutaneous absorption of the glucocorticoid, alclometasone dipropionate, is approximately 15 times greater from the ointment product than the cream product. However, their apparent potency to induce blanching appears equivalent in the VC assay (Table 9.5).[45]

SUMMARY

A substantial body of data exists to support the fact that the *in vitro* measurement of percutaneous absorption in excised human skin is a valid method by which to predict absorption in the living state. Studies specifically designed to quantify the relationship between *in vitro* and *in vivo* data have shown excellent correlation between the two. When the essential parameters under which *in vitro* studies are conducted are tightly controlled so that they adequately duplicate *in vivo* conditions, the average IVIV ratio approximates 1 (0.96, range 0.58–1.28). Two critical components necessary for good IVIV correlation are the use of skin from identical body sites and vehicles of identical composition and dose. Both are factors that are well known, but not always suitably respected.

Clinical studies also support the validity of the excised skin model by demonstrating the accuracy of predictions obtained *in vitro* with respect to formulation development and clinical outcome, particularly in the areas of transdermal delivery and topical bioavailability/BE. The results of several prospective studies, in which a number of test and reference formulations were shown to be equally bioavailable in the *in vitro* model, have all been validated when subsequent clinical evaluation found the test and reference products to be bioequivalent. Taken collectively, the conclusion of a large number of studies is that data obtained in the excised skin model consistently and accurately reflect absorption in living man, whether the comparator end point is a rigorous quantifiable metric such as total absorption or a clinical end point such as the VC score or therapeutic efficacy. In some cases, greater sensitivity of the *in vitro* model over clinical end point studies has been unambiguously documented. A full discussion of the detailed factors to be considered when conducting an *in vitro* diffusion experiment and some recommendations about the most suitable methodologies for optimizing IVIV correlation are further discussed in Chapter 5.

REFERENCES

1. WINSOR T, BURCH GE. Differential roles of layers of human epigastric skin on diffusion rate of water. *Arch Intern Med* 1944; 74: 428–436.
2. BURCH GE, WINSOR T. Rate of insensible perspiration (diffusion of water) locally through living and through dead human skin. *Arch Intern Med* 1944; 74: 437–444.
3. ONKEN HD, MOYER CA. The water barrier in human epidermis. *Arch Dermatol* 1963; 87: 584–590.
4. FRANZ TJ. Percutaneous absorption: On the relevance of *in vitro* data. *J Invest Dermatol* 1975; 64: 190–195.
5. FELDMANN RJ, MAIBACH HI. Absorption of some organic compounds through the skin in man. *J Invest Dermatol* 1970; 54: 399–404.

6. Franz TJ. The finite dose technique as a valid *in vitro* model for the study of percutaneous absorption in man. In: Simon GA, Paster A, Klingberg MA, Kaye M, eds. *Skin: Drug Application and Evaluation of Environmental hazards. Current Problems in Dermatology.* Karger, Basel, Switzerland, 1978; 58–68.

7. Bartek MJ, LaBudde JA. Percutaneous absorption *in vivo*. In: Maibach HI, ed. *Animal Models in Dermatology.* Churchill-Livingstone, New York, 1975; 103–120.

8. Bronaugh RL, Franz TJ. Vehicle effect on percutaneous absorption: *In vivo* and *in vitro* comparisons. *Br J Dermatol* 1986; 115: 1–11.

9. Franz TJ. Percutaneous absorption of benzene. *Adv Mod Environ Toxicol* 1984; 6: 61–70.

10. Feldmann RJ, Maibach HI. Percutaneous penetration of steroids in man. *J Invest Dermatol* 1969; 52: 89–94.

11. Maibach HI, Feldmann RJ. Systemic absorption of pesticides through the skin of man. In: Occupational Exposure to Pesticides, Report to the Federal Working Group on Pest Management from the Task Group on Occupational Exposure to Pesticides, Appendix B, U.S. Government Printing Office, Washington DC, 1975, pp 120–127.

12. Bronaugh RL, Maibach HI. Percutaneous absorption of nitroaromatic compounds: *In vivo* and *in vitro* studies in the human and monkey. *J Invest Dermatol* 1985; 84: 180–183.

13. Bucks DAW, McMaster JR, Maibach HI, Guy RH. Bioavailability of topically administered steroids: A "mass balance" technique. *J Invest Dermatol* 1988; 91: 29–33.

14. Carmichael NG, Nolan RJ, Perkins JM, Dabies R, Warrington SJ. Oral and dermal pharmacokinetics of triclopyr in human volunteers. *Hum Toxicol* 1989; 8: 431–437.

15. Bucks DAW, Guy RH, Maibach HI. Percutaneous penetration and mass balance accountability: Technique and implications for dermatology. *J Toxicol Cut and Ocular Toxicol* 1990; 8: 439–451.

16. Hotchkiss SAM, Hewitt P, Caldwell J. Percutaneous absorption of nicotinic acid, phenol, benzoic acid and triclopyrbutoxyethyl ester through rat and human skin *in vitro*: Further validation of an *in vitro* model by comparison with *in vivo* data. *Food Chem Toxicol* 1992; 30: 891–899.

17. Ramsey JD, Woollen BH, Auton TR, Batten TR, Leeser PL. Pharmacokinetics of fluazifop-butyl in human volunteers. II. Dermal dosing. *Hum Exp Toxicol* 1992; 11: 247–254.

18. Wester RC, Maibach HI, Melendres J, Sedik L, Knaak J, Wang R. *In vivo* and *in vitro* percutaneous absorption and skin evaporation of isophenos in man. *Fund Appl Toxicol* 1992; 19: 521–526.

19. Wester RC, Sedik L, Melendres J, Logan F, Maibach HI, Russell I. Percutaneous absorption of diazinon in humans. *Food Chem Toxicol* 1993; 31: 569–572.

20. Ramsey JD, Woollen BH, Auton TR, Scott RC. The predictive accuracy of *in vitro* measurements for the dermal absorption of a lipophilic penetrant (fluazifop-butyl) through rat and human skin. *Fund Appl Toxicol* 1994; 23: 230–236.

21. Dick D, Ng KM, Sauder DN, Chu I. *In vitro* and *in vivo* percutaneous absorption of ^{14}C-chloroform in humans. *Hum Exp Toxicol* 1995; 14: 260–265.

22. Franz TJ, Lehman PA, Franz SF, Guin JD. Comparative percutaneous absorption of lindane and permethrin. *Arch Dermatol* 1996; 132: 901–905.

23. Beckley-Kartey SAJ, Hotchkiss SAM, Capel M. Comparative *in vitro* skin absorption and metabolism of coumarin (1,2-benzopyrone) in human, rat and mouse. *Toxicol Appl Pharmacol* 1997; 145: 34–42.

24. Dick IP, Blain PG, Williams FM. The percutaneous absorption and skin distribution of lindane in man. II. *In vitro* studies. *Hum Exp Toxicol* 1997; 16: 652–657.

25. Wester RC, Hui X, Hartway T, Maibach HI, Bell K, Schell MJ, Northington DJ, Strong P, Culver BD. *In vivo* percutaneous absorption of boric acid, borax, and disodium octaborate tetrahydrate in humans compared to *in vitro* absorption in human skin from infinite and finite doses. *Toxicol Sci* 1998; 45: 42–51.

26. Griffin P, Mason H, Heywood K, Cocker J. Oral and dermal absorption of chlorpyrifos: A human volunteer study. *Occup Environ Med* 1999; 56: 1–10.

27. Griffin P, Payne M, Mason H, Freedlander E, Curran AD, Cocker J. The *in vitro* percutaneous penetration of chlorpyrifos. *Hum Exp Toxicol* 2000; 19: 104–107.

28. VAN DE SANDT JJ, MEULING WJ, ELLIOTT GR, CNUBBEN HH, HAKKERT BC. Comparative *in vitro–in vivo* percutaneous absorption of the pesticide propoxur. *Toxicol Sci* 2000; 58: 15–22.

29. FORD RA, HAWKINS DR, MAYO BC, API AM. The *in vivo* dermal absorption and metabolism of [4-^{14}C]coumarin by rats and by human volunteers under simulated conditions of use in fragrances. *Food Chem Toxicol* 2001; 39: 153–162.

30. CNUBBEN NH, ELLIOTT GR, HAKKERT BC, MEULING WJA, van de SANDT JJ. Comparative *in vitro–in vivo* percutaneous penetration of the fungicide ortho-phenylphenol. *Regul Toxicol Pharmacol* 2002; 35: 198–208.

31. BENECH-KIEFFER F, MEULING WJA, LECLERC C, ROZA L, LECLAIRE J, NOHYNEK G. Percutaneous absorption of Mexoryl SX® in human volunteers: Comparison with *in vitro* data. *Skin Pharmacol Appl Skin Physiol* 2003; 16: 343–355.

32. VAN DE SANDT JJM, VAN BURGSTEDEN JA, CAGE S, CARMICHAEL PL, DICK I, KENYON S, KORINTH G, LARESE F, LIMASSET JC, MAAS WJM, MONTOMOLI L, NIELSEN JB, PAYAN JP, ROBINSON E, SARTORELLI P, SCHALLER KH, WILKINSON SC, WILLIAMS FM. *In vitro* predictions of skin absorption of caffeine, testosterone, and benzoic acid: A multi-centre comparison study. *Regul Toxicol Pharmacol* 2004; 39: 271–281.

33. HUEBER-BECKER F, NOHYNEK GJ, MEULING WJA, BENECH-KIEFFER F, TOUTAIN H. Human systemic exposure to a [^{14}C]-*para*-phenylenediamine-containing oxidative hair dye and correlation with *in vitro* percutaneous absorption in human or pig skin. *Food Chem Toxicol* 2004; 42: 1227–1236.

34. MODJTAHEDI BS, MAIBACH HI. *In vivo* percutaneous absorption of benzene in man: Forearm and palm. *Food Chem Toxicol* 2008; 46: 1171–1174.

35. LEHMAN PA, RANEY SG, FRANZ TJ. Percutaneous absorption in man: *In vitro–in vivo* correlation. *Skin Pharmacol Physiol* 2011; 24: 224–230.

36. WESTER RC, MAIBACH HI. Regional variation in percutaneous absorption: Principles and applications to human risk assessment. In: Bronaugh RL, Maibach HI, eds. *Percutaneous Absorption: Drugs-Cosmetics-Mechanisms-Methodology.* Taylor & Francis, New York, 2005; 85–93.

37. GIBALDI M, PERRIER D. *Pharmacokinetics,* 2nd ed. Marcel Dekker, New York, 1982; 321.

38. SHAW JE, CHANDRASEKARAN SK, MICHAELS AS, TASKOVICH L. Controlled transdermal delivery, *in vitro* and *in vivo.* In: Maibach HI, ed. *Animal Models in Dermatology.* Churchill Livingstone, New York, 1975; 138–146.

39. HADGRAFT J, BEUTNER D, WOLFF H. *In vivo-in vitro* comparisons in the transdermal delivery of nitroglycerin. *Int J Pharm* 1993; 89: R1–R4.

40. ROY SD, MANOUKIAN E, COMBS D. Absorption of transdermally delivered ketorolac acid in humans. *J Pharm Sci* 1995; 84: 49–52.

41. ROHATAGI S, BARRETT JS, MCDONALD LJ, MORRIS EM, DARNOW J, DISANTO AR. Selegiline percutaneous absorption in various species and metabolism by human skin. *Pharm Res* 1997; 14: 50–55.

42. ROHR UD, ALTENBURGER R, KISSEL T. Pharmacokinetics of the transdermal reservoir membrane system delivering β-estradiol: *In vitro/in vivo*-correlation. *Pharm Res* 1998; 15: 877–882.

43. VENKATESHWARAN S. *In vitro-in vivo* correlation for transdermal delivery. IBC International Conference on Transdermal Drug Delivery, Coronado, 1997, pp 15–16.

44. FRANZ TJ, LEHMAN PA, RANEY SG. The cadaver skin absorption model and the drug development process. *Pharm Forum* 2008; 34: 1349–1356.

45. FRANZ TJ, LEHMAN PA, RANEY SG. Use of excised human skin to assess the bioequivalence of topical products. *Skin Pharmacol Physiol* 2009; 22: 276–286.

46. FRANZ TJ, PARSELL DA, HALUALANI RM, HANNIGAN JF, KALBACH JP, HARKONEN WS. Betamethasone valerate foam 0.12%: A novel vehicle with enhanced delivery and efficacy. *Int J Dermatol* 1999; 38: 628–632.

47. FDA, CDER. Summary Basis of Approval: NDA 20-934, Luxiq (betamethasone valerate) foam. Clinical Pharmacology Biopharmaceutics Review. 28 February 1999. Available at: http://www.accessdata.fda.gov/drugsatfda_docs/nda/99/20934.cfm (accessed January 20, 2011).

Chapter 10

Risk Assessment

Jon R. Heylings

INTRODUCTION

This chapter will consider how dermal absorption and risk assessment has developed over the years and some of the debates, primarily on the *in vitro* methodology, that are ongoing on how experimental data are used in the human risk assessment process. The focus of attention, based largely on the author's own experience, will relate mainly to the safety of industrial chemicals and, more specifically, crop protection products. However, recognizing that the rest of this book covers the dermal absorption of chemicals used in pharmaceutical and personal care products, where dermal exposure is intentional, the author has also attempted to cover various aspects of risk assessment as it relates to a broad range of chemical products that come into contact with human skin, either intentionally or unintentionally.

Across all sectors of industry the key regulatory challenge has been centered on what is the appropriate experimental methodology that should be used for predicting dermal absorption in man. With regard to human risk there is universal agreement that prediction of systemic exposure to any chemical should not be underestimated. However, just how rigorous should we be in our pursuit of the most accurate prediction? We should always bear in mind that the experimental models provide an estimate of dermal absorption, as it relates to man. No toxicological-based test provides complete certainty of an effect in man for a given exposure, so when it comes to relating a hazard-based endpoint to exposure via the dermal route, sensible evidence-based decisions are needed that minimize the risk that a given chemical substance will be unsafe to the human population.

HISTORICAL PERSPECTIVE

The models used to estimate dermal absorption in man have evolved considerably between the 1970s and 2000s to encompass a variety of nonanimal approaches that

Transdermal and Topical Drug Delivery: Principles and Practice, First Edition. Edited by Heather A.E. Benson, Adam C. Watkinson.
© 2012 John Wiley & Sons, Inc. Published 2012 by John Wiley & Sons, Inc.

183

have been used alongside, or even replaced, conventional toxicity testing in animals. Interestingly, the incorporation of the emerging models by the various industry groups into their own risk assessment processes has been far from uniform. Indeed, having represented the interests of various European Union (EU) and Organisation for Economic Cooperation and Development (OECD) groups over the years, the author has found this lack of harmonization across the various regulatory bodies worldwide for what is essentially the same methodology, an interesting and challenging experience. A classic example of this occurred with the development of OECD Test Guideline 428, an *in vitro* percutaneous absorption method designed to be used in the risk assessment process for industrial chemicals, pesticides, and cosmetic ingredients, as well as assessing the risk following the dermal exposure to chemicals during manufacture, such as drug intermediates. The first OECD draft guideline using the *in vitro* model was proposed around 1992. This gained wide support from the chemical and personal care sectors of industry through the 1990s and also from the various pesticide agencies in the EU. Most of the laboratories conducting *in vitro* dermal absorption studies had been following other published guidance from the European Centre for Ecotoxicology and Toxicology of Chemicals,[1] the European Centre for the Validation of Alternative Methods,[2] and for cosmetics products, the European Cosmetics Association (COLIPA) guidance.[3] Indeed, the OECD guideline produced in the late 1990s was used as a "draft" test guideline for the next 10 years by many EU regulatory authorities for dermal absorption studies as part of the product registration process.

DEVELOPMENT OF THE OECD TEST GUIDELINES FOR DERMAL ABSORPTION

In 1992, the intention was to provide OECD member states with a single harmonized approach for the assessment of dermal absorption. This new test guideline would include industrial chemicals, cosmetic products, and pesticides. The original proposal from the United Kingdom outlined an *in vitro* and an *in vivo* test method. Over the next 5 years, a number of expert groups met, reviewed, and tried to resolve the issues that prevented the establishment of a new test guideline. These mainly centered on the *in vitro* method and the lack of formal validation. A number of workshops and OECD steering committees and expert groups met and continued to work to resolve the issues on how the *in vitro* method should be used in risk assessment. In 1997, the Toxicology Expert Group of the European Crop Protection Association (ECPA) volunteered to assist with the preparation of a draft OECD guidance document for dermal absorption, in addition to the revision of the draft OECD test guidelines. A subgroup of technical experts from ECPA was formed to undertake this task. Further versions of the draft test guideline emerged. In 2000, an OECD Expert Group was appointed to resolve the final few remaining issues. This group included experts from the U.S. Environmental Protection Agency (EPA), Health Canada, U.S. Food and Drug Administration (FDA), ECPA, and the OECD Secretariat. Finally, in May 2001, a consensus was reached by the Joint Meeting of the Chemicals Committee and Working Group on Chemicals, Pesticides and Biotechnology; the OECD Test Guidelines 427[4] and 428[5] for dermal absorption *in vivo* and *in vitro*, respectively, were approved. In addition, an OECD Guidance Document on dermal absorption[6] with further detail on how to conduct the method was also published. There is a good synopsis of the history of this particular test guideline and animal welfare developments in general that was published by a member of the OECD Secretariat.[7]

Despite the existence of OECD test guidelines, there are still differences in the way in which studies on the dermal absorption of pesticides is both conducted and interpreted between North America and other OECD member states. These differences, and the attempts to harmonize the approaches for dermal absorption and risk assessment, have been the subject of ongoing discussions and workshops.[8] One of the major issues is the reluctance of North America to accept *in vitro* dermal absorption studies in the regulation process for pesticide-containing products by the Office of Pesticides Programs (OPPS), part of the U.S. EPA, due to the lack of formal validation. This is despite the overwhelming evidence presented in various publications and reviews that *in vitro* data, as used in the EU for over 20 years for pesticide products, provide a useful approach to the prediction of dermal absorption in man.[1,2,5,8] Indeed, all areas of industry, with the exception of pesticides in North America, endorse the *in vitro* approach in OECD 428, and do not use animal studies to determine dermal absorption values. For example, the *in vitro* approach, using nonviable human skin, is used in the human risk assessment process for industrial chemicals, as endorsed by the EPA,[9] but *in vitro* methods were not permitted for pesticide products by the same agency.[10] It therefore remains surprising that in North America the regulation of industrial chemicals and also personal care products, which are intended to be applied to the skin, utilize the *in vitro* dermal absorption approach, but the *in vitro* method was not deemed acceptable by other parts of the agency that regulate pesticide-containing products.

Perhaps one of the difficulties for some regulatory authorities to accept the *in vitro* approach relates to the aspect of predictive accuracy. In conventional validation of a hazard-based test the objective is to develop an *in vitro* model that is robust and predicts *in vivo* with an acceptable degree of accuracy. In the pesticide dermal absorption field, a quantitative assessment of the likely systemic exposure of an active ingredient from a formulated product is being made, as opposed to the generation of a positive or negative result. Prediction of percutaneous absorption using *in vitro* approaches is not about the development of a like-for-like replacement model; it is to provide a conservative approach where the *in vitro* study is unlikely to underestimate skin absorption compared with an *in vivo* approach. Furthermore, skin absorption is one area of the toxicological sciences where human models are accepted practice. Therefore, the key scientific aspect of any "validation" is the prediction of human absorption from human skin models. Providing the *in vitro* human model does not underestimate absorption in man, it should have a pivotal role in the regulatory process for assessing the dermal absorption potential of chemicals.

RISK ASSESSMENT RELATING TO PESTICIDES WITHIN THE EUROPEAN UNION

The dermal route is the most likely exposure route for almost all pesticide-containing products. The assessment of percutaneous absorption is therefore an important part of the safety evaluation of pesticide products. Within the EU, data on the absorption of the active ingredient through the skin are obligatory for inclusion in Annex I of Directive 91/414 of the European Community. Inclusion of active substances in Annex I is only possible if the crop protection products containing them can be used with acceptable risk to humans.[11] Evaluation of risk to populations who may be exposed to pesticides (e.g., manufacturers, workers, spray operators, and bystanders) is essential in order to authorize the use of these products in the market.

Exposure to pesticides primarily occurs via occupational exposure during the handling and normal use of crop protection products. Following skin contact, the active ingredient has the potential to be absorbed through the skin and may become systemically available. As part of the overall risk assessment process, the toxicological profile of the active ingredient and the extent of exposure are determined. The assessment of percutaneous absorption under relevant field exposure conditions is then used to predict whether the amount of the active ingredient that could be absorbed has any likely adverse health consequences.

The systemic dose that is considered to be safe for exposed individuals is derived from the results of toxicological investigations, and the acceptable operator exposure level (AOEL) is established. The quantitative estimate for skin exposure for a particular type of application is derived from experimental data for the specific formulation or a similar type of application, or may be based on a theoretical model such as the European Predictive Operator Exposure Model (EUROPOEM).[12] The result of such an assessment is wide ranging; in many cases, the data generated in percutaneous absorption studies will determine whether the product can be registered for a specific application. It may determine that the risk from dermal contact is negligible even if the entire dose applied to the skin was systemically available, or the safety may depend on a low percentage skin absorption being demonstrated. Alternatively, it may determine that specific personal protective equipment or engineering controls are required in order to minimize or prevent dermal exposure. The assessment may determine that there is a significant risk for human health and the product will not be registered for the specific use.

Dermal absorption studies for pesticide products should be performed in accordance with the OECD Test Guidelines 427 (*in vivo*) and 428 (*in vitro*) and their associated Guidance Document No. 28.[4-6] Data from these studies allow the comparison of the external exposure, derived from separate operator exposure models, with the AOEL. The AOEL is the acceptable systemic dose, based on the toxicity of the active ingredient and is expressed in milligrams per kilogram per day. If the evaluations, including the dermal absorption value, exceed the AOEL then the product would not be approved for the specific use under consideration.

The OECD guidelines for dermal absorption provide the basic framework for the practical methods used to assess the skin absorption of chemicals and the products that contain them. As such, the guidelines are not specific to a particular industry or regulatory area. They are intended to cover the general principles of the tests and to provide information on where additional guidance can be sought. For crop protection products, more specific guidance can be found in separate documents, including European Commission (EC) Health and Consumer Protection Directorate General (DG SANTO) 222/2000 rev.7.[13] This describes the process for assessing dermal absorption of pesticides, based on the OECD guidelines, plus how the data are used in the risk assessment process for pesticide products. This guidance used in the EU has a tiered approach for occupational risk assessment in which dermal absorption and exposure assessment are integrated. Although the OECD includes as its members the United States and Canada, there are different approaches within North America's system for pesticide regulation. For example, the U.S. EPA has a separate Health Effects Test Guideline OPPTS (Office of Prevention, Pesticides and Toxic Substances) 870.7600[10] for pesticides. This covers *in vivo* studies only.

The current regulatory procedure for evaluating human *in vivo* skin absorption within Europe is well documented.[13] As a first step, the potential human exposure is assessed, then if the theoretical total amount present on skin were absorbed, and the AOEL were not exceeded, no further evaluation is needed. The physicochemistry of the active ingredient may be taken into account to justify less than 100% absorption as the default absorption factor, but currently the regulations do not account for realistic absorption percentages without experimental evidence.

The traditional approach to provide experimental evidence involves the performance of an *in vivo* rat skin absorption study with the agrochemical formulation, commonly of the commercial concentrate formulation and of the typical in-use spray dilutions. Rat skin is generally far more permeable than human skin.[1,2,14] To make an assessment of the equivalent human *in vivo* absorption, *in vitro* studies performed with the same formulations in both rat and human skin allow a correction factor to be applied to the rat *in vivo* result. Thus, a prediction of the human *in vivo* percentage absorption can be made. This procedure is commonly performed for a representative formulation. It is well known that changes to formulations can have effects on skin absorption. For example, adjuvants can enhance absorption and other components can reduce absorption. Agrochemical companies sometimes have a range of similar formulations which are adapted for specific pests, local climates, or specific use patterns. So it is common practice to use *in vitro* tests to compare such formulations with the "reference" formulation that was tested *in vivo*, such that a correction factor can be derived to produce an estimate of human *in vivo* absorption for a range of relatively similar formulations.

A flow diagram was suggested by Heylings and Esdaile,[15] which shows a proposed tiered approach and the various stages required to demonstrate safety as related to skin exposure to an agrochemical product. This diagram (Fig. 10.1) is a proposed scheme, based on the principal current regulatory requirements and the experience of the authors, but it must be noted that different regulatory authorities have different opinions on which studies are acceptable in the regulatory process.

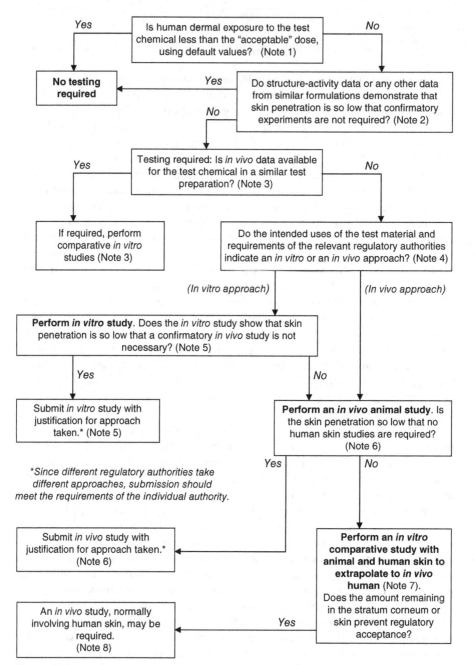

Figure 10.1 A proposed decision tree for performance of *in vivo/in vitro* studies for an agrochemical with unknown dermal absorption.

Notes:

(1) The theoretical maximum dermal exposure to the test chemical in a specified time period should be estimated. This will rely on the default absorption percentage, which is often 100% unless a lower value can be justified. Exposure = dermal dose per individual × default percentage absorption/body weight, expressed as milligrams per kilogram per day or milligrams per kilogram per hour. If this value is lower than the "acceptable" exposure limit and the regulatory authority accepts the calculations, then no percutaneous absorption testing should be required.

(2) In some cases it is possible to demonstrate that the skin penetration of a chemical will be near zero. Examples include large molecules such as polymers, large charged ions, or chemicals in a physical form such as large insoluble crystal structures. In other cases it may be possible to make

Figure 10.1 (*Continued*)

appropriate structure-activity predictions by mathematical calculation, based on the physicochemical characteristics. Where a robust prediction can be made, which is sufficiently conservative or where the safety margin is sufficiently large, the evaluation should be acceptable to regulatory authorities. Evaluations of this nature should be justified on a case-by-case basis, but acceptability will be affected by the knowledegability of the individual regulatory authority. It is recognized that predictions of penetration from multicomponent formulations is more complex than predictions for pure chemicals or simple solutions.

In some cases, there will be existing information about the penetration characteristics for a similar formulation. Where the formulations are adequately similar, it can be assumed that the penetration characteristics will be similar, and hence if the margins of safety are large enough, no further experimental work should be required.

(3) In cases where adequate *in vivo* data exist for a similar formulation but that the differences between the formulations may influence the penetration characteristics, the usual approach will be to perform bridging studies. Evaluation of skin penetration *in vitro* can be used to assess relative penetration between similar formulations or similar chemicals (as flux, percentage absorption, or K_p values). *In vitro* studies can also be used to predict relative penetration for the same formulation between different exposure conditions on similar skin. For example, skin penetration of test chemical from formulation "A" *in vivo* is known to be 10% of the applied dose per 24 hours in man. In an *in vitro* study using rat skin, formulation "A" gave 30% penetration at 24 hours and formulation "B" gave 15% penetration at 24 hours. Hence, the extrapolated *in vivo* human skin penetration rate over 24 hours for formulation "B" is $(10\% \times 15/30) = 5\%$.

(4) Certain regulatory authorities have specific requirements to avoid *in vivo* experimentation whenever an alternative can be justified. Other authorities prefer the use of live animals in safety evaluation studies. Hence, although the choice of study type should include an ethical approach with a reduction of animal use wherever possible, the regulatory bodies do have the right to specify specific studies for inclusion in regulatory submissions.

(5) *In vitro* evaluation under correct conditions can give a conservative estimate of *in vivo* skin penetration of a chemical from a dermal exposure, normally as milligrams per square centimeter per hour or per day. If this evaluation shows that the potential systemic exposure would not exceed the "acceptable" dose, then *in vivo* experimentation will not be required. It should be noted that *in vitro* studies using rat skin give absorption characteristics higher (often five or 10 times higher) than the *in vivo* human absorption values.

(6) Evaluation of skin penetration *in vivo* can be used to assess skin penetration in the test species, under the specific conditions of exposure used in the study. The rat is the species of choice for many regulatory authorities. It must be noted that the rat has relatively permeable skin compared to that of humans. The protective external layer of the rat against its normal environment is the layer of hair; for humans, it is the SC, hence in the rat the SC is relatively permeable. Some species (such as the pig) have skin permeability characteristics close to that of man; where a more accurate prediction of human skin penetration is required, consideration should be given to use of such models. A correctly performed *in vivo* skin penetration study will give a conservative estimate of the amount of chemical which could become systemically available from dermal exposure, normally on a 24-hour basis. Where the *in vivo* data show an adequate safety margin, no further experimentation should be required.

(7) In many cases an *in vivo* rat dermal absorption study will be required for a new chemical or active ingredient. Where a better estimate of absorption through human skin is required, a common approach is to perform a comparative assay of *in vitro* absorption in animal versus human skin. When these data are combined with animal *in vivo* data, they allow the prediction of *in vivo* human absorption, provided that the exposure conditions were adequately similar.[2,11,25]

That is, skin penetration *in vivo* in man is extrapolated from:

$$\frac{\text{rat } in \, vivo \times \text{human } in \, vitro}{\text{rat } in \, vitro}.$$

(8) Human volunteer studies or worker exposure studies with markers of exposure may be scientifically justified if they can be performed with full ethical approval; however, a number of the regulatory authorities discourage or refuse to accept human volunteer studies for political reasons. A study with human skin grafted onto nude mice[14] is likely to provide good quality data with human skin to justify the lack of systemic absorption of chemical from the skin compartment. In some cases, it may be possible to demonstrate the lack of absorption from the skin over time with a rat *in vivo* model; although the relatively high permeability of rat skin can make this difficult, *in vivo* studies in other species such as the pig may be more appropriate.

GOOD PRACTICE ACROSS ALL INDUSTRY SECTORS

The focus of the rest of this chapter is to provide information on some of the current issues on dermal absorption that are being debated and relate directly to risk assessment and the overall registration process. Much of the detailed methodology of the *in vitro* and *in vivo* models has been dealt with elsewhere in this book. The following issues are under current debate between regulatory bodies and industry groups around the globe. These issues span the sectors of industry that have a need to generate dermal absorption data for the registration or approval process for their products.

Complex Formulations

The applied dose of the test preparation for skin absorption studies should mimic the "in use" conditions.[6] Normally the preparation will be made with a radiolabeled active ingredient in order to trace the absorption. Some formulations are highly complex in nature. Therefore, it is critical that the added radiolabeled chemical is in the same form and compartment as the cold active ingredient. This can require specialist formulation knowledge for certain formulation types; for example, for oil-in-water or water-in-oil emulsions, suspension concentrates, granules, and powders, it can be difficult to ensure the radiolabeled material is homogenously distributed. In many other cases there will be no radiolabeled form of the active ingredient and the percutaneous absorption study will rely on a cold analytical method to measure the test chemical. Historical studies used to focus on measuring the flux of the chemical through skin, and measurement in the receptor fluid was all that was required to calculate likely human exposure. With the advent of OECD 428, where a mass balance recovery of the test chemical is required, this provides a greater challenge for the experimentalist since the test chemical needs to be measured in the various compartments associated with the skin. This includes the skin wash, the tape-stripped stratum corneum (SC), the residual epidermis, and in some cases, in carbon filter traps above the skin when the test chemical is volatile. For risk assessment purposes, the analytical method needs to be validated to good laboratory practice (GLP), and to meet guideline standards, a mass balance recovery of $100\% \pm 10\%$ should be achieved for radiochemical studies. A recovery between 80% and 120% is regarded as acceptable for nonradiolabeled studies, although any shortfall should be justified. It is general practice to include any "missing" dose in a mass balance study as potentially in the systemic compartment in order to make the risk assessment as conservative as possible.

The dermal absorption of test substances (or formulated products containing the test substance) that are in a solid form at the temperature of the skin surface normally requires a vehicle or carrier to allow it to penetrate into the SC. Dry solid large particles or granules are very poor platforms for dermal absorption. Fine particles and dusts (depending on the actual particle size) will absorb any surrounding moisture on the skin surface and will therefore have more surface contact and a greater ability to penetrate into the skin. When *in vitro* or *in vivo* dermal absorption studies are designed to assess the risk from contact with solids, it is important to examine the actual real-life exposure scenario. This includes a number of aspects such as the particle size and the potential exposure period. For example, if the material at the top of a container is a lumpy granule but is a fine dust at the bottom of the same container due to settling, it is prudent to test the finer dust material since it is likely to have a greater opportunity to release and deliver the active onto and into the skin. The OECD Test Guidelines 427 and 428 suggest that moistening of the solid should be undertaken for *in vitro* and *in vivo* dermal absorption studies. In order to better simulate typical exposure it would be more useful and relevant to compare the neat material with a simulated sweat type of application. This would involve preparing a ground-down version of the solid in this sweat medium that is then applied to the skin as a paste. This would provide a conservative assessment of dermal absorption relative to the neat solid and represent a worst-case scenario that may occur during handling of the chemical or product.

For products that are volatile at room temperature, or likely to be lost from the skin via evaporation during their normal use, it is important to measure the amount of the applied dose that is lost during *in vitro* and *in vivo* studies. This is a key element of the mass balance, and in situations where this has not been quantified by trapping the test substance in the void above the skin surface, the study is compromised and the "missing" fraction of the dose would therefore be assumed to have been absorbed. The usual procedure for studies with volatile test substances is to place a charcoal filter above the donor chamber (*in vitro*) or skin device (*in vivo*), and to extract the compound from the matrix at the end of the exposure period. With some of the more volatile pesticide products, such as soil fumigants, a significant proportion of the applied dose may be lost from the skin surface by evaporation.

Skin Integrity Measurement

Human skin is the preferred model for the assessment of dermal absorption of pesticide products. Indeed, it is regarded as the "gold standard" for such assessments.[8] The OECD Test Guideline 428[5] is quite specific about the need for measurement of the skin barrier integrity prior to studies. Skin tissue from humans is procured, transported, stored, prepared, and handled in potentially so many different ways that some uniform assessment of the quality of each specimen is very important. Surprisingly, over the many years of operation of the *in vitro* percutaneous absorption method there have been only a few systematic evaluations of the skin barrier integrity across species, skin preparation type (e.g., epidermal membranes, dermatomed skin, etc.), and the integrity method being used.[16,17] Traditionally, tritiated water flux was used as the primary method to determine skin integrity and particularly if any gross physical damage had been caused to the specimen such as those that may be caused by instruments during dissection and preparation. More recently, the electrical resistance (ER) and, in some case, transepidermal water loss (TEWL) assessments have replaced the tritiated water flux approach, largely due to the gains in efficiency, cost, and safety.[17] The ER and TEWL methods are just as useful as tritiated water for measuring barrier damage and the former is very simple and allows damaged specimens to be identified and replaced quickly. One of the key considerations here is what actually constitutes "normal" skin when determining values by these simple barrier integrity checks. This is particularly important with human skin. Obviously, specimens that appear grossly abnormal or are physically damaged during preparation should not be used. However, values of tritiated water flux, ER, or TEWL have their own broad distributions across different human donors and within donors. This inherent variability can be controlled to a certain extent by use of skin from the same anatomical site. Abdominal skin is generally regarded as the most useful and widely used anatomical site for human skin studies and is recommended in various guidance documents in this field.[1,2,8,13] It has an intermediate SC thickness and follicle density. Other factors, as mentioned above, can broaden the distribution of skin integrity values in human skin beyond just biological variability. Indeed, certain tissue banks that provide human skin sometimes have whole batches with "abnormal" integrity values and others, perhaps with more careful adherence to preparation, storage, and shipping, have consistently better integrity values. This is obviously not due to inherent variability across the population; it is due to quality control. These features are only easy to detect and monitor in laboratories that have a high turnover of *in vitro* percutaneous absorption studies, maintain skin integrity databases, and utilize multiple skin banks. Poor quality tissues would be more difficult to identify in small one-off research projects, particularly in less experienced laboratories.

If we make the assumption that quality control of human skin specimens from procurement to point of use is satisfactory, we still have the issue of intrinsic biological variability and what constitutes acceptable values of tritiated water, ER, and TEWL for *in vitro* skin absorption experiments. It is recognized that the skin flux of chemicals will vary across a group of replicates, more so in the diverse target human than in the relatively homogeneous animal skin taken from the same strain, sex, body weight, and so on. Therefore, we must not narrow down "acceptable" human skin specimens to, for example, those of very low permeability to water. Specimens must be of acceptable quality and representative of the population.

The methods for assessing skin integrity in OECD 428 are described but no suggested cut-off values for normal skin are specified in the OECD guidance. The paper by Davies et al. (2004) published after the OECD test guideline,[17] has studied a wide range of species and skin preparation types comparing tritiated water and ER as skin integrity measures. In this paper there are suggested cut-off values that this specific laboratory recommends to accept or reject specimens mounted in static diffusion cells for use in percutaneous absorption studies (Table 10.1). It is critical that new laboratories entering into the field of *in vitro* percutaneous absorption understand all these potential issues relating to the barrier integrity of their skin samples. Since the SC is the most important component of these studies, its function must be

Table 10.1   Acceptance Values for T_2O Permeability Coefficient and Electrical Resistance (ER) Using Standard Diffusion Cells for Various Skin Preparations

Species	Skin type	T_2O permeability (cm/h)	ER ($k\Omega/cm^2$)	ER ($k\Omega$)[a]
Human	Epidermis	<1.5	3.94	>10
	Whole	<1.5	3.94	>10
Rat	Epidermis	<2.5	0.98	>2.5
	Whole	<2.5	1.18	>3.0
Pig	Epidermis	<4.5	1.18	>3.0
	Whole	<4.5	1.57	>4.0
Mouse	Whole	<1.2	6.33	>5.0
Rabbit	Whole	<13	0.35	>0.8
Guinea pig	Whole	<2.0	1.97	>5.0

[a] Static diffusion cells as used by Syngenta Central Toxicology Laboratory (CTL) and Dermal Technology Laboratory (DTL): skin area = 2.54 cm^2, with the exception of mouse with area = 0.79 cm^2.

representative of *in vivo* conditions. Otherwise the interpretation of the dermal absorption potential of the test chemical would be compromised.

Receptor Fluid and Solubility of the Test Chemical

The OECD Test Guideline 428[5] permits a range of receptor fluids (RFs) that can be used for *in vitro* percutaneous absorption studies. The primary reason for this is the wide-ranging physicochemical properties of the test substances that are being measured. The key principle here is that the test substance must be adequately soluble in the chosen RF. If the solubility of the test substance exceeds 10% of its saturated concentration during a study, then the diffusion (and therefore the quantity of material in the receptor) may be underestimated since sink conditions have not been maintained. This is stated in the OECD Guidance Document[6] and is a key element relating to the interpretation of these studies. For example, if a lipophilic test substance is used with an aqueous receptor, then it is likely that the test substance with a poor aqueous solubility will tend to partition into the skin tissue rather than into the RF. Hence, measurements of the chemical in the RF would underestimate the absorption rate, due to improper test conditions related to RF solubility. This effect can have a greater impact when full-thickness skin is used, compared with epidermal membranes; thicker tissues can have a greater effect on the distribution of the test substance. If the RF does not adequately solubilize the test substance, then a proportion of the dose applied to the skin surface that remains in the tissue following surface decontamination at the end of the exposure period should be included as absorbed.

Many laboratories undertaking *in vitro* percutaneous absorption studies pay insufficient attention to the skin:receptor partitioning effects that are key to the *in vitro* method. Where test substances are freely water soluble, there is not much of a problem and saline-based receptors should be acceptable. However, when test substances are less water soluble, investigators often incorporate surfactants or other additives to the aqueous receptor to "improve" the solubility of the chemical under study. It clearly states in the OECD guidance that the solubility in the receptor should be established and that it is not a rate-limiting step.[6] For the more lipophilic test substances, even those that penetrate the skin relatively easily, the addition of "solubilizers" such as polyethylene glycol, albumin, and so on to the receptor may not be adequate to maintain the sink conditions. One option, rather than supplement a physiological medium with solubilizers, is to select an appropriate solvent system that ensures that partitioning from skin to receptor is not rate limiting. Many laboratories use ethanol: water mixtures that are permitted in OECD 428, as a universal receptor approach to achieve this.[18,19] Skin absorption is a passive process and does not rely on active biochemical processes. The rate and extent of absorption is determined by the ability of the test substance to diffuse through the skin barrier, the SC, which is a nonliving tissue. Clearly, if the objective of the study involves assessment of skin metabolism and not just diffusion, then only a physiological receptor can be used. This is carefully spelled out in the OECD Test Guideline 428.[5] It is important to recognize that the OECD guideline is primarily designed to assess the risk from systemic exposure to the chemical in question by measuring the quantity of the chemical that can diffuse from the surface of the skin and into the RF. When a solvent-based receptor is used, which invariably aids the partitioning of the test material from skin to receptor, it is unlikely that the amount of test substance absorbed will be underestimated. There are other advantages of the universal receptor approach when it comes to measurement of the test substance. Specific cold analytical methods are compatible with ethanol: water mixtures, whereas other solubilizing additives can interfere with a number of nonradiolabeled methods of analysis.

OECD guidance on the *in vitro* method for percutaneous absorption also states that the choice of receptor medium should not affect skin preparation integrity. Guidance is given elsewhere in this chapter and in other published reports about the various methods for assessing skin integrity and the advantages/disadvantages of each approach.[17] Naturally, if a simple physiological receptor solution of isotonic saline is used, then this is less likely to cause any changes to the tissue that could indirectly affect dermal absorption. However, use of solubilizers and solvents are more likely to act as absorption enhancers and increase the absorption of the test chemical. Therefore, in the context of risk assessment, any increase in overall skin absorption caused by a solvent system would be deemed as conservative. It should be pointed out that studies comparing *in vitro* and *in vivo* absorption that have utilized solvent receptors have shown that the *in vitro* approach generally overpredicts *in vivo* absorption.[1,18,19] If the effect of the receptor on the skin barrier is an important aspect of the study, the skin integrity can also be measured following exposure to the test chemical. This is useful in the context of study performance or where potentially irritant adjuvants are used in products together with the test substance being measured.[20] Skin integrity checks in untreated controls undertaken at the end of the exposure period can also be used to demonstrate that the receptor medium does not cause barrier disruption in its own right.

Reference Chemicals

The consensus is that the *in vitro* percutaneous absorption method can predict *in vivo* absorption when evaluating the potential systemic exposure of chemicals and formulated products following dermal application.[5,8] However, since the *in vitro* method was not subjected to a formal validation program, there are still a number of key issues relating to the methodology that do not have sufficient published scientific evidence to make the method universally acceptable by all regulatory authorities dealing with pesticide registration. The OECD guidance directs any new laboratory to demonstrate their competency with the *in vitro* technique by providing data on specific reference chemicals. The reference chemicals named in the OECD guidance are benzoic acid, caffeine, and testosterone. These widely studied compounds cover a range of polarities since this particular physicochemical property can have a major influence on skin absorption. The skin integrity characteristics of human skin that was sourced, prepared, and stored in different laboratories (Syngenta Central Toxicology Laboratory [CTL] in the United Kingdom and TNO in The Netherlands) was compared. The permeability coefficient for tritiated water was very similar in the two labs with values of 1.0×10^{-3} cm/h (CTL) and 1.1×10^{-3} cm/h (TNO) for groups of six normal human skin samples. This study determined how transferable two independent methods of measuring *in vitro* percutaneous absorption was by comparing data for tritiated water flux and that of the three reference chemicals benzoic acid, caffeine, and testosterone. A standard protocol was used to study the reference chemicals under GLP in the two laboratories using different diffusion skin cell equipment. The chemicals were applied in a universal application vehicle (1 mg/mL in a 50% ethanol in physiological saline vehicle). The application rate was 100 μL/cm^2 ($\equiv$ 100 μg penetrant/cm^2) and the donor chambers were occluded for the entire exposure period (24 hours) to maximize absorption of the test penetrants.

The two laboratories routinely use the *in vitro* percutaneous absorption method and have many years experience of it. As shown in Table 10.2, the permeability to the three test chemicals was also very similar in the two labs, indicating robustness of the method. A wider study (Evaluations and Predictions of Dermal Absorption of Toxic Chemicals [EDETOX]) involving many labs that had less experience with *in vitro* percutaneous absorption showed where the potential pitfalls that can lead to variability are, but nevertheless there was reasonable concordance across labs.[21]

Data Interpretation

Generally for dermal absorption studies on crop protection products, the application is finite (low volume) rather than infinite (high volume), and the results of the study tend to be presented as percentage absorbed, rather than flux. The reason for this

Table 10.2 Interlaboratory Comparison of Reference Chemicals Using Human Epidermal Membranes

Test chemical	TNO	CTL	TNO	CTL
	Absorption after 24 hours (%)		Max. absorption rate ($\mu g/cm^2/h$)	
Caffeine	6 ± 1.1	8 ± 1.3	0.3 ± 0.04	0.5 ± 0.08
Testosterone	36 ± 3.7	21 ± 4.7	1.7 ± 0.19	1.2 ± 0.27
Benzoic acid	63 ± 1.8	69 ± 3.0	5.3 ± 0.45	3.4 ± 0.15

Mean values (± standard error of the mean) for $n = 10$ observations in each case.
CTL, Syngenta Central Toxicology Laboratory; TNO, TNO Nutrition and Food Research Institute.

type of data presentation is that the majority of the regulatory authorities prefer this format; it is more readily applicable to their safety calculation procedures.

Following both *in vivo* and *in vitro* studies, there is sometimes a high proportion of test chemical remaining in the SC and/or underlying skin at the end of the study. This is particularly the case with more highly lipophilic substances, or with chemicals that bind to skin components (e.g., amines). This fraction is not classed as absorbed (the OECD definition of absorbed dose is the test substance reaching the RF or systemic circulation within a specified period of time).[5] However, in the interpretation of data by regulatory authorities, the SC/skin fraction may be included as potentially absorbable unless there is good evidence that it is not absorbable.[11] The reason for this approach is to ensure a conservative risk assessment.

In cases where the risk assessment is not acceptable following this conservative approach, it is important to have more information about the fate of the chemical found in the skin layers. This is best achieved by incorporating a tape-stripping technique into the study protocol. This has been shown to be a good predictor of the skin distribution of chemicals in man.[22] For studies involving crop protection products, the so-called dislodgeable dose that can be washed off the skin following dermal exposure using normal soap/water sponge-type decontamination is followed by a technique that usually involves taking five strips of the SC sequentially. The test substance is then measured in each strip and presented for each skin sample. This allows the regulatory authority to look at the profile of penetration into the SC and to include or exclude the dose present in this layer as potentially systemically available, or a proportion of the tape strips. There is a current debate as to whether the first two tape strips should be regarded as unabsorbed since the test material may simply be adsorbed onto the skin surface and not actually in the tissue itself. Different designs of skin diffusion cells make the surface decontamination easy or difficult. Conventional large surface area glass static diffusion cells can be fully dismantled and the skin surface can be thoroughly washed with soap and water using a dissolvable natural sponge.[22] Other smaller flow-through devices make the skin washing process more difficult so the dislodgeable fraction may be underestimated in such devices and a higher dermal absorption value may result if the whole of the skin tissue is assumed to be an "absorbable" compartment.

The diffusion of a chemical through skin is a complex, dynamic process. Although the processes are governed by the physicochemistry of the test substance and the structure of the skin layers, it is difficult to describe the whole process in mathematical terms. Mathematical models do exist and relate to various aspects of conditions of skin absorption,[23] but there are no useful models to cover the most common exposure scenarios that involve formulated products where the mixture may contain emulsifiers and surface-active adjuvants in addition to the active chemical.

During *in vivo* and *in vitro* dermal absorption studies, the test chemical will be in one or more of these compartments:

a. dislodgeable from the skin surface at the end of exposure

b. remain associated with the application or protection system, or as contamination on the surface of the skin outside the treated area

c. remain bound to the skin surface at the treatment site (difficult to remove)

d. remain in the SC

e. remain in the epidermis

f. remain in the dermis or deeper tissue layers

g. be absorbed (present in the RF or systemic circulation)

The fractions (a), (b), and (c) are clearly not absorbed, and the fraction (g) is clearly absorbed. For the other fractions the question is, what would be the fate of the fraction if the study duration was beyond the exposure period being studied? If it would be sloughed off the skin surface by the normal desquamation of the skin layers, then it would not be absorbed. If it diffuses into the dermis, then it would be absorbed. In most cases, there is no experimental evidence to substantiate this. However, in studies with human volunteers, it is common to find that the majority of the residue in the SC is lost by desquamation.[24] Similarly, in rodent studies on pesticide products, where rats have been carefully bandaged daily to trap desquamated skin, it is common to find a significant portion of the SC fraction is lost and not absorbed. In a model with human skin grafted onto nude mice, it was shown that even with a highly lipophilic molecule (lindane), the majority of the SC fraction was lost by desquamation.[14]

In the case of *in vitro* studies, the study is commonly terminated at 24 hours (due to the slow degeneration of skin integrity *in vitro*). Therefore, it is more difficult to be certain of the potential fate of chemical remaining at the treated site because the time profile over several days can only be studied *in vivo*. The solubility of the test item in the RF is an important factor affecting the amount of residue in the skin. For materials of low lipophilicity, the partitioning of the test item into the RF from the skin is not a problem. In these cases, the amount of test item remaining in the SC/skin is generally relatively small, except when chemicals bind to the skin layers. For more lipophilic chemicals, the use of a more lipophilic RF will favor partitioning into the RF from the skin. This is designed to model the physiological situation of the capillary circulation *in vivo*, which would remove chemicals reaching the epidermis–dermis interface by diffusion into the circulating blood. Therefore, for more lipophilic chemicals, either a more lipophilic RF must be used, or the skin fraction must be included with the absorbable dose.

For *in vivo* studies, the daily measurements of excreted test chemical gives an estimate of the elimination profile with time. When this shows that all or almost all elimination is complete, then we can be confident that no or almost no more chemical is being absorbed from the application site. However, if the elimination process is slow, then this demonstrates that either the chemical is still becoming available to the systemic circulation at the application site or that the elimination characteristics from the various internal compartments are slow. Data from the elimination characteristics following administration via another route can help to clarify which of these factors are relevant.

Agencies regulating pesticide products will take a conservative approach, often including the SC/skin fraction into the absorbable dose. Therefore, the study design should allow for this and where a significant skin residue remains, appropriate data should be produced to show the likely fate of the skin dose. An example of this would be for a chemical that binds to skin: A rat *in vivo* study can show that after the exposure period, no further chemical becomes available systemically, and a significant percentage of the amount in the SC is lost by desquamation daily. This evidence can be sufficient to exclude the SC/skin residue in the absorbable dose in risk assessment calculations.

REFERENCES

1. ECETOC. Percutaneous Absorption. European Centre for Ecotoxicology and Toxicology of Chemicals (ECETOC) Monograph No. 20, Brussels, 1993.
2. Howes D, Guy R, Hadgraft J, et al. Methods for assessing percutaneous absorption, report and recommendations of ECVAM Workshop Report 13. *Alternatives To Laboratory Animals* 1996; 24: 81–106.
3. Diembeck W, Beck H, Benech-Kieffer F, et al. Test guidelines for *in vitro* assessment of dermal absorption and percutaneous penetration of cosmetic ingredients. *Food and Chemical Toxicology* 1999; 37: 191–205.
4. OECD. OECD 427 Guideline for the Testing of Chemicals. Skin Absorption: In Vivo Method. Organisation for Economic Cooperation and Development, Paris, 2004. Adopted April 13, 2004.
5. OECD. OECD 428 Guideline for the Testing of Chemicals. Skin Absorption: In Vitro Method. Organisation for Economic Cooperation and Development, Paris, 2004. Adopted April 13, 2004.
6. OECD. OECD Guidance Document Number 28 for the Conduct of Skin Absorption Studies. Organisation for Economic Cooperation and Development, Paris, 2004.
7. Koeter HBWM. Dialogue and Collaboration: A personal view on laboratory animal welfare developments in general, and on ECVAM's first decade in particular. *Alternatives to Laboratory Animals* 2002; 30(Suppl. 2): 207–210.
8. IPCS. Dermal Absorption. Geneva, World Health Organization, International Programme on Chemical Safety No. 235. Environmental Health Criteria, 2006.
9. U.S. EPA. Proposed test rule for *in vitro* dermal absorption rate testing of certain chemicals of interest to Occupational Safety and Health Administration; Proposed rule. *Federal Register* 1999; 64(110): 31073–31090.

10. U.S. EPA. Health Effects Test Guidelines. OPPTS 870.7600. Dermal Penetration. U.S. Environmental Protection Agency, 1998; 1–12.
11. EC. Commission Directive 94/79/EC Amending Council Directive 91/414/EEC Concerning the Placing of Plant Protection Products on the Market. Official Journal of the European Communities No. L 354, 21 December 1994.
12. VAN HEMMEN JJ. EUROPOEM, a predictive occupational exposure database for registration purposes of pesticides. *Applied Occupational and Environmental Hygiene* 2001; 16: 246–250.
13. EC. Guidance Document on Dermal Absorption. SANCO/222/2000 rev. 7. European Commission, 2004; 1–15.
14. CAPT A, LUZY AP, ESDAILE D, et al. Comparison of the human skin grafted onto nude mouse model with *in vivo* and *in vitro* models in the prediction of percutaneous penetration of three lipophilic pesticides. *Regulatory Toxicology and Pharmacology* 2007; 47: 274–287.
15. HEYLINGS JR, ESDAILE DJ. Percutaneous absorption of pesticides. In: Roberts MS, Walters KA, eds. *Dermal Absorption and Toxicity Assessment*, 2nd ed. Informa Healthcare, New York, 2007; 575–591.
16. FASANO WJ, MANNING LA. Rapid integrity assessment of rat and human epidermal membranes for *in vitro* dermal regulatory testing: Correlation of electrical resistance with tritiated water permeability. *Toxicology In Vitro* 2002; 16: 731–740.
17. DAVIES DJ, WARD RJ, HEYLINGS JR. Multi-species assessment of electrical resistance as a skin integrity marker for *in vitro* percutaneous absorption studies. *Toxicology In Vitro* 2004; 18: 351–358.
18. SCOTT RC, BATTEN PL, CLOWES HM, et al. Further Validation of an *In vitro* method to reduce the need for *in vivo* Studies for measuring the absorption of chemicals through rat skin. *Fundamental and Applied Toxicology* 1992; 19: 484–492.
19. RAMSEY JD, WOOLLEN BH, AUTON TR, et al. The predictive accuracy of *in vitro* measurements for the dermal absorption of a lipophilic penetrant (fluazifop-butyl) through rat and human skin. *Fundamental and Applied Toxicology* 1994; 23: 230–236.
20. HEYLINGS JR, DIOT S, ESDAILE DJ, et al. A prevalidation study on the *in vitro* skin irritation function test (SIFT) for prediction of acute skin irritation *in vivo*: Results and evaluation of ECVAM phase III. *Toxicology In Vitro* 2003; 17: 123–138.
21. WILLIAMS FM. EDETOX evaluations and predictions of dermal absorption of toxic chemicals. *International Archives of Occupational and Environmental Health* 2004; 77: 150–151.
22. TREBILCOCK KL, HEYLINGS JR, WILKS MF. *In vitro* tape stripping as a model for *in vitro* skin stripping. *Toxicology In Vitro* 1994; 8: 665–667.
23. POTTS RO, GUY RH. Predicting skin permeability. *Pharmaceutical Research* 1992; 9: 663–669.
24. RAMSEY JD, WOOLLEN BH, AUTON TR, et al. Pharmacokinetics of fluazifop-butyl in human volunteers II: Dermal dosing. *Human and Experimental Toxicology* 1992; 11: 247–254.
25. SCOTT RC, CARMICHAEL NG, HUCKLE KR, et al. Methods for measuring dermal penetration of pesticides. *Food and Chemical Toxicology* 1993; 31: 523–529.

Part Two

Topical and Transdermal Product Development

Chapter 11

An Overview of Product Development from Concept to Approval

Adam C. Watkinson

INTRODUCTION

This chapter is by no means exhaustive. Whole books are available that discuss pharmaceutical development; indeed, whole books are available that discuss what might appear to the outsider to be the smallest details of pharmaceutical development. This chapter simply serves as a brief introduction to the process of developing new pharmaceutical products and makes reference to a few specific examples where transdermal products raise specific issues. The chapters that follow this are written by the true experts.

IDEAS AND MONEY

Harvey Firestone (1868–1938) was the founder of the Firestone Tire and Rubber Company, one of the first global makers of car tires and a leading industrialist in the United States in the early twentieth century. He is credited with the following quote:

> *Capital isn't so important in business. Experience isn't so important. You can get both these things. What is important is ideas. If you have ideas, you have the main asset you need, and there isn't any limit to what you can do with your business.*

This suggests that, if an idea is good enough, it will attract funding. This may have been the case in the late nineteenth and early twentieth centuries but, particularly in today's financial environment, is not necessarily true now. There are so many more well-educated and informed people who are so connected in today's world that

Transdermal and Topical Drug Delivery: Principles and Practice, First Edition. Edited by Heather A.E. Benson, Adam C. Watkinson.
© 2012 John Wiley & Sons, Inc. Published 2012 by John Wiley & Sons, Inc.

there are many, many more ideas out there seeking funding. This is why it is important to differentiate these ideas into those that relate to pure science and those that relate to something that can be sold at a profit. In this respect, it is important to understand the distinction between "science" or "research" and a product concept. A product concept, more often than not, originates from an understanding of the market and its unmet needs rather than a deep understanding of some esoteric branch of science. The notion that "eureka moments" are responsible for successful product concepts is dubious at best and the thought that the ideas behind successful product concepts materialize out of nowhere is downright naïve. If there is a key moment of realization involved, it is usually based on a very large investment of time and effort beforehand and often requires a deep understanding of the field in which it also arises as a prerequisite. Once a market need has been identified, qualified, and quantified, then science and research can be given direction and purpose. As examples, these markets might be as broad as "a cure for cancer" or as narrow as "the alleviation of a specific drug side effect by changing the delivery route." The point being that, given an objective or "target product profile," research efforts can be directed appropriately.

The expectations and motivations of those funding the development of concepts into products will usually shape the nature of the direction and purpose of research. Shareholders in private or public companies will be focused on adding value and shaping exit strategies to reap some of this value for themselves. Conversely, governments and charitable organizations may be focused on solving wider health issues in a manner not designed to make them richer but, in the case of the former, perhaps to save money or resources and in the case of the latter, maybe to simply save lives or make them more bearable. The pharmaceutical industry per se is more focused on the former approach simply because of where the majority of its funding comes from. Industry involvement in government and charity-funded work is usually motivated by something that adds to their bottom line—"What's in it for me?" being a not unreasonable question for them to ask of our leaders and aid organizations. The matter of funding pharmaceutical product development (the metamorphosis of a concept into a product) is not a topic for this chapter to dwell too much on; suffice to say, it usually comes from one of the three sources mentioned above (investors, governments, or charitable organizations) and the source of funding will usually determine the nature of the product being developed.

PROTECTING INVESTMENTS

It takes a lot of money to develop a pharmaceutical product. It doesn't really matter how much exactly (the figure seems to increase year on year), but it is always a lot. The ultimate promise that a successful product must meet is that it will sell well enough to justify the investment required to develop and market it. The return required to satisfy this need is defined by the investor but one thing is certain: that return will be reduced spectacularly if the product can be copied cheaply and undercut in price. There are several strategies available to organizations to protect their investments against such attacks, or at least to delay them for a while.

The main strategies for protection in the pharmaceutical industry are the judicious use of patents and regulatory exclusivity periods. A patent is a set of exclusive rights granted (by a national government) to an inventor or their assignee in exchange for public disclosure of their invention. The exclusive rights are granted for a limited time (a minimum of 20 years from the date of filing of the patent) and do not necessarily mean that the patentee can exploit the invention (as it may rely partially on the inventions of others) but that no one else can do so without their permission. The original purpose of patents was to encourage innovation and spread understanding of new ideas such that innovation proliferates more rapidly than may happen if inventions were simply unpublished secrets. The modern patent system in Europe can be traced back to the fifteenth-century Republic of Venice, while the first U.S. Congress adopted a patent act in 1790 and granted its first patent in the same year. To obtain a patent, an invention must be (1) novel, (2) not obvious, (3) useful, and (4) adequately disclosed in the patent application to enable practice of the invention. Patents in the pharmaceutical arena are commonly based on drug molecule structure, treatment of specific diseases, methods of drug delivery, descriptions of medical devices or formulations, or methods of manufacturing. Such patents prevent generic alternatives from entering the market until the patents expire, and thus maintain the often high prices of medication. For a blockbuster drug, each month of exclusivity could be worth $100 million or more. Despite the term of a patent being 20 years, in the pharmaceutical world this is never the period of exclusivity it confers on a product because the development process takes so long and patentees must file early in this process to ensure protection. U.S. patent law was changed by the 1984 Hatch–Waxman Act (the Drug Price Competition and Patent Term Restoration Act) to try and ease these problems by extending periods of exclusivity to compensate for the time lost during clinical trials and the regulatory approval process.[1] The act also created incentives for generic companies to rapidly enter the market on patent expiry via the ANDA (Abbreviated New Drug Application) process and subsequent legislation has granted companies extended exclusivity for marketing drugs with orphan status and for providing data on the use of the product in pediatric indications. At the time of writing there is no abbreviated process to approve biotechnology products and discussions about so-called biosimilar products are ongoing. There is much debate about the patent system as it relates to pharmaceutical products and Barton and Emanuel provide an interesting perspective on much of it.[2]

DRUG DISCOVERY, FORMULATION, AND TOXICOLOGY TESTING

Broadly, these are the phases of development that a new product must negotiate prior to entering into human clinical trials. Depending on the product and/or eventual indication, there are potentially many different types of testing required at this stage. For most transdermal and topical products to date, this has largely involved formulating existing drugs into patches or topical formulations (not a trivial exercise by any means), *in vitro* skin permeation testing, toxicology testing, irritation and sensitization testing, and possibly the use of *in vivo* animal models for assessing drug delivery per se. If the development program involves switching an oral drug to a transdermal form then the matter of potentially flatter plasma levels versus the peaks and troughs of oral delivery must be considered. If efficacy of an oral product is associated with achieving a certain C_{max}, then it is unlikely that a transdermal presentation is a good idea as overall exposure would need to be higher. However, if matching up area under the curve (AUC) values is what is required, then the rationale for a switch to transdermal is often simpler. Drugs with narrow therapeutic windows are especially suited in these cases but the variability associated with transdermal delivery per se must also be considered. Most of these stages of development are the subject of subsequent chapters in this book so they will not be covered in any depth here.

CLINICAL TRIALS

Once a drug or formulation has been created and passed through the stages described briefly above, the next phase of its journey toward the market involves ensuring it is safe and efficacious in its intended patient population. Entering into human clinical trials is a very serious business and, quite rightly, they are regulated very tightly by government agencies (regulatory authorities) across the globe.

Until recently, Phase I trials were where a clinical development program began. In fairly recent times, a novel approach to the assessment of drug pharmacokinetics (PK) in man has seen increasing use. So-called Phase 0 studies use very low doses (the trials are often referred to as microdosing trials) to establish whether the drug behaves in human subjects as was expected from pre-clinical studies. Because the doses used are so low there is usually not such a large safety element to such trials as for those that follow.

Phase I trials are typically conducted in small groups (perhaps 12–24) of healthy volunteers with doses of drug that have been carefully selected during pre-clinical development. Phase I trials are usually conducted in a clinical trial unit where the volunteers are kept under medical supervision. The less that is known about the drug under test and the more potential there are for side effects, the greater the level of medical supervision that will be required. Most trials are designed to assess the PK associated with a particular drug or formulation and therefore involve frequent blood sampling over appropriate periods of time. In the first instance, a single-dose study is usually conducted, and when the drug is new, a single-ascending-dose study will be performed to safely raise the dose to the predicted therapeutic levels. Data from this can be used to model the PK of multiple doses and assist in the design of an appropriate multiple-dose study that may involve subjects taking the drug over a period of several days or longer. Depending on the number of formulations to be tested these trials may be cross-over trials or utilize parallel groups of subjects to save time. As well as basic PK data, Phase I trials are used to gain an initial understanding of the safety, tolerability, and pharmacodynamics of a drug.

For drugs undergoing bioequivalence testing, Phase I-type trials are all that are required from a clinical and regulatory perspective. A regulatory authority will stipulate how "similar" the PK of a new formulation must be to be considered the same as an already approved product. In the European Union (EU) and the United States, if the 90% confidence intervals of the relative mean PK parameters (C_{max}, $AUC_{(0-t)}$, and $AUC_{(0-\infty)}$) of the new product and reference are within 80%–125%, then the two are considered bioequivalent. For oral drugs, "food effects" must sometimes be examined by conducting these comparisons in both fed and unfed states. Such testing is not required for transdermal drugs, but in recent times other Phase I-type testing has been required for drugs delivered through the skin. Table 11.1 summarizes some of the assessments that have been conducted with transdermal products as a requirement for their registration. Some of these are done at different times postdose also, for example the effect of washing the application site of a gel might be studied at 1, 6, and 12 hours after application of the formulation. Depending on the regulatory review (and drug involved), such studies may not be required but the product label may have to contain statements to the effect that the studies have not been conducted and that the patient should avoid a particular circumstance, for example taking a sauna or going swimming. It is not uncommon for studies such as these to be requested by regulatory authorities during the regulatory review process. The question of drug transfer is certainly an issue that is on the U.S. Food and Drug Administration's (FDA) current agenda and has resulted in a black box warning on all U.S. nonocclusive transdermal testosterone products to be aware of the dangers. This is an excellent example of where pharmacovigilance in the form of Periodic Safety Update Reports (PSURs; reports that capture adverse events associated with a products use in the market) has captured

Table 11.1 Examples of Additional Phase I Type Studies Required by Regulatory Authorities for Transdermally Administered Products

Occlusive transdermal systems (patches)	Nonocclusive transdermal systems (gels, solutions, etc.)
Effect of bathing/showering on patch adhesion and drug delivery	Effect of washing the application site on drug delivery
Effect of physical exertion (exercise) on patch adhesion and drug delivery	Demonstration of effective removal of drug from skin surface
Effect of elevated external temperature on patch adhesion and drug delivery	Assessment of drug exposure in third parties that contact the dosed skin of the patient
	Assessment of effectiveness of interventions (e.g., clothing) to reduce drug transfer
	Assessment of any interaction with cosmetic products such as antiperspirants on drug delivery

an issue (transfer) and how it has changed the labeling of a number of products after their launch.

Phase II trials are performed on larger groups (20–300) and are designed to assess the dose of drug required (Phase IIA) and the efficacy of the drug (Phase IIB). Many trials combine both of these objectives. The larger number of subjects involved in these trials also allows a little more to be learned about drug safety and potential toxicity. Prior to Phase II, it is sensible to fix any formulation issues that may have arisen during the initial Phase I trials. As far as transdermals are concerned, two of the main issues observed in Phase I are skin irritation and poor patch adhesion to the skin. As most transdermal development programs to date have utilized known drugs, it is not usually the efficacy of the drug that is in question but the ability of the formulation to deliver it effectively and safely. It is therefore a much more reasonable approach to sort out these issues in Phase I than later in the development program. Indeed, because of the known efficacy of most drugs delivered transdermally, it is not unusual to look at their development programs and see only a small Phase II or even no formal Phase II study at all. If the relationship between the PK and efficacy is reasonably well established, some programs jump from Phase I to Phase III. In these instances, it is even more important to have ironed out any product performance issues prior to moving the product forward from Phase I. Drug development has a habit of "running away with itself" and companies must be careful not to unwittingly take products into Phase II or beyond when they have flaws (perhaps an adhesion problem for a patch, for example). It is not necessarily wrong to do this, but the developer must be aware that the product will need to be fixed and studies possibly rerun at not insignificant cost. Many anecdotal examples of patches being taken into Phase II and beyond with known adhesion issues exist and one thing is for sure, the market will find you out if a flawed product is ever launched.

Phase III studies are randomized controlled trials conducted in multiple centers and often in multiple countries. Large numbers of patients are typically involved (150–4000 or more depending upon the medical condition in question) because these are the ultimate yardstick by which a regulatory authority will assess the safety and efficacy of a product. Phase III trials are very complex and long (they can take years to complete) and it is wise to obtain regulatory buy-in to their design prior to their commencement (more on this topic later) so that the large expenditure required to fund them is suitably de-risked, to some extent at least. Phase III trials may have additional components that purely address safety rather than efficacy. These may be termed "safety extension studies" and involve a proportion of subjects recruited to a Phase III trial continuing on the medication beyond the efficacy section of the trial such that further data can be collected on the longer-term (or greater patient exposure) safety of the product. While not required in all cases, it is typically expected that there be at least two successful Phase III trials, demonstrating a drug's safety and efficacy, in order to obtain approval from the appropriate regulatory agencies such as the FDA (United States) or the European Medicines Agency (EMA) (EU), for example.

If they deem it appropriate, regulatory bodies can ask companies to conduct further trials after the launch of a product. These postmarketing surveillance trials involving pharmacovigilance (safety surveillance) are often referred to as Phase IV trials. Safety surveillance is designed to detect any rare or long-term adverse effects in a larger patient population and over a longer time period than is possible during the development process of a product. Phase IV trials are also conducted as "marketing studies," the results of which can be used to further back claims for products.

Sietsema (2005) has written an excellent practical review about strategic clinical development planning, trial design, and of the accompanying regulatory process.[3]

CHEMISTRY, MANUFACTURING, AND CONTROLS

Chemistry, manufacturing, and controls (CMC) is the part of pharmaceutical development that deals with the nature of the drug substance and the drug product. CMC focuses, in very great detail, on the manner in which both the drug substance and product are made, and the manner by which the manufacturing process is shown to be in control. The area is very diverse and very heavily regulated, with many guidelines from regulatory bodies in circulation and in development. In many ways this area is always changing, with regulators continually trying to improve the way things are done and controlled. Probably the simplest way to give the reader a flavor for the breadth of the CMC area is to look at the different sections that come under its banner in a New Drug Application (NDA) filing. These are as follows:

Drug Substance

- Name, structure, properties
- Manufacturing process and process controls (from Drug Master File)
- Controls of critical steps and intermediates
- Development and validation of manufacturing process
- Characterization
- Impurities
- Specifications
- Analytical procedures
- Validation of analytical procedures
- Batch analysis data and comparison
- Justification for specifications
- Reference standards or materials
- Packaging/container closure system
- Stability conditions and data (pre- and postapproval)

Drug Product

- Description and composition
- Components (i.e., actives and inactives, excipients)

- Manufacturing process development
- Container closure system
- Microbiology attributes (e.g., sterility, endotoxins, bioburden, preservative efficacy, etc.)
- Compatibility (e.g., extractables, leachables, etc., from primary and secondary contact materials)
- Manufacturer(s)
  - Batch formula
  - Manufacturing process and process controls
  - Controls of critical steps and intermediates
  - Process validation
- Excipient controls (for each excipient)
  - Specifications
  - Analytical procedures
  - Validation of analytical procedures
  - Justification of specifications
- Drug product controls
  - Specifications
  - Analytical procedures
  - Validation of analytical procedures
  - Batch analysis data and comparison
  - Characterization of impurities
  - Justification of specifications
- Reference standards or materials
- Stability conditions and data (pre- and postapproval)
- Executed batch records
- Method validations package
- Literature references

As the above lists show, a lot of attention to detail is required in this area and all aspects of the product and a justification for how it came to be what it is will be required. This can take the form of a development history that discusses and rationalizes the changes made to the product during its development. It is impossible to overstate the importance of getting this portion of development correct and ensuring drug and excipient sources are appropriate for the markets they are entering.

REGULATORY AFFAIRS

As the two major markets for pharmaceuticals are the EU and the United States, this section only covers the regulatory processes in these areas. There are several excellent texts[4,5] that describe the multifaceted process of FDA submission in the United

States in great and practical detail, so the purposes of this section will be served by a brief description of only the major points. Chapter 12 also contains a lot of information that pertains specifically to the regulatory aspects of transdermal and topical development programs.

The three most common types of submission to the FDA for product approval are all types of NDA:

- 505(b)(1) Applications
- 505(b)(2) Applications
- ANDAs

A 505(b)(1) application contains full reports of investigations of safety and effectiveness all conducted by or for the applicant, or the applicant has obtained a right of reference or use for the investigations. A 505(b)(2) application is one in which some or all of the investigations were not conducted by or for the applicant and for which the applicant has not obtained a right of reference or use. The investigations not conducted by the applicant are usually either described in published literature or are the result of prior review by the FDA of supporting data related to the drug in question. The 505(b)(2) approach is most suited to situations where the application involves changes to previously approved drugs (e.g., changes in dosage, route of administration, indication, formulation, and strength). The ANDA was intended to make the review process for generic versions of already approved drug products more efficient by reducing review time and effort. ANDA applications are termed "abbreviated" because they are not required to include pre-clinical and clinical data to establish safety and efficacy but are based on the simplified concept of bioequivalence.

The regulatory process usually begins with a pre-IND (an IND is a file held by FDA containing all information about an Investigational New Drug) meeting and is followed by several other meetings and milestones that correspond to the stage of development reached.

- Pre-IND meeting
- Open (or file) IND
- End of Phase I meeting
- End of Phase II meeting
- Pre-NDA meeting (End of Phase III)
- File NDA
- FDA review of NDA
- Label negotiations
- Approval

In the United States, it is possible to agree with the FDA on certain study designs and very specific end points via a process called the Special Protocol Assessment (SPA). The important outcomes and interpretation of particular pivotal studies (e.g., carcinogenicity studies or Phase III studies) can be agreed in advance of their conduct, which, as long as the agreed criteria are satisfied, can make for an easier review process. However, reaching initial agreement with the FDA on the study design and its interpretation is an open-ended process that can take some time to complete.

In the EU and many other parts of the world, the IND is replaced by a slightly different document known as the Clinical Trial Authorisation (CTA), and although there are some differences between the two approaches they largely serve the same purpose. The main difference is that a new CTA must be submitted per clinical protocol while an IND is opened per product and new protocols added to it.

The system for approval of a product in the EU is perhaps less straightforward than that in the United States and offers a sponsor company a number of options in terms of regulatory processes.

- National procedure
- Mutual recognition
- Decentralized procedure
- Centralized procedure

A national approval procedure takes place in an individual EU country after which a marketing authorization is granted for that particular country only. Approval is based on the successful review of a marketing application by the relevant country's regulatory authority.

Mutual recognition means that EU countries may approve the decision made by another EU country. The sponsor submits their application to the country chosen to carry out the review, which then approves or rejects the application. The other countries have to decide within 90 days whether they approve or reject the decision made by the original country. If a country cannot approve the application on grounds of potential risk to health or to the environment, a prereferral procedure is begun. If the countries fail to reach an agreement during this 60-day procedure, a referral to the Committee for Medicinal Products for Human Use (CHMP) for arbitration may be made through its secretariat at the EMA.

The CHMP is composed of:

- A chair, elected by serving CHMP members
- One member nominated by each of the EU countries
- One member nominated by each of the European Economic Area–European Free Trade Association (EEA-EFTA) countries Iceland and Norway
- Up to five co-opted members, chosen among experts to gain additional expertise in a particular scientific area.

The decentralized procedure is used for products that have not yet received authorization in an EU country. The sponsor may request one or more concerned member states to approve a draft assessment report, summary of product characteristics, labeling, and package leaflet as proposed by a chosen reference member state in 210 days. If a member state cannot approve the assessment report and other documents, a prereferral and then referral (as for the mutual recognition process) to an arbitration process involving the CHMP is begun and resolution achieved as a result.

The Centralised Procedure is an approval process for a medicinal product intended for use in all EU countries and may be obtained by applying to the EMA. Within the EMA, the CHMP prepares an opinion preceding formal approval by the Commission. The assessment work for the application is done by any of the EU countries. On the basis of the opinion from the CHMP, the commission (or the council) issues the formal decision to authorize a product in the centralized procedure. There are some product types for which a centralized procedure is mandatory and these include those derived from biotechnology processes, those for HIV/AIDS, cancer, diabetes, neurodegenerative ailments, autoimmune diseases, and also those for orphan diseases.

Additionally, in Europe, there is a requirement to come to an agreement with regulators about the status of a product with respect to its use in pediatric populations. Since 2007 it has been a requirement that a sponsor needs to have a Paediatric Investigation Plan (PIP) in place and, at the time of filing the Marketing Authorisation Application (MAA), have conducted the studies in it, or to have agreed to defer the performance of these studies or to have been granted a waiver for their requirement.

It is vital to maintain a good relationship with any regulatory body and if it is intended that a product will be marketed in the EU and the United States, it is important to balance and meet the requirements of both. Ultimately, the process of regulatory approval in the United States results in a negotiation around the exact form of the labeling that accompanies a product on launch. A good relationship with the regulatory bodies in question can make for a smoother negotiation process. Statements and assertions contained in pharmaceutical product labeling have to be carefully justified and reflect the content of the regulatory submission and/or acceptable published data. It is not unusual to have to negotiate this label content substantially and for in-depth discussions to be held over what may appear to be small points on wording and meaning. In the EU, this is perhaps less the case, where products will have preexisting core SPC (Summary of Product Characteristics) and PILs (patient information leaflets) and the negotiation is about what is added to these. In all cases, the labeling of a pharmaceutical product is much more than a medication guide; it is a legal document asserting methods for the safe use of the product along with any accompanying risks its use may have. Engaging with regulators in a pragmatic and sensible manner usually gets good results as long as your arguments make sense and are supported by appropriate data.

The preceding section has attempted to capture the complexities of the regulatory process in no more than a few pages and it does not do justice to the amount of work involved in even the simplest regulatory submission. However, hopefully it is a starting place for those setting out on the long road to regulatory approval. A more detailed discussion of the regulatory process (particularly in the

United States) as it pertains to dermal and transdermal delivery is to be found in Chapter 12.

PRODUCT LAUNCH AND BEYOND

It is by no means all over when a product is approved. When all the backslapping of those who developed it is finished, there is a lot of work to be done by those involved in launching and maintaining a product's presence in the market. Areas such as reimbursement, product launch, sales and marketing, citizen's petitions, and patent litigation are obviously all complex undertakings requiring increasingly detailed input from legal experts.

Citizen's petitions, for example, are a mechanism for interested parties to attempt to influence the way the FDA does business. They may suggest that the FDA issue, change, or cancel a regulation, or to take other action. The agency receives about 200 petitions yearly. These petitions are also used by innovator companies in attempts to hinder the launch of generics. Citizen's petitions were filed at the FDA in 2004 objecting to the registration of generic versions of Duragesic (Johnson & Johnson, New Brunswick, NJ) on several grounds. These petitions were filed by Alza, Johnson & Johnson, and related parties (those with an interest in maintaining Duragesic sales) and also two practicing physicians concerned about increased potential for drug abuse associated with generic versions of Duragesic. Companies such as Noven and Mylan that were developing generic forms of fentanyl patches submitted comments to the FDA in opposition to the citizen's petitions, and all four petitions were denied by the FDA in early 2005. Some of the generic patches were not straight copies of Duragesic (a reservoir patch with a rate-controlling membrane) and one of the innovator's objections was to matrix patches that did not contain rate-limiting membranes. This was couched in terms that suggested the dosage forms were therefore not the same. The FDA judged that all transdermal patches are essentially the same dosage form (classified by them as "film, extended release") and that the control in delivery from a matrix patch was essentially the same as from Duragesic and therefore rejected this part of the petition. The FDA also stated that they believe both reservoir and matrix systems have the same abuse potential, all other things being equal. Citizen's petitions have also been filed objecting to the registration of generic versions of a clonidine patch. All these petitions were filed to block the registration of products via the ANDA route where bioequivalence (equal blood levels) is all that is required for registration. There are now several generic clonidine patches on the U.S. market that were approved in 2009 and 2010.

The regulatory process does not end after approval but becomes an ongoing relationship with the authorities, whereby safety monitoring and reporting is the responsibility of the holder of the marketing license. PSURs must be compiled and provided to regulatory authorities for review and these can result in label changes depending on their content. Label changes can also result from findings involving products of a similar type, that is, class labeling changes. The conduct of Phase IV studies may be precipitated by findings in the market or result from regulatory demands also.

CONCLUSION

The process of pharmaceutical development is a long and complex one. It can also be a very expensive business but one that, if completed successfully, can reap great benefits for those involved. Corporations and their shareholders may enjoy financial benefits, academics and governments may earn the admiration of their peers, and societies, sometimes at least, get the medicines and treatments they need. There is, however, a more personal element to the successful development of a new drug product and that is the satisfaction for those involved of working in a multidisciplinary team and to have done it. It's quite a special feeling.

REFERENCES

1. MOSSINGHOFF GJ. Overview of the Hatch-Waxman act and its impact on the drug development process. *Food and Drug Law Journal* 1999; 54: 187–194.
2. BARTON JH, EMANUEL EJ. The patents-based pharmaceutical development process rationale, problems, and potential reforms. *J Am Med Soc* 2005; 294(16): 2075–2082.
3. SIETSEMA WK. *Strategic Clinical Development Planning*. FDA News, Falls Church, VA, 2005.
4. Pisano DJ, Mantus DS (eds.). *FDA Regulatory Affairs—A Guide for Prescriptions Drugs, Medical Devices and Biologics*, 2nd ed. Informa Healthcare, New York, 2008.
5. WEINBERG S. *Guidebook For Drug Regulatory Submissions*. John Wiley & Sons Inc, Hoboken, NJ, 2009.

Chapter 12

Regulatory Aspects of Drug Development for Dermal Products

William K. Sietsema

OVERVIEW OF DRUG DEVELOPMENT AND REGULATORY PROCESS

Development of any new pharmaceutical product is generally divided into a series of phases, beginning with the discovery phase. This is followed by a pre-clinical phase, during which the product's toxicological, pharmacological, pharmacokinetic, and pharmacodynamic properties are examined in experimental animals. Next is Phase I, which involves examination of the safety, pharmacokinetics, and pharmacodynamics, frequently in healthy volunteers. This is followed by Phase II, in which the dose range of the new product is examined so that one can select the minimally effective, optimally effective, and maximally effective doses for further study. In Phase III, a definitive proof of efficacy is provided and the safety is further examined so that a risk/benefit profile can be considered. During these phases, there continues to be an examination of the product's toxicological properties and there is an evolution of the chemistry, manufacturing, and controls used in its preparation, along with production scale-up to enable commercialization. This overall development process is shown graphically in Figure 12.1.

Throughout the development process, it is useful to seek scientific advice from regulatory agencies which will be asked to approve the product. In the United States, there is a well-defined series of advice meetings which begins with a pre-Investigational New Drug (IND) meeting and can continue with an end-of-Phase I, an end-of-Phase II (perhaps even an end-of-Phase IIA meeting), and a pre-New Drug Application (NDA) meeting.[1,2] For Europe, the European Medicines Agency (EMA) allows scientific advice meetings as well as presubmission meetings, which serve a

Transdermal and Topical Drug Delivery: Principles and Practice, First Edition. Edited by Heather A.E. Benson, Adam C. Watkinson.

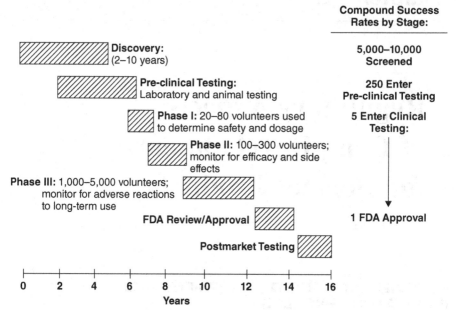

Figure 12.1   Overview of drug development process. Source: Adapted from: WK Sietsema. Strategic Clinical Development Planning. FDAnews. Washington, DC, 2005.

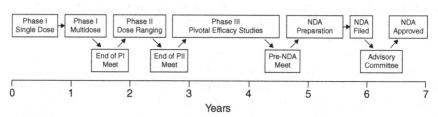

Figure 12.2   Typical sequence of advice meetings, illustrated for the United States.

similar role.[3,4] The Australian Therapeutic Goods Association (TGA) also has a formal procedure for meetings.[5]

A typical sequence of these meetings for the United States is shown in Figure 12.2. In practice, meetings in Europe or Australia or other regions may be held in parallel so that a development program can meet the needs of multiple regions. There is even a pilot program for joint scientific advice meetings between the United States and Europe.[6]

The United States, Europe, and Australia all encourage these meetings with regulatory agencies so that development programs can be designed to better meet the needs of regulators.

REQUIREMENTS FOR CONDUCTING CLINICAL TRIALS

All geographic regions have regulations related to the conduct of clinical trials with unapproved products. In the United States, it is necessary to file an IND before a human clinical trial can be initiated.[7] The IND includes information related to the pharmacology and toxicology of the product, the chemistry, manufacturing, and controls, and the proposed clinical protocol and any clinical results obtained to date.[8] Once the IND has been submitted, the U.S. Food and Drug Administration (FDA) has 30 days to review the information and to decide whether to allow the proposed investigation to proceed. It is also necessary to have approval from an institutional review board (IRB) before the investigation can proceed.

Other geographies have similar procedures. In Australia, there are two schemes under which clinical trials involving unapproved products may be conducted: the Clinical Trial Exemption (CTX) scheme and the Clinical Trial Notification (CTN) scheme.[9,10] Under a CTN, the protocol and other information about the clinical trial is submitted to a Human Research Ethics Committee, which reviews the information for scientific validity, safety, and ethical concerns and approves the conduct of the trial. Under a CTX, information about the product is submitted to the TGA, which reviews for safety, and to the Human Research Ethics Committee, which reviews for scientific validity and ethical concerns.

In Europe, it is necessary to request a Clinical Trial Authorisation (CTA).[11] This request for a CTA is made to the competent authority for each country in which a clinical trial is to be conducted. A CTA generally includes the application form, a clinical protocol, an investigator's brochure, and a summary of what is known about the product, in the form of an Investigational Medicinal Product Dossier (IMPD). Ethics committee approval is also required before human research can be conducted in the European Union.

PHARMACEUTICS

The pharmaceutics of dermal products can be quite different from those of products administered by other routes. The other ingredients included in the formulation will depend on whether the product is intended to have a systemic action, as may be the case with a transdermal scopolamine formulation for prevention of seasickness, or to work locally, as may be the case with lidocaine for local anesthesia. For systemic action, controlled absorption with delivery to the systemic circulation is desired, so often the formulation may include absorption-enhancing substances. For local action, systemic effects may not be desired and excipients may be chosen so as to avoid systemic absorption. In either case, there will be great interest in making certain that the formulation remains on the skin, without exposure to other parts of the body or other persons.

The EMA has issued a guidance document on development pharmaceutics that provides some discussion on items to consider in development of a medicinal formulation, such as physicochemical characteristics of the ingredients, compatibility between components, homogeneity, and performance characteristics.[12] A short section of this guidance addresses special issues with transdermal systems, such as consideration of reservoir properties, adhesion to the skin, and release testing.

HOW DELIVERED AMOUNTS ARE SPECIFIED

With an oral dose form, the dose is generally specified in weight units, such as milligrams. This would not be suitable for many dermal products, particularly if the goal of the product is to achieve systemic absorption. It would also be difficult to compare differing dermal products of the same active ingredient since the amount of active ingredient in the formulation may be the same but the relative absorption could be different.

Accordingly, transdermal products often express the strength as a weight unit "delivered" or absorbed per unit time, for example, micrograms per hour or milligrams per day. This approach is more useful to the prescribing physicians, particularly when there is a need to calculate some equivalency to another formulation, whether it be another transdermal formulation or a formulation with a different route of administration. A good example of this is the transdermal delivery of fentanyl. Many of the transdermal fentanyl products express delivery in micrograms per hour and there may be elaborate charts or formulae to aid in estimating equivalency to other dosage forms or other opioid products.[13]

Another common difference observed with transdermal products is to express the dosage strength as an area of the patch. This is because the delivery of active ingredient across the skin is proportional to the surface area, so an increase in dose level is often associated with an increase in the patch size.[14]

PHARMACOKINETIC EVALUATION OF DERMAL DOSAGE FORMS

Pharmacokinetic evaluation of dermal dosage forms can be quite different from other dosage forms, depending on the drug delivery objectives.

If the product is meant to treat a dermatological disease, it may not be intended to reach the systemic circulation, thus traditional pharmacokinetic methods of measuring the drug concentration in blood may not be useful, other than to assess the quantities which unintentionally reach the systemic circulation. For these dermal products, it may be more relevant to measure drug concentration in tissue biopsies taken from the site of administration.

Additionally, whereas the half-life of a substance in blood will depend on rates of elimination, primarily via metabolism or excretion in the liver or kidney, the half-life of a dermal application may depend heavily on the rate of its exit from the skin, either due to absorption into the body, or washing of the application site, or more rarely metabolism within the skin. Indeed, skin can serve as a reservoir for the substance, creating a sort of sustained-release mechanism. The pharmacokinetics of such a process can be difficult to model.[15]

When the dermal application is intended to reach the systemic circulation, then blood levels of the active agent are considered the "standard" for assessing pharmacokinetics. However, the modeling of pharmacokinetics can be challenging, as the skin often acts as a reservoir. In this case the absorption phase can be prolonged over many days.

A guidance document that discusses some pharmacokinetic issues with transdermal products has been issued by the EMA.[16] Although it does not specifically address the difficulties of modeling pharmacokinetic data from transdermal delivery, it does mention that the effect of changing site of application should be examined if a product is intended to be applied to different areas of the body. The guidance also mentions that it is necessary to evaluate in human subjects the potential for irritation and sensitization at the site of application, as well as the possibility for phototoxicity or photosensitivity.

BIOAVAILABILITY AND BIOEQUIVALENCE OF TRANSDERMAL PRODUCTS

For transdermal products which are intended to deliver an agent into the systemic circulation, the general approach to measuring bioavailability and bioequivalence can be similar to that used for products administered orally.[17] However, there are some additional considerations. An EMA guidance indicates that for transdermal drug delivery forms, bioequivalence should be evaluated after single and multiple dosing.[16] The reason for this is that skin can serve as a reservoir, thus bioequivalence should be studied under steady-state conditions, which require multiple dosing.

On the other hand, for certain types of topical solutions for treatment of dermatological diseases, U.S. regulations allow bioequivalence to be waived.[18]

It is well known that the absorption of an agent through skin can differ dramatically by the skin area to which it is applied, for example, abdomen compared to thigh or arm. For this reason, it is essential that when bioequivalence is being evaluated, that the same body area should be used for all products being tested.[16]

Furthermore, due to the varying characteristics of different types of transdermal devices, there is a concern about repeatability of a demonstration of bioequivalence if the release mechanisms are different for two transdermal dosage forms being compared. In this case, the bioequivalence study should be replicated in order to demonstrate the reliability of the result.[16]

Finally, for demonstration of bioequivalence of two transdermal dosage forms, the EMA emphasizes that in addition to considering the pharmacokinetics, one should also demonstrate the comparability of other characteristics, including adherence, irritation and sensitization, phototoxicity, and the general adverse-event profile.[16]

The FDA does not have a general guidance document for bioequivalence of transdermal formulations. However, bioequivalence requirements are thoroughly described in the Code of Federal Regulations.[19]

DEMONSTRATING BIOEQUIVALENCE FOR LOCALLY ACTING DERMAL PRODUCTS

For substances not intended to reach the systemic circulation, the approach to establishing bioequivalence by measuring systemic concentrations may not be sound. In these cases, a pharmacodynamic or clinical end point approach may be more reliable. This concept is discussed in the EMA guidance[17] and is also discussed in the U.S. Code of Federal Regulations.[20]

The FDA does have a guidance that focuses specifically on topical dermatological corticosteroids.[21] These agents can provide a vasoconstrictive effect, which has been found to be a useful pharmacodynamic end point for establishing bioequivalence. The guidance document goes into great detail on the conduct of an assay, sometimes referred to as the skin blanching method. This assay is also discussed in an EMA publication.[22]

Additionally, there is a general guidance document for bioequivalence of topical dermatological formulations, which includes a detailed discussion of a skin-stripping method for establishing comparability.[18]

TRANSFERENCE STUDIES

Often, a key concern with a dermal product is the potential for the active ingredient to be exposed to subjects other than the intended recipient. This is not so much a concern for patch formulations but can be a serious concern for gels, creams, and sprays. Concern about such transference will be elevated for acutely hazardous substances such as fentanyl.

The mechanism of transference is generally as simple as skin-to-skin contact, for example a parent hugging a child, but can also extend to contamination of surface areas with which subjects may come in contact, including clothing, bedding, and even carpeted areas if contaminated skin cells are shed over long periods of time. For spray formulations, there may be concern about airborne contamination.

At this time, there are no specific guidance documents on transference. However, the FDA and other regulatory agencies expect transference data for any dermal products for which there is a possibility of transference and where such transference could create an acute or chronic hazard to human subjects. Examples of transference data can be found in the package inserts for products such as AndroGel®[23] and EstroGel®[24] and in a paper by Mazer et al. which compares transference potential for a patch versus a gel formulation of testosterone.[25]

Transference studies are generally conducted using a pharmacokinetic end point. The product is applied to the intended recipient and the potential for transference is determined by having an unintended recipient make contact by rubbing the area of application. Transference potential may be examined at short and long time points after application, and in the presence and absence of clothing.

WASHING STUDIES AND INTERFERENCE FROM OTHER APPLIED PRODUCTS

Since the effectiveness of a transdermal product may be decreased if the active ingredient is washed off the skin, most regulatory agencies will expect to see some data on the effect of washing the skin at short and long time points after application. This is of most concern for gel, cream, and spray formulations. The information is generally based on pharmacokinetic studies and is often reflected in the package insert or summary of product information. For example, if washing at short time points after applications suggests that effectiveness of the product is reduced, the patient would be instructed not to wash for some period of time after application. An example of this can be found in the U.S. EstroGel package insert.[24] Examples of study designs can be found in the papers by Schumacher et al.[26] and Rolf et al.[27]

Regulatory agencies may also wish to know what will be the effect of application of other substances such as sunscreen, lotions, or even deodorant on the absorbed dose. This can readily be examined in a simple crossover study in which subjects apply the product either by itself, or in combination with some potentially interfering product. The end point will most likely be pharmacokinetic measures to evaluate any increase or decrease in absorption that is observed.

LOCAL TOLERANCE TESTING REQUIREMENTS IN EXPERIMENTAL ANIMALS AND HUMANS

With topical products, there is a particular concern about local tolerance. Accordingly, suitable studies evaluating local tolerance should be conducted in experimental animals prior to exposing human subjects. The EMA has a guidance document which outlines some of the considerations in such testing.[28] Local tolerance in experimental animals is also mentioned in International Conference on Harmonisation (ICH) M3(R2), which emphasizes that such testing can be included in standard toxicology studies and should not require separate studies.[29] The topic of irritation and sensitivity testing is considered in further detail in Chapter 16.

Most regulatory agencies will also expect to see some evaluation of the potential for local irritancy in humans. This can often be accomplished with appropriate irritancy testing as a secondary measure in one or more pivotal studies. Under certain circumstances, where a pivotal study is not conducted for registration of a new product, it may be necessary to conduct a special study to evaluate the potential for human irritancy. Irritancy of skin is most often evaluated by some variation of the Draize criteria[30,31] or by an irritancy response scale[32] and in addition, there are recommended scales in the FDA guidance on lidocaine products.[37]

PHOTOSAFETY TESTING REQUIREMENTS

For active ingredients which are photoreactive, it is expected that the potential for photoirritation or photoallergy be examined. The FDA has issued a guidance document which outlines methods of assessing these issues.[33] The EMA has a similar guidance document.[34] Keep in mind that inactive excipients may also be photoreactive and may require safety testing.[35]

ASSESSMENT OF ADHESION PROPERTIES

Patch formulations often have difficulty with adhesion characteristics due to the vast variation in skin to which patches are applied. This is made particularly difficult with the wide usage of skin creams and liquid soaps which may contain oils, fats, and waxes that interfere with adhesion. It can be quite challenging to formulate a patch that will remain on the skin for its intended duration of use but can still be removed without damaging the skin.

Regulatory agencies expect that patch adhesion will be evaluated during the development program.[36] The FDA does not have a specific guidance which addresses adhesion of dermal patch products, however the concept is discussed in some detail in a draft guidance on lidocaine patches.[37]

Generally, a measure of adhesion is included in each clinical trial conducted with the product. There is often a question in the patient's daily diary which assesses each day whether a patch product is fully adhered, or whether the patch has started to come loose. A sample diary page is shown in Figure 12.3.

LABELING ASPECTS OF TRANSDERMAL PRODUCTS

Various regulatory agencies have certain expectations on labeling of transdermal products. A draft EMA guidance on content of a Summary of Product Characteristics specifies that for transdermal patches, quantitative information should be provided about the content of active substance within each patch, the mean dose delivered per unit time, and the area of the releasing surface.[38] It is also expected that the Summary of Product Characteristics list all the ingredients of the patch, including the adhesive, the release liner, and the backing material.

The FDA does not specifically include any discussion of dermal products in the general labeling guidance documents. However, dermal products may be mentioned in guidance documents for certain product classes. For example, the guidance document on noncontraceptive estrogen products recommends including the information shown in Figure 12.4 in the package insert.

The same guidance document specifies that for transdermal products, adhesion characteristics should be specified in the package insert.[39]

For Australia, the general guidance for labeling indicates that the product information should specify the quantity of active ingredient, along with the quantity of active ingredient released per unit of time.[40]

PATCH ADHESION

Time of assessment of patch adhesion : |___|___| : |___|___|
(24hr clock)

Did you apply any additional tape to the
patch in this 24 hour period ?   Yes ☐   No ☐

How well did the patch stick in this 24 hour period ? *(tick one box only):*
Please give the actual achieved adhesion, even if tape was used, for example.

0 ☐₀   90% adhered (essentially no lift off of the skin)

1 ☐₁   75% to less than 90% adhered (some edges only lifting off
        of the skin)

2 ☐₂   50% to less than 75% adhered (less than half of the system
        lifting off of the skin)

3 ☐₃   less than 50% adhered but not detached (more than half the
        system lifting off of the skin without falling off)

4 ☐₄   patch detached (patch completely off the skin)

Figure 12.3 Sample diary page for a transdermal patch, showing a typical approach to assessing patch adhesion.

PEDIATRIC USE OF TRANSDERMAL FORMULATIONS

It is worth highlighting that transdermal formulations can be a preferred method of administration for certain pediatric populations. Transdermal formulations may be easy to apply, and may be favored in populations who are unable to swallow or who are averse to an injection. Absorption may be enhanced relative to adults because the stratum corneum, particularly in newborns, is thinner than adults, and more highly perfused, thus favoring drug absorption. The younger pediatric groups also have a higher surface : weight ratio than adults.

1. The rate and extent of absorption (e.g., C_{max}, T_{max}, C_{avg}, AUC, fluctuation index, and parent/metabolite ratio) generated during the clinical pharmacology and biopharmaceutical studies.
2. Data for all the anatomical application sites that will be proposed in the prescribing information.
3. Dose proportionality data for the proposed dosing range.
4. Tables and figures, including baseline-unadjusted levels of estradiol and metabolites. In the event that baseline-adjusted levels are more appropriate, this fact should be clearly indicated.
5. The nominal mean *in vivo* delivery rate.

Figure 12.4   Recommended data to include in U.S. package inserts for transdermal formulations of estrogen-containing products.[39] AUC, area under the curve; C_{max}, maximum concentration; T_{max}, time of maximum concentration; C_{avg}, average concentration.

However, development of pediatric transdermal formulations can also be demanding because there may variability of absorption by site of administration, and absorption characteristics of the skin may vary by age group, thus requiring careful evaluation of age-dependent absorption. These challenges are discussed in some detail in an EMA reflection paper on formulations of choice for pediatric populations.[41]

SPECIAL CONSIDERATIONS FOR TOPICAL PRODUCTS FOR TREATMENT OF PSORIASIS

The EMA has published a guidance document on development of products for the treatment of psoriasis.[42] This publication is particularly useful because it provides insights into the needs of regulators for many types of dermatological diseases. For example, it is recommended to study the absorption and pharmacokinetics of dermatological formulations on both healthy and diseased skin, in order to determine whether differences exist in the product performance. Additionally, the effect of frequency of applications on amount of drug retained as a reservoir in the skin should be examined. Absorption and pharmacokinetics from various application sites and in various age groups should be examined. And as with any program, population pharmacokinetics is expected to play a key role in identifying outlier high and low absorbers and the potential consequences.

SPECIAL CONSIDERATIONS FOR TOPICAL DERMATOLOGICAL CORTICOSTEROIDS

Prescription and over-the-counter corticosteroids are widely used for dermatological applications and their absorption through the skin has been extensively studied. Accordingly, there is considerable guidance on the development of these products. There is an EMA guidance which provides a detailed perspective on the types of

- Skin atrophy, which becomes often irreversible, producing clinical thinning of the skin
- Telangiectasia, purpura, striae
- Rosacea-like and perioral dermatitis with or without skin atrophy
- Rebound, which may lead to steroid "dependence"
- Impairment of healing
- Effects on the eye: increased risk of glaucoma, cataract, and exacerbation of mycosis and of herpes simplex
- Systemic effects, resulting from suppression of the hypothalamo–pituitary–adrenal axis
- Miscellaneous events such as depigmentation, hypertrichosis, and so on.

Figure 12.5   Potential adverse reactions from topical corticosteroids.[43]

data needed for approval of such products.[43] The EMA suggests an evaluation of the effect of several factors on the extent of dermal absorption and clinical efficacy, including the concentration of the active ingredient, the characteristics of the formulation being used to apply the active ingredient, the site of application, the condition of the skin (e.g., damaged or undamaged), and the conditions of application (e.g., occluded or not occluded).

The potential for local adverse reaction should be evaluated, with particular attention to the events outlined in Figure 12.5.

SPECIAL CONSIDERATIONS FOR TOPICAL LIDOCAINE PRODUCTS

The FDA guidance on topical lidocaine products also provides a useful case study of the expectations of a regulatory agency for successful approval of a locally acting, topical product.[37]

This guidance provides detailed expectations, including the number of studies required, study designs, requirements for blinding, and what to measure. There are examples of scoring systems to use for local irritation, and a discussion on how to display patch adhesion data. Of particular interest is advice on tables and listings to be provided as part of the submitted data (see Fig. 12.6).

SPECIAL CONSIDERATIONS FOR TOPICAL FENTANYL PRODUCTS

Fentanyl has enjoyed wide use as a transdermal product for the treatment of painful conditions. However, fentanyl is also a potentially very hazardous medication, as disastrous consequences could result from overexposure or unintended exposure to health-care workers or family members. Due to an increasing interest in the development of generic transdermal fentanyl products, the FDA has issued a guidance which outlines expectations for these products.[44]

1. Center/site, subject number
2. Race, sex, age
3. Adverse events, reason for discontinuation
4. Analysis populations for each patch:
   - Test product per-protocol population for irritation analysis (yes/no), reason for exclusion
   - Reference product per-protocol population for irritation (yes/no), reason for exclusion
   - Test product per-protocol population for sensitization (yes/no), reason for exclusion
   - Reference product per-protocol population for sensitization (yes/no), reason for exclusion
   - Test product per-protocol population for adhesion (yes/no), reason for exclusion
   - Reference product per-protocol population for adhesion (yes/no), reason for exclusion
5. Patch removed due to strong skin irritation reaction (yes/no)
6. Time from first patch application to removal for unacceptable irritation
7. Cumulative number of patches removed for unacceptable irritation
8. Cumulative number of detached patches
9. Reinforced with tape (yes/no)
10. Number of days until reinforcement with tape
11. New patch application due to detachment (yes/no)
12. Date of a new patch application due to detachment
13. Time from application to detachment
14. Designation of skin sensitization (yes/no)
15. Per each visit if data exist
    - Visit number, date of visit, days from baseline
    - Reason for exclusion from each per-protocol population per visit
    - Time from patch application to detachment for both test and reference products
    - Irritation scores for each product
    - Sensitization scores for each product
    - Adhesion scores for each product
    - Identity of the evaluator
    - Adverse events
    - Reason for discontinuation

Figure 12.6   Tables and listings requested by the FDA for evaluation of topical lidocaine products.[37]

The guidance recommends three studies: one to assess pharmacokinetics, another to examine the effect of an overlay on product performance, and a third to assess the potential for irritation and sensitization. As for the lidocaine guidance, the FDA provides a detailed listing of the data analyses they expect to receive.

SUMMARY

Dermal products may be intended to provide systemic exposure for treatment of systemic disease, for example, transdermal testosterone or estrogen for hormonal replacement, or they may be intended to provide local exposure to treat a dermatological disease, for example, postherpetic neuralgia or psoriasis. In either case, regulatory agencies expect that such products be fully characterized with regard to their local and systemic pharmacokinetic and pharmacodynamic properties, and that they be evaluated for their potential toxicological effects and other adverse events. Products designed for topical administration may differ from other products in the way dose levels are expressed, since in most cases only a portion of the administered dose is absorbed.

One particular challenge for dermal products intended for local exposure is the demonstration of bioequivalence; some regulators will expect to see a demonstration of clinical efficacy for such products, which requires larger trials, thus making development more expensive. Development of topically applied products may also require special studies, such as to evaluate transference, or the effect of washing the skin after application, or the effect of coapplication with lotions and antiperspirants. If the product is a patch, the adhesion properties must be examined as an element of any pivotal studies to support registration.

Although dermally applied products have their own unique challenges, there are also unique advantages, so there is no doubt that dermally applied products will play an important role in health care for the foreseeable future.

REFERENCES

1. Food and Drug Administration. Guidance for Industry. Formal Meetings between the FDA and Sponsors or Applicants. United States Department of Health and Human Services. Food and Drug Administration. Centers for Drug and Biologics Evaluation and Review, Washington, DC, May 2009. Available at: http://www.fda.gov/downloads/Drugs/GuidanceComplianceRegulatoryInformation/Guidances/UCM153222.pdf (accessed August 8, 2011).
2. Food and Drug Administration. Guidance for Industry. End-of-Phase 2A Meetings. United States Department of Health and Human Services. Food and Drug Administration. Centers for Drug and Biologics Evaluation and Review, Washington, DC, September 2008. Available at: http://www.fda.gov/downloads/Drugs/GuidanceComplianceRegulatoryInformation/Guidances/ucm079690.pdf (accessed August 8, 2011).
3. European Medicines Agency. EMEA Guidance for Companies Requesting Scientific Advice or Protocol Assistance. European Medicines Agency, London, January 22, 2009. Available at: http://www.emea.europa.eu/pdfs/human/sciadvice/426001en.pdf (accessed August 8, 2011).
4. European Medicines Agency. Draft EMEA Guidance on Pre-Submission Meetings for initial Marketing Authorisation Applications for Human Medicinal Products in the Centralised Procedure. London, January 12, 2007. Available at: http://www.emea.europa.eu/htms/human/presub/38271206en.pdf (accessed August 8, 2011).
5. Therapeutic Goods Administration. Australian Regulatory Guidelines for Prescription Medicines. Appendix 5. Conduct of Meetings between TGA and Sponsors. Therapeutic Goods Administration, Department of Health and Ageing, Canberra, Australia, June 2004. Available at: http://www.tga.gov.au/pdf/pm-argpm-ap05.pdf (accessed August 8, 2011).
6. Food and Drug Administration. SOPP 8001.6: Procedures for Parallel Scientific Advice with European Medicines Agency (EMEA); Pilot. United States Department of Health and Human Services. Food and Drug Administration, Center for Drug Evaluation and Research, Washington, DC, June 3, 2009. Available at: http://www.fda.gov/BiologicsBloodVaccines/GuidanceComplianceRegulatoryInformation/ProceduresSOPPs/ucm061218.htm (accessed August 8, 2011).
7. Food and Drug Administration. Guidance for Industry. Content and Format of Investigational New Drug Applications (INDs) for Phase 1 Studies of Drugs, Including Well-Characterized, Therapeutic,

Biotechnology-derived Products. United States Department of Health and Human Services, Food and Drug Administration, Centers for Drug and Biologics Evaluation and Research, Washington, DC, November 1995. Available at: http://www.fda.gov/downloads/Drugs/GuidanceComplianceRegulatoryInformation/Guidances/ucm074980.pdf (accessed August 8, 2011).

8. Code of Federal Regulations. Title 21–Food and Drugs. Chapter I—Food and Drug Administration, Department of Health and Human Services. Part 312—Investigational New Drug Application. Washington, DC, April 1, 2009. Available at: http://www.access.gpo.gov/nara/cfr/waisidx_09/21cfr312_09.html (accessed August 8, 2011).

9. Therapeutic Goods Administration. *The Australian Clinical Trial Handbook. A Simple, Practical Guide to the Conduct of Clinical Trials to International Standards of Good Clinical Practice (GCP) in the Australian Context.* Therapeutic Goods Administration, Department of Health and Ageing, Canberra, Australia, 2006. Available at: http://www.tga.gov.au/pdf/clinical-trials-handbook.pdf (accessed August 8, 2011).

10. Therapeutic Goods Administration. Access to Unapproved Therapeutic Goods via the Special Access Scheme. Therapeutic Goods Administration, Department of Health and Ageing, Canberra, Australia, November 2009. Available at: http://www.tga.gov.au/pdf/access-sas-guidelines.pdf (accessed August 8, 2011).

11. European Commission. Detailed guidance on the request to the competent authorities for authorisation of a clinical trial on a medicinal product for human use, the notification of substantial amendments and the declaration of the end of the trial. European Commission. Enterprise Directorate—General. Single market: Management & legislation for consumer goods Pharmaceuticals: Regulatory framework and market authorizations. Revision 3. Brussels, Belgium. March 30, 2010. http://ec.europa.eu/health/files/eudralex/vol-10/2010_c82_01/2010_c82_01_en.pdf (accessed August 8, 2011).

12. European Medicines Agency. Note for Guidance on Development Pharmaceutics. European Medicines Agency, London, England, January 28, 1998. Available at: http://www.emea.europa.eu/pdfs/human/qwp/015596en.pdf (accessed August 8, 2011).

13. Duragesic Fentanyl Transdermal System. US Prescribing Information. February 2008. Available at: http://www.duragesic.com/duragesic/shared/pi/duragesic.pdf (accessed August 8, 2011).

14. Climara Estradiol Transdermal System. US Prescribing Information. January 3, 2008. Available at: http://www.accessdata.fda.gov/drugsatfda_docs/label/2008/020375s026lbl.pdf (accessed August 8, 2011).

15. SINGH P, ROBERTS MS. Dermal and underlying tissue pharmacokinetics of lidocaine after topical application. *Journal of Pharmaceutical Sciences* 1994; 83(6): 774–782.

16. European Agency for the Evaluation of Medicinal Products. Note for Guidance on Modified Release Oral and Transdermal Dosage Forms: Section II (Pharmacokinetic and Clinical Evaluation). The European Agency for the Evaluation of Medicinal Products, Human Medicines Evaluation Unit, London, England, July 28, 1999. Available at: http://www.emea.europa.eu/pdfs/human/ewp/028096en.pdf (accessed August 8, 2011).

17. European Agency for the Evaluation of Medicinal Products. Note for Guidance on the Investigation of Bioavailability and Bioequivalence. The European Agency for the Evaluation of Medicinal Products, Human Medicines Evaluation Unit, London, England, December 14, 2000. Available at: http://www.emea.europa.eu/pdfs/human/qwp/140198en.pdf (accessed August 8, 2011).

18. Food and Drug Administration. Guidance for Industry. Topical Dermatological Drug Product NDAs and ANDAs—*In Vivo* Bioavailability, Bioequivalence, *In Vitro* Release, and Associated Studies. United States Department of Health and Human Services, Food and Drug Administration, Center for Drug Evaluation and Research, Washington, DC, June 1998. Available at: http://www.fda.gov/ohrms/dockets/98fr/980388gd.pdf (accessed August 8, 2011).

19. Code of Federal Regulations. Bioavailability and Bioequivalence Requirements. United States Code of Federal Regulations. 21 CFR 320, Washington, DC, April 1, 2009. Available at: http://www.access.gpo.gov/nara/cfr/waisidx_09/21cfr320_09.html (accessed August 8, 2011).

20. Code of Federal Regulations. Types of Evidence to Measure Bioavailability or Establish Bioequivalence. United States Code of Federal Regulations. 21 CFR 320.24, Washington, DC, April 1, 2009. Available at: http://edocket.access.gpo.gov/cfr_2009/aprqtr/pdf/21cfr320.24.pdf (accessed August 8, 2011).

21. Food and Drug Administration. Guidance. Topical Dermatologic Corticosteroids: *In vivo* Bioequivalence. United States Department of Health and Human Services, Food and Drug Administration, Office of Generic Drugs, Division of Bioequivalence, Washington, DC, June 2, 1995. Available at: http://www.fda.gov/downloads/Drugs/GuidanceComplianceRegulatoryInformation/Guidances/ucm070234.pdf (accessed August 8, 2011).
22. European Medicines Agency. Questions and Answer on Guideline Title: Clinical Investigation of Corticosteroids Intended for Use on the Skin. European Medicines Agency, Committee for Medicinal Products for Human Use, London, England, November 16, 2006. Available at: http://www.emea.europa.eu/pdfs/human/ewp/2144106en.pdf (accessed August 8, 2011).
23. AndroGel® US Prescribing Information. Abbott Laboratories, Abbott Park, IL. March 2011. http://www.rxabbott.com/pdf/androgel_PI.pdf (accessed August 8, 2011).
24. EstroGel® US Prescribing Information. Ascend Therapeutics, Herndon, VA. January 2008. Available at: http://www.estrogel.com/PDFs/EstroGel-Prescribing-Info.pdf (August 8, 2011).
25. MAZER N, FISHER D, FISCHER J, COSGROVE M, BELL D, EILERS B. Transfer of transdermally applied testosterone to clothing: A comparison of a testosterone patch versus a testosterone gel. *The Journal of Sexual Medicine* 2005; 2(2): 227–234.
26. SCHUMACHER RJ, GATTERMEIR DJ, PETERSON CA, WISDOM C, DAY WW. The effects of skin-to-skin contact, application site washing, and sunscreen use on the pharmacokinetics of estradiol from a metered-dose transdermal spray. *Menopause* 2009; 16(1): 177–183.
27. ROLF C, KEMPER S, LEMMNITZ G, EICKENBERG U, NIESCHLAG E. Pharmacokinetics of a new transdermal testosterone gel in gonadotrophin-suppressed normal men. *European Journal of Endocrinology* 2002; 146(5): 673–679.
28. European Agency for the Evaluation of Medicinal Products. Note for Guidance on Non-Clinical Local Tolerance Testing of Medicinal Products. The European Agency for the Evaluation of Medicinal Products, Evaluation of Medicines for Human Use, London, England, March 1, 2001. Available at: http://www.emea.europa.eu/pdfs/human/swp/214500en.pdf (accessed August 8, 2011).
29. International Conference on Harmonisation. ICH Harmonised Tripartite Guideline. Guidance on Nonclinical Safety Studies for the Conduct of Human Clinical Trials and Marketing Authorization for Pharmaceuticals M3(R2). International Conference on Harmonisation, Brussels, Belgium, June 11, 2009. Available at: http://www.ich.org/fileadmin/Public_Web_Site/ICH_Products/Guidelines/Multidisciplinary/M3_R2/Step4/M3_R2__Guideline.pdf (accessed August 8, 2011).
30. DRAIZE JH, WOODWARD G, CALVERY HO. Methods for the study of irritation and toxicity of substances applied topically to the skin and mucous membranes. *The Journal of Pharmacology and Experimental Therapeutics* 1944; 82: 377–390.
31. VINARDELL MP, MITJANS M. Alternative methods for eye and skin irritation tests: An overview. *Journal of Pharmaceutical Sciences* 2008; 97(1): 46–59.
32. KIRKLAND CR, YELVERTON CB, FLEISCHER AB JR, CAMACHO FT, FELDMAN SR. Gel vehicles are not inherently more irritating than creams. *Journal of Drugs in Dermatology* 2006; 5(3): 269–272.
33. Food and Drug Administration. Guidance for Industry. Photosafety Testing Requirements. United States Department of Health and Human Services, Food and Drug Administration, Center for Drug Evaluation and Research, Washington, DC, May 2003. Available at: http://www.fda.gov/ohrms/dockets/98fr/99d-5435-gdl0002.pdf (accessed August 8, 2011).
34. European Agency for the Evaluation of Medicinal Products. Note for Guidance on Photosafety Testing. The European Agency for the Evaluation of Medicinal Products, Evaluation of Medicines for Human Use, London, England, June 27, 2002. Available at: http://www.emea.europa.eu/pdfs/human/swp/039801en.pdf (August 8, 2011).
35. Food and Drug Administration. Guidance for Industry. Nonclinical Studies for the Safety Evaluation of Pharmaceutical Excipients. United States Department of Health and Human Services, Food and Drug Administration, Center for Drug Evaluation and Research, Washington, DC, May 2005. Available at: http://www.fda.gov/downloads/Drugs/GuidanceComplianceRegulatoryInformation/Guidances/ucm079250.pdf (August 8, 2011).
36. International Conference on Harmonisation. ICH Harmonised Tripartite Guideline. Pharmaceutical Development Q8 (R2). International Conference on Harmonisation, Brussels, Belgium, August 2009.

Available at: http://www.ich.org/fileadmin/Public_Web_Site/ICH_Products/Guidelines/Quality/Q8_R1/Step4/Q8_R2_Guideline.pdf (accessed August 8, 2011).

37. Food and Drug Administration. Draft Guidance on Lidocaine. United States Department of Health and Human Services, Food and Drug Administration, Office of Generic Drugs, Washington, DC, May 2007. Available at: http://www.fda.gov/downloads/Drugs/GuidanceComplianceRegulatoryInformation/Guidances/ucm086293.pdf (accessed August 8, 2011).

38. European Medicines Agency. Proposal for a Revision of the European Commission Guideline on Summary of Product Characteristics (Draft). Doc. Ref. EMEA/663087/2009. European Medicines Agency, Committee for Medicinal Products for Human Use, London, England, October 22, 2009. Available at: http://www.ema.europa.eu/docs/en_GB/document_library/Regulatory_and_procedural_guideline/2009/12/WC500027105.pdf (accessed August 8, 2011).

39. Food and Drug Administration. Guidance for Industry. Non-contraceptive Estrogen Drug Products for the Treatment of Vasomotor Symptoms and Vulvar and Vaginal Atrophy Symptoms—Recommended Prescribing Information for Health Care Providers and Patient Labeling. United States Department of Health and Human Services, Food and Drug Administration, Center for Drug Evaluation and Research, Washington, DC, November 2005. http://www.fda.gov/downloads/Drugs/DrugSafety/InformationbyDrugClass/UCM135336.pdf (accessed August 8, 2011).

40. Therapeutic Goods Administration. Guidance on Therapeutic Goods Order No. 79. General Requirements for the Labelling of Medicines. Australian Government, Department of Health and Ageing, Therapeutic Goods Administration, Canberra, Australia, January 2008. Available at: http://www.tga.gov.au/pdf/archive/consult-label-medicines-080118-guide.pdf (accessed August 8, 2011).

41. European Medicines Agency. Reflection Paper: Formulations of Choice for the Paediatric Population. European Medicines Agency, Committee for Medicinal Products for Human Use, London, England, July 28, 2006. Available at: http://www.emea.europa.eu/pdfs/human/paediatrics/19481005en.pdf (accessed August 8, 2011).

42. European Medicines Agency. Guideline on Clinical Investigation of Medicinal Products Indicated for the Treatment of Psoriasis. European Medicines Agency, Committee for Medicinal Products for Human Use, London, England, November 18, 2004. Available at: http://www.emea.europa.eu/pdfs/human/ewp/245402en.pdf (accessed August 8, 2011).

43. European Medicines Agency. Clinical Investigation of Corticosteroids Intended for Use on the Skin. European Medicines Agency, Committee for Medicinal Products for Human Use, London, England, February 1987. Available at: http://www.emea.europa.eu/pdfs/human/ewp/3cc26aen.pdf (accessed August 8, 2011).

44. Food and Drug Administration. Draft Guidance on Fentanyl. United States Department of Health and Human Services, Food and Drug Administration, Office of Generic Drugs, Washington, DC, May 2009. Available at: http://www.fda.gov/downloads/Drugs/GuidanceComplianceRegulatoryInformation/Guidances/UCM162427.pdf (accessed August 8, 2011).

Chapter 13

Toxicological and Pre-clinical Considerations for Novel Excipients and New Chemical Entities

Andrew Makin and Jens Thing Mortensen

INTRODUCTION

To support clinical trials, and ultimately registration of novel drugs to be applied to the skin for topical treatment or intended to permeate the skin and elicit a systemic effect, a well-designed regulatory nonclinical safety program must be conducted. Such a program should address all potential hazards associated with the product, including local and systemic toxicity, caused either by the active new chemical entity (NCE) or by any excipients used in the formulation. As for any other drug candidate intended for systemic or local effect, the nonclinical safety program should address at least the following areas: general acute and repeat-dose toxicity, genotoxicity, carcinogenicity, reproductive and juvenile toxicity, local toxicity and safety pharmacology, as well as primary and secondary pharmacodynamics. Pharmacokinetic aspects should be described, including local and systemic exposure to the active compound (and excipients, if relevant). Specific hazards that are particularly important for dermally applied drugs include local skin irritation, allergic skin sensitization, and photosafety.

In general, the "pivotal" nonclinical studies conducted and used in the risk assessment of the drug product should be conducted according to the rules of good laboratory practice (GLP). In reality, the majority of safety studies will be conducted according to the GLP rules. Exceptions to this rule are certain dose-finding, pharmacokinetic or specific mechanistic studies. Also, for some old compounds the

Transdermal and Topical Drug Delivery: Principles and Practice, First Edition. Edited by Heather A.E. Benson, Adam C. Watkinson.
© 2012 John Wiley & Sons, Inc. Published 2012 by John Wiley & Sons, Inc.

nonclinical safety studies were conducted many years ago, before the introduction of GLP, and such studies may be included in the safety documentation for a new product. It should be remembered, though, that it is the responsibility of the developing company to document the scientific quality of the data submitted and justify their use in the safety evaluation.

The more strategic regulatory aspects of the development program for a dermal drug are described in detail in Chapter 12 of this book. However, the composition of the nonclinical safety program for a dermally applied drug should follow the general guidance given in the internationally accepted International Conference on Harmonisation (ICH) M3(R2) guideline (Nonclinical Safety Studies for the Conduct of Human Clinical Trials and Marketing Authorization for Pharmaceuticals),[1] as well as the more specific guidance given in the other ICH nonclinical safety guidelines (in particular, ICH-S1–S7).[2–12] In addition to the international ICH guidelines, regional guidance is available from the U.S. Food and Drug Administration (FDA)[13] or the European Medicines Agency (EMA)[14] on some subjects relevant for dermal drugs, specifically local tolerance testing, photosafety, fixed combination products, and excipients.

This chapter will focus on the practical aspects of designing a suitable nonclinical safety program for a dermal drug. We will discuss the various types of studies required for investigating the safety of both NCEs and excipients, as well as nonclinical support of fixed combination products. Choice of species for the toxicology studies and useful *in vitro* models will be discussed. Finally, we will present a typical nonclinical program to support the entire development and life cycle of a dermal drug.

GENERAL TOXICOLOGY

NCEs intended for dermal application should be investigated for general toxic effects, similar to all other drugs. Standard repeat-dose toxicology studies in laboratory animals will normally be suitable for the purpose. As stated in the earlier mentioned ICH M3(R2) guideline, these studies should be conducted in two relevant species (rodent and nonrodent), and the treatment length should be at least as long or, in the later stages of clinical development, longer than the intended treatment time in human patients, up to a maximum of 6 or 9/12 months for rodents and nonrodents, respectively. The route(s) of administration should mimic the intended clinical use, but also secure that all relevant potential systemic toxic reactions are disclosed. The reversibility of the toxic changes should be examined by adding recovery groups to the relevant toxicology studies, in good time before these adverse effects could potentially occur in clinical trials. As for all other NCEs the nonclinical program for a dermal drug will most probably be built up in parallel with the clinical trial program in Phase I, II, III clinical trials, or marketing supporting "packages," to ensure that the required type and length of nonclinical studies to support the next clinical trial program is available in good time (Tables 13.1–13.4).

The dose levels used in the studies should be set to reveal both local and systemic toxicity of the NCE without causing severe life-threatening toxicity in the

Table 13.1 Dermal Phase I Clinic Supporting Nonclinical Program

Study type	Comments
SC/oral MTD/DRF study in the rat 4-week SC/oral toxicity study in the rat	Intended to provide data on general toxicology profile of test compound. Use route that ensures good bioavailability in the animals and best mimics pharmacokinetic profile and metabolism in humans. The SC route may be best choice, if a vehicle that does not induce local reaction after repeated SC injections is available.
Dermal MTD/DRF study in the minipig 4-week dermal toxicity study in the minipig	Minipig considered default choice for dermal nonclinical studies.
Bacterial reverse mutation assay Mouse lymphoma assay Bone marrow micronucleus test in the mouse/rat	*In vivo* micronucleus assay may be postponed until before Phase II clinic.
Local irritation study in minipigs or rabbits	May be omitted if vehicle is used in dermal toxicology studies is identical to clinical vehicle
Phototoxicity assay *in vitro* or *in vivo*	
Skin sensitization test	Use LLNA if possible
CNS safety pharmacology (modified Irwin screen in mice)	Use route that ensures systemic bioavailability: dermal if possible, otherwise SC or oral
Cardiovascular safety pharmacology study in the minipig (telemetry study)	
Respiratory safety pharmacology study in the rat (plethysmograph study)	
Pharmacokinetics/metabolism	Consider metabolite profiling in animal and human liver cells, plasma protein binding, CYP450 inhibition, ADME studies, and so on. Pharmacokinetic information can usually be extracted from toxicokinetic measurements in toxicology studies and combined with non-GLP pharmacokinetic data

MTD, maximum tolerated dose; DRF, dose range finding; CNS, central nervous system; ADME, absorption, distribution, metabolism, and excretion.

animals. It is also very important to investigate the potential toxic effects of the vehicle, since the vehicle is very often an integrated and important part of the mode of action of dermally applied drugs. The vehicle is intended to carry the active drug into or through the skin, and therefore often has the potential to override the natural defense mechanisms of the skin, which is essentially an organ designed to keep out foreign substances and organisms from the body. Sometimes the final vehicle to be used clinically has not been decided upon at the time when the dermal repeat-dose

Table 13.2   Dermal Phase II Clinic Supporting Nonclinical Program

Study type	Comments
13-week dermal/SC/oral toxicity study in the rat	Include reversibility groups, if not
13-week dermal toxicity study in the minipig	included in 4-week toxicology studies.
Fertility study in rats	Use route of administration that ensures
Preliminary DRF embryofetal study in rats	systemic bioavailability
Embryofetal toxicity study in rats	
Preliminary DRF study in nonpregnant rabbits	
Preliminary DRF embryofetal study in rabbits	
Embryofetal toxicity study in rabbits	
Pharmacokinetics/metabolism	Consider quantitative whole-body autoradiography (QWBA) and mass balance studies

DRF, dose range finding.

Table 13.3   Dermal Phase III Clinic Supporting Nonclinical Program

Study type	Comments
26-week SC/oral toxicity study in the rat	
39-week dermal toxicity study in the minipig	
13-week dermal carcinogenicity dose-finding study in the mouse	Consult with regulatory agencies before dose levels for carcinogenicity
13-week oral carcinogenicity dose-finding study in the rat	studies are finally determined.
13-week dermal photo(co)carcinogenicity dose-finding study in the hairless mouse	Only if a photo(co)carcinogenicity study is considered necessary
Pharmacokinetics/metabolism	Consider pharmacokinetic studies for clarification and mechanistic interpretation, and so on.

Table 13.4   Dermal Marketing Supporting Nonclinical Program

Study type	Comments
104-week dermal carcinogenicity study in the mouse	
104-week oral carcinogenicity study in the rat	
52-week dermal photo(co)carcinogenicity study in the hairless mouse	Only to be conducted if photosafety evaluation for chronic use cannot be handled based on short-term tests and existing knowledge.
Pre- and postnatal study in the rat	Use route of administration that ensures systemic bioavailability
Pharmacokinetics/metabolism	Consider relevant pharmacokinetic studies for clarification and mechanistic interpretation, etc.

toxicology studies must be conducted, or due to technical reasons this vehicle cannot be used unmodified in the toxicology studies (e.g., because high enough concentrations of the NCE suitable for toxicity testing cannot be achieved in the clinical vehicle). In these cases it would be prudent to use an experimental vehicle that has as many as possible of the intended properties of the clinical vehicle, with respect to consistency, skin penetration, preservatives, and so on. The combination of test species, the route of administration, and the appropriate dose levels to be used in these pivotal repeat-dose toxicology studies for dermal drugs will be discussed later in this chapter. But as always the choice should be based on scientific considerations that include exposure, metabolism, and the possibility of investigating both local and systemic toxicity, altogether with the aim of generating robust safety data for an appropriate hazard and risk assessment of the dermal drug, in relation to the intended clinical use. Generally, the toxicology studies should be conducted according to standard protocols and should include all the usual parameters that one would expect to see in a nonclinical safety study (clinical observation, feed intake and growth performance, ophthalmoscopy, electrocardiography, toxicokinetic and exposure data, clinical pathology, and macroscopic and microscopic examination of organs).

The highest exposure to the active NCE compound—and to the excipients—will most probably occur in the skin. Toxic reactions of the skin—either caused by the NCE or by one or more excipients in the vehicle—are a very common reason for failure of dermal drug candidates. It should be remembered that the skin has some metabolic capacity in the form of CYP450 and other enzymes that might act by either detoxifying the drug, or in some cases by generating toxic metabolites. It is therefore important to be especially careful with inclusion of parameters in the toxicology studies that will detect and describe toxic effects to the skin and its appendages. Since, in contrast to most other target organs, the skin is visible to the eye, this can to a large degree be accomplished by careful clinical examination of the skin during the study, combined with routine microscopic examination of the skin after study termination. However, inclusion of more quantitative methods of measurement of the skin's condition could be considered, for example, transepidermal water loss (TEWL), colorimetric measurement of skin erythema, ultrasonographic examination of skin structure and thickness, immunological or immunohistochemical measurement of local biomarkers (cytokines) of skin damage, and so on.

Specific single-dose toxicity studies are normally not very useful, since the required information on systemic and local toxicity after acute exposure to high doses can often be extracted from a well-conducted program of repeat-dose toxicity studies using a combination of dermal and systemic routes, or from specific local tolerance studies. The latter will be particularly useful for an evaluation of the adverse effects of the final pharmaceutical formulation of the drug, including various excipients that will be used in the clinical trial.

GENOTOXICITY

NCEs and excipients intended for dermal treatment should be examined for their genotoxic potential, similar to NCEs intended for any other route of treatment of human patients, to prevent exposure of human volunteers and patients to drugs that could theoretically be carcinogenic, teratogenic, or cause other types of irreversible damage associated with changes of the genes or chromosomes. In this connection it is important to consider if there are impurities present in the formulated dermal drug product, either formed during the synthesis of the NCE, by reaction of the NCE with excipients in the vehicle, or during storage of the drug, that could be genotoxic. Impurities that will occur above certain levels in the finished product will have to be investigated for potential genotoxic potential in addition to potential general toxicity of the impurity.

Traditionally and according to existing ICH guidelines,[5,6] an NCE should be investigated *in vitro* for its potential to cause mutations in cultured bacteria and for mutations/chromosome damage in cultured mammalian cells. Additionally, the NCE should be examined *in vivo* for its potential to cause chromosome damage, usually in the bone marrow of rodents exposed to the test compound. This battery of genotoxicity tests has been criticized for being too sensitive and lacking in specificity, thereby picking up too many compounds that have later on proved not to be a carcinogenic hazard to humans. The ICH guideline for genotoxicity testing of NCEs is currently under revision with the intention of recommending a more relevant and predictive genotoxicity testing battery for pharmaceuticals, but the final outcome of this ICH process was not known at the time of writing this chapter.

CARCINOGENICITY

Similar to all other drugs for chronic treatment of human patients, all NCEs for dermal treatment—and novel excipients without sufficient relevant safety data used in the dermal formulation—should be tested for carcinogenic effect in two rodent species before marketing of the drug.[2-4] The most common combination of carcinogenicity studies for dermal drugs is a 2-year dermal carcinogenicity study in mice, combined with a 2-year oral carcinogenicity study in the rat. This combination of study designs will ensure that both the general carcinogenic hazard associated with systemic exposure to the drug is addressed (by oral administration to rats), as well as the skin tumor hazard (dermal administration to mice where the exposure of the skin to the test article is the highest obtainable). However, it is difficult to avoid oral ingestion of a test article when treating the skin of the mice since occlusion cannot practically be used over a 2-year treatment period, so inevitably there will be a mixed local skin and systemic oral exposure in this study.

As stated in ICH guidelines,[4] one of the 2-year carcinogenicity studies could be replaced by a short-term model in genetically modified mice. For dermal drugs, the most relevant validated, alternative short-term carcinogenicity model is a 6-month dermal carcinogenicity study in the Tg.AC mouse. The Tg.AC model is a transgenic mouse model that works by activation of the oncogenic zetaglobin-promoted v-Ha-ras transgene. It is possible to induce a tumorigenic response within 6 months when dosed topically with nongenotoxic carcinogens, using skin papillomas as phenotypic indication of a tumorigenic response. The model has been criticized for not being specific enough and it has been feared that unspecific stimuli, for example, nicks of the skin during clipping of the hair or unspecific irritative effects of the vehicle, might induce a false positive result.[15–17] For this reason, before including alternative models in the carcinogenicity testing program it is probably recommended to discuss this issue with relevant regulatory authorities in order to ensure that all available knowledge and experience is taken into consideration.

REPRODUCTIVE TOXICITY

New drug products intended for topical use should be investigated for effects on the reproductive system similar to all other novel drug products.[10] Relevant reproductive toxicology studies investigating male and female fertility, embryo–fetal development, pre- and postnatal effects, and juvenile toxicity should be investigated before including male volunteers, women of childbearing potential, pregnant women, and children into clinical trials, according to general guidelines for the area. The route of administration should ideally be dermal using the exact same vehicle as in the clinic, since this will best mimic the behavior of both the NCE and the excipients in the vehicle. However, very often sufficiently high systemic exposure of the reproductive organs and the embryos or fetuses to the NCE cannot be achieved after dermal application. If sufficient systemic exposure cannot be achieved after dermal application to the animals to reliably detect potential reproductive function hazards and to conduct an appropriate risk assessment, alternative routes of administration must be considered, for example, the subcutaneous (SC) or oral route. In this context it will be important to take the exposure and potential differences in the metabolic pattern between the dermal and other routes of administration into consideration, when performing the reproductive risk assessment.

SAFETY PHARMACOLOGY

Generally, a standard battery of safety pharmacology tests to assess unwanted pharmacological effects of the NCE on the so-called vital systems (cardiovascular, respiratory, and central nervous systems) is required before the start of Phase I clinical trial.[11] According to ICH guideline S7A, "Safety pharmacology studies may not be needed for locally applied agents (e.g., dermal or ocular) where the pharmacology of the test substance is well characterized, and where systemic exposure or distribution to other organs or tissues is demonstrated to be low." Taken literally, this statement would mean that for very many dermal drugs, safety pharmacology studies would not be required. However, it is the experience that there may not always be agreement between sponsors and regulators to which degree a compound—even if old—is "well characterized," and what should be understood by "low systemic exposure or distribution to other organs". Also, since many NCEs intended for dermal treatment are very potent within their pharmacological class (e.g., anti-inflammatory, antiproliferative, anti-infective) and might also be considered for systemic treatment, it may be prudent to conduct the standard battery of safety pharmacology studies addressing potential unwanted effects on the cardiovascular, respiratory, and central nervous systems, before initiating a Phase I clinical trial, in order to reduce the overall risk for the drug candidate and to optimize the design of these clinical trials. The route of exposure in the animals should ideally be similar to the intended clinical route (dermal). However, similar to the discussion under reproductive studies, it is important that a sufficiently high systemic exposure is achieved in the animals to make the studies meaningful, and alternative routes of administration (SC, oral, etc.) should be considered for these safety pharmacology studies. The exposure pattern (pharmacokinetics) and metabolic properties of the test compound should be considered when performing the risk assessment.

LOCAL SKIN IRRITATION

Since local skin irritancy has been the cause of failure of many dermal drug product candidates, it is extremely important to consider and investigate new dermal drug products for a potential local irritant effect to the skin. It should be remembered that local skin irritancy can be caused not only by the active NCE, but just as well by any of the often many excipients used for different purposes in dermal vehicles (solubilizers, emulgents, preservatives, stabilizers, penetration enhancers, moisturizers, etc.). Each of these chemicals could be harmful to the skin in their own right, or they could work in concert to cause irritancy or other harmful effects to the skin. It is therefore important to consider the need and function of each excipient in the vehicle, to search for all known safety information on each excipient, and ideally to conduct appropriate nonclinical safety studies with the exact same formulation as intended for clinical treatment.[18]

Since there is often a need to test a range of potential formulations of a new dermal drug candidate for skin irritation before selecting the most promising formulation, it is recommended and should be considered good practice to use suitable *in vitro* methods for initial screening and characterization of the potential formulations for skin penetration and skin irritancy in order to avoid excessive use of experimental animals. Fortunately, there are now several validated, or at least robust and commonly used, *in vitro* methods available for the purpose. Methods to characterize and test the skin-penetrating properties of dermal products are thoroughly described in Chapters 2–10 in this book. Methods for sensitivity and irritation testing are described in Chapter 19 of this book. Some methods that could be of particular interest for the nonclinical safety evaluation are Franz-type diffusion cells for measurement of transdermal penetration of the test compound, and 3D-reconstituted skin models (e.g., SkinEthic®) for evaluation of skin damage.[19]

Once the most suitable combination(s) of NCE, composition of the vehicle, and strength have been selected, most probably based on theoretical considerations in combination with an array of *in vitro* measurements of skin-penetrating properties and local skin irritancy, the most promising drug candidate(s) must be tested for skin irritation in animals before conducting clinical trials in humans. Very often this can be done as part of the general dermal repeat-dose toxicology studies in suitable animal species discussed above and in more detail later in this chapter. However, sometimes specific stand-alone skin irritation studies in animals are necessary; for example, if the final to-be-marketed composition of the dermal vehicle has not been decided upon, when the repeat-dose toxicology studies must be conducted; or a dermal drug product is being developed as a line extension to an existing drug product (i.e., the active drug is being reformulated in a different vehicle to suit different patients' preferences or treatment of different parts of the body, such as inverse skin folds, face, or scalp areas vs. the general body surface or limbs). These studies should be conducted in relevant animal species that are known to be predictive for dermal treatment of humans (discussed later in this chapter), and they should include relevant observations: clinical observations including erythema, edema, and thickness of the skin, as well as progression, severity, and reversibility of these changes over time. More objective methods of measurement, for example, TEWL, colorimetric measurement of skin color, ultrasonographic measurement of skin structure, and potential measurement of relevant biomarkers of skin damage by immunohistochemistry or immunological methods should be considered in order to further clarify the potential causes of any changes observed.

As a curiosity, and especially for dermal products intended for treatment of the face and scalp, dermal products must also be evaluated for potential irritancy to the eye, since the product could accidentally come into contact with the eye. From an animal welfare point of view, eye irritation studies are controversial and should be avoided whenever possible. We believe that the risk of eye irritancy could very often be assessed from existing dermal irritancy data and that the risk could in most cases be managed with suitable labeling of the drug. Fortunately, some potentially useful alternative *ex vivo* methods are now becoming available. One example of such a method is the bovine corneal opacity and permeability (BCOP) assay.[20] This assay is probably best at predicting moderate to severe eye irritants or corrosives, and is not suitable for formulations. But the method may nevertheless be useful. Unfortunately, it has been the experience that some regulatory agencies do not recognize risk management for eye irritancy by labeling based on existing data or *in vitro* data, but require animal testing of the actual product, regardless.

ALLERGIC SKIN SENSITIZATION

Allergic contact dermatitis is a hazard that may be associated with the active NCE, but perhaps more commonly with the various excipients used in the dermal drug formulations. Therefore, for the nonclinical evaluation of a new drug formulation for allergenic potential, existing data for every excipient considered for the formulation should be carefully scrutinized. Relevant sources of information are pharmacopoeias, the safety database RTECS (Registry of Toxic Effects of Chemical Substances, http://www.symyx.com/products/databases/bioactivity/rtecs/index.jsp), and the FDA's list of inactive ingredients (http://www.accessdata.fda.gov/scripts/cder/iig/index.cfm). Also, computer databases of quantitative structure-activity relations (QSAR) should be consulted. For example, the QSAR database DEREK (http://

www.lhasalimited.org) is known to be useful in predicting the risk of potential contact sensitizing properties of chemical compounds.

There are a few animal models available for nonclinical testing for allergic skin sensitization, if needed. The classic guinea pig maximization test (GPMT) is a very sensitive and robust test that will, in the hands of experienced scientists, produce reliable results.[21] There are two important drawbacks to the GPMT:

1. The test is not suitable for testing pharmaceutical formulations, since according to the protocol the test compound must be injected intradermally at the highest nonirritant concentration as part of the procedure for induction of the potential allergy, and this is not practical for ointments, creams, foams, or many other dermal drug forms.

2. The protocol prescribes intradermal injection of Freund's complete adjuvant (FCA), which inevitably will lead to necrotizing sores at the injection site in some animals; this is clearly an animal welfare issue and alternative methods should be considered.

An alternative to the GPMT is the Buehler test, in which potential skin sensitization is induced by repeated dermal exposure to the test article. This protocol is useful for formulated products, and is often used for such products in place of the GPMT, although it is not as sensitive as the GPMT.

A very useful and highly recommended protocol for skin sensitization testing that should be the default choice if applicable is the local lymph node assay (LLNA) in mice.[22] In this assay, potential skin sensitization is induced by repeated topical application of the test article to the ear of the mouse, and induction of sensitization is evaluated quantitatively by measurement of uptake of a radioactive DNA marker in the lymphocytes in the draining lymph node as a measure of the cellular activity of the lymph node. This method is recommended since it is simple, cheap, quantitative, may be used for formulations, and is not overly harmful to the animals. The drawbacks are that the assay is not sensitive for certain classes of test compounds (e.g., certain metal ions), and that it is difficult to ensure absorption of water-soluble test compounds through the ear skin. Modifications of the LLNA that might overcome some of these problems, for example, by alternative routes of administration, are currently under investigation.

At the time of writing, the LLNA is not fully validated for complex mixtures such as dermal formulations, and therefore while it is a useful indicator of potential sensitizing effects, it is not always accepted by all regulatory authorities.

Finally, it should be remembered that testing for contact sensitizing potential for new dermal pharmaceutical products is most often also included as part of the Phase I clinical trial safety battery (local irritancy, contact dermatitis, phototoxicity, photoallergy).

PHOTOSAFETY

Since topically applied drugs are normally exposed to sunlight, it is important to consider if the NCE or any of the excipients in the formulation may be photoreactive, which may lead to the induction of phototoxicity. FDA/Center for Drug Evaluation and Research (CDER) and EMA/Committee for Medicinal Products for Human Use (CHMP) have both issued guidelines on nonclinical photosafety testing.[23,24] Although there are similarities in the recommended approach from the two agencies, there are also differences. In general, EMA/CHMP recommends *in vitro* methods (photocytotoxicity and photogenotoxicity) to a higher degree than FDA/CDER, who puts more emphasis on animal studies or clinical investigation. Both guidelines have very useful decision trees for the photosafety risk assessment. Both the FDA and EMA recommend a risk assessment-based approach to photosafety evaluation of dermal drugs based on all available evidence, rather than a formal and stringent test procedure based approach.

Under all circumstances, the initial step in a photosafety evaluation of a drug or drug substance would be to examine if the drug absorbs electromagnetic radiation in the ultraviolet (UVB or UVA) or visible ranges (wavelengths between 270 and 700 nm). If the drug does not absorb radiation in this range of wavelengths, the risk of phototoxic reactions is considered small. Photostability testing and examination of possible structure-activity relationship may be helpful in determining if a particular chemical structure may be photoreactive and have phototoxic liabilities. Additionally, in order to be phototoxic, the drug should of course distribute to the skin or eyes to become irradiated by sunlight or artificial light. Needless to say that this is almost always the case for dermally applied drugs.

The next step in the evaluation of drug substances that absorb UV or visible light could be an *in vitro* phototoxicity test, that is, the validated 3T3 neutral red uptake (NRU) assay.[25] Basically this is a cytotoxicity test in which it is investigated if the test substance becomes more cytotoxic after irradiation with simulated sunlight, compared to nonirradiated test compound. The assay may be very useful, but it has become evident that in the current design it is very sensitive and not overly specific, and it produces far more positive results compared to later *in vivo* testing in animals or clinical testing in humans. Also, results from the 3T3 NRU assay do not seem to correlate well with other *in vitro* phototoxicity assays, for example, photogenotoxicity tests in bacteria, and drug formulations cannot be tested in this assay. At the moment and although officially validated, within safety evaluation of pharmaceutical drugs the 3T3 NRU phototoxicity assay is probably most suitable for screening and ranking purposes. Initiatives have been taken to revise the conditions and design of the assay and the photosafety testing strategy, intending to make the process more predictive.

Nonclinical testing in animals for primary, nonallergic phototoxicity (acute photoirritation) should be conducted only if the above methods are not considered sufficient for the risk evaluation. It should be considered to conduct testing for photoirritation as part of the clinical safety testing in humans. If done, the animal testing is traditionally conducted in mice, rats, or guinea pigs. Basically, it is examined if irradiation of test article-treated skin with suberythemal doses of simulated sunlight causes the test article to become more irritating to the skin, when compared to nonirradiated skin treated with the test article.

Photoallergy is an acquired, immunologically mediated reaction to a drug or chemical initiated by the formation of photoproducts when that drug or chemical is exposed to light. Although animal models using guinea pigs are described in the literature, it is probably fair to say that there are no reliable and predictive models available at the time. Therefore, photoallergy testing of new dermal drugs is normally not required; however, it should be considered to address this issue in humans during the clinical development of the drug.

Dermal drugs that are intended for long-term treatment should be assessed for the risk of causing or accelerating sunlight-associated skin cancer (photocarcinogenicity). Short-term assays for evaluation of photogenotoxicity have been described, but none have been thoroughly validated, and these tests, although useful for specific or screening purposes, should probably be interpreted with caution. The most established model for photocarcinogenesis is the 1-year photo(co)carcinogenicity model in hairless mice. In this model it is investigated if the test drug enhances UV-induced skin tumor formation: the mice are treated dermally with the test article and receive simulated sunlight 5 days a week for 40 weeks. After 52 weeks the accumulated occurrence of UV-induced skin tumors in drug-treated groups versus untreated (but UV-irradiated) groups is compared as an expression of the test drug's potential to enhance UV-induced skin tumor formation. The model may be useful, since it reasonably mimics the use pattern of dermal drugs and the patients' everyday behavior. However, the model is purely descriptive, gives no mechanistic information, and it has been reported to be overly sensitive to vehicle effects (increased UV penetration into the thin skin of the hairless mice that might not be relevant for humans). Also, the model is not optimal from an animal welfare point of view. Attempts to replace the testing for potential drug-induced skin cancer in the photo(co)carcinogenicity model in hairless mice with measurement of biomarkers in the skin of animals or humans thought to predict long-term UV-induced skin damage (effect of test drug on minimal erythemal dose of UV, sunburn cell number, p53 alterations, DNA dimer formation, etc.) have been done, but have not proved to be successful so far.[26]

EXCIPIENTS

The preceding sections have focused on the pharmacologically active NCE in the dermal drugs. Excipients are mentioned whenever relevant. It should be remembered that the excipients will constitute the major part of any drug product and might have safety issues of their own. Examples of excipients particularly relevant for dermal drugs are solvents, emulsifiers, waxes, preservatives, and permeation enhancers. Although these excipients are not intended to be pharmacologically active, some of them are intended to interfere with living tissue, for example, to enhance absorption of the NCE. Other excipients are known to cause allergic skin sensitization or irritation (e.g., formaldehyde-releasing preservatives), or to be endocrine hormone disruptors (e.g., parabens). Many other mechanisms of toxic effects of excipients are imaginable and should be considered and assessed.

In principle, all the excipients used in a drug formulation should be assessed and documented for potential harmful toxicological effects in a similar manner as the active NCE. The FDA has issued a very useful guideline on this subject, where a tiered approach is recommended.[27] For many well-known excipients that have been used for dermal drug products through many years, the information may be available in pharmacopoeias, chemical products safety databases, or from the producer. Some excipients may have been used in food products and may have attained GRAS status (generally recognized as safe), or may be found at FDA's inactive ingredients list. One should be aware, though, that if an excipient is used for a new purpose, administered via a new route or at higher concentrations than previously, then the overall safety of the excipient to the patient should be assessed for this new intended use and exposure and so on. The regulatory agencies may very well require supplementary safety information and potentially nonclinical testing in animals if the existing safety data is not considered sufficient.

If a new excipient is being used in a dermal formulation it should, in principle, be safety tested in a manner completely similar to an NCE. In this case it is therefore very important to plan ahead and consider including the new excipient in the nonclinical safety studies that are to be conducted anyway. This can often be done by adding extra excipient-treated groups to the toxicology studies. In this case it can also be very important to define the final formulation of the dermal drug as early as possible and conduct the toxicology studies with this specific formulation. This will save both time and money.

LIFE CYCLE MANAGEMENT

Once a new dermal drug product has been launched it is very common, in a process called line extension, to extend the range of products available to the patient by developing new drug forms (e.g., cream, lotion, spray, and gel in addition to an ointment formulation), or by developing fixed combination products containing the NCE in combination with another active substance.

For line extensions consisting of an NCE in a new formulation at the same concentration, and for the same clinical indication, the nonclinical safety program required is mostly limited to investigation of effects on the skin: local skin irritation, allergic skin sensitization, and photosafety are probably the most important areas that may need evaluation or testing, together with relevant investigation of comparative systemic exposure to the active compound from the various formulations. However, if the clinical indication and thereby the use of the product is changed, a more thorough nonclinical testing program might be needed.[28] For example, if a dermal drug product intended for treatment of the skin of the body is reformulated for use on the face or scalp, or body areas with very thin skin, or for new patient populations (e.g., children), supplementary toxicology and pharmacokinetic studies may be needed. As previously mentioned, a drug intended for application to the face will probably need to be assessed or tested for its potential to cause eye irritation. A drug that was originally intended for dermal treatment of adult patients and further developed into a drug form intended for treatment of children will need to be assessed for local irritancy and so on, as described above, but will also need to be investigated for potential harmful effects to young individuals (juvenile toxicity).

Fixed combination products containing two or more well-known active compounds in the same vehicle are sometimes developed within the dermal area for the convenience of patients who need dermal treatment with several active drugs. When determining a suitable nonclinical program to support clinical trial and registration of fixed combination products, the existing nonclinical safety data for each of the active compounds should be evaluated for gaps. Missing data may need to be generated (e.g., genotoxicity data if the compounds are very old) to complete the safety evaluation of each active compound. It should be remembered that long clinical experience with a compound may be more relevant than testing in animals (e.g., general toxicity, local tolerance, allergic skin sensitization), while some other toxicological hazards cannot easily be evaluated from human clinical observations (genotoxicity, reproductive toxicity, carcinogenicity).

In general, a nonclinical safety program for a fixed combination product with two well-known active compounds would probably be centered on a 3-month bridging toxicology study in a suitable animal species. The study should include groups of animals that are treated with each of the active compounds alone, as well as with the combination, and relevant vehicle or untreated control groups. It is important to consider if there are signs of pharmacological, pharmacokinetic, or toxicological interactions between the active compounds. Are there indications of synergistic effects? Or do the active compounds "only" have additive effects? If interaction between the active compounds is suspected, specially designed pharmacology or toxicology studies may assist in describing the mechanism and extent.

Both FDA/CDER and EMA/CHMP have issued very useful guidelines on nonclinical safety evaluation of fixed combination products and these guidelines should be consulted for definition of the most optimal safety evaluation program for a fixed dose combination.[29,30]

ANIMAL MODELS

Animal models are used in development of drug products, including products intended for dermal application, for two primary purposes. One is for safety testing (i.e. evaluation of potential adverse events) and the other is to screen compounds for potential efficacy. The models used include both *in vivo* and *in vitro/ex vivo*. In general terms, it is most essential to have some consistency throughout a drug development program, so that all the various studies can be linked together and outcomes can be related to each other. For this reason models chosen should as much as possible be relevant to humans. In the following part of this chapter, we look at what models are available and provide an overview of a development program that meets the requirements of the existing legislation.

SPECIES SELECTION

Species selection for *in vivo* dermal testing is an interesting area. It is a regulatory requirement that nonclinical toxicology studies are performed in two species, one

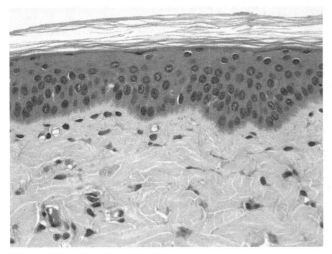

Figure 13.1   Normal minipig skin.

of which is a nonrodent. It is also important that the species used should be appropriate for the drug and route of administration. Rats are unquestionably the most commonly used rodent species in safety studies on all types of drug, regardless of therapeutic area or route of administration, and therefore they should also be considered for testing of dermal products. From the range of nonrodent species that is available, the minipig or pig should be the first choice. The reason for this is that of all the experimental species in current use, the structure and nature of porcine skin is the most similar to that of humans (Fig. 13.1).

The similarity is shown in both the physical characteristics (thickness, density of hair growth) and in the finer structure (close adherence to the underlying structures, rete ridges, presence of Langerhans cells, etc.).[31] It is very much the case that regulatory authorities expect to see that the minipig or pig has been used in any package of studies intended for regulatory submission. Several authors have reviewed the usefulness of pigs and minipigs as models of human dermal exposure, both *in vivo* and *in vitro*.[32–34]

It should be noted that when discussing minipigs and pigs, we consider them to be essentially alike. Minipigs as used in laboratories are the result of years of selective breeding to give an animal that is smaller and more easily handled than "standard" domestic pigs. Minipigs are genetically identical to domestic pigs and retain all of the characteristics of their larger counterparts. Therefore the comments made in this chapter could be applied to both types of pig.

As mentioned previously, the rat would normally be selected as the rodent species in regulatory safety testing of NCEs. However, taking into consideration the purpose of the nonclinical safety studies, one of the key outcomes is to be able to get a prediction of likely adverse effects in humans and to define a dose–response relationship. The nature of many products for dermal application is that they are often intended to work at or close to the site of application. Therefore it is normal

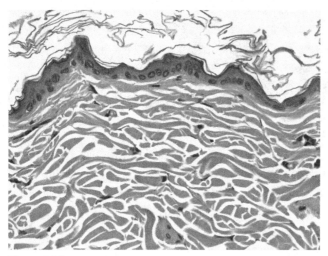

Figure 13.2 Normal rat skin.

that systemic exposure, measured as presence of parent drug or metabolites in blood, is low in terms of the peak levels (C_{max}), but that this low level would be prolonged, and that therefore the total exposure (area under the curve, AUC) could still be quite high.

Figure 13.2 shows an example of normal rat skin. One can immediately see that the characteristics are different from that of the minipig, for example, the epidermis is much thinner, giving different absorption characteristics. Some of the earlier chapters in this book give a more detailed description of skin penetration of drugs, however it should be noted that drugs basically pass the epidermis by passive diffusion, therefore the differences between the epidermises of the different species will affect the rate at which they absorb drugs.

If the intended site of action of the drug in this case is the skin, it can be seen that in the case of the rodent the duration of exposure at the site of application would be short, and probably unrepresentative of the human situation. In animals with skin characteristics such as those found in rats, mice, and rabbits, an approach that we often use, and one that is accepted by regulatory authorities, is to use the rat to give information on systemic exposure and to use the clinical dose route only in the minipig. We recommend using the SC route for dosing in the rat although others use other routes (intravenous [IV], oral, etc.). In these cases, where the dose route is not dermal, the dose formulation should be appropriate to the dose route, for example, a solution for injection, and we would not advocate using the clinical formulations. Therefore, when interpreting findings and comparing between routes, any toxic effects that might be due to a combination of the parent drug and excipients or carriers in the vehicle(s) used should be considered. We suggest use of the SC route in the rodent species if a suitable vehicle is available because in our opinion this gives the advantage of presenting a kind of "worst-case scenario" which is representative of what would happen if all of the drug substance was to become systemically available after reaching the subcutis (e.g., if the dose formulation had been applied to broken skin). We would like to stress the importance of using a vehicle for SC injection that does not cause local irritation at the injection site, also after repeated injections. Due to the chemical structure and poor solubility in aqueous vehicles of many NCEs, this is often not easily achievable. Some people, however, use the oral route and this is perfectly acceptable, though the systemic exposure would be expected to be lower following oral administration compared to SC, and the contributory effects of drug metabolism in the liver after oral dosing should also be considered. Therefore, it is important to measure not just the parent drug in blood, but also to look for metabolites.

EXPOSURE

In the evaluation of toxic effects, and therefore the evaluation of the safety of products and their potential to do harm to humans, it is important to be able to look at the relationship between toxicity and exposure to the drug (or metabolites). This emphasizes the need for the selected models to be relevant. Other chapters in this book deal with the various efficacy and *in vitro* models that are commonly used for testing safety and efficacy in the development of new products for dermal administration; however, in the context of the present chapter, the reader should bear in mind that all stages of the process are linked. But in the final evaluation, there is no value in estimating potential human effects if the model used gives an unrealistic view of the risks.

One of the most interesting and important considerations when planning nonclinical programs with products intended for human dermal application is the question of intended exposure. We have already seen that the choice of species, and the different skin characteristics of the species available, can have an effect on the systemic exposure to the applied drug product. Perhaps even before selecting the species and formulation one should think about the intended site of action of the product. Many products that are applied to the skin are intended to have an activity at that site, but several are not. For instance there are drugs (e.g., hormones, nicotine, etc.) that are applied to the skin in patches, but are intended to have a systemic effect. Here the patch and the skin in combination act as a depot, slowly releasing the drugs into the systemic circulation. Other drugs are intended to act at the surface of the skin, for example topical antibiotics, and so absorption is not important for their pharmacological activity, although their safety in the case of potential systemic exposure should still be investigated. In all cases the nonclinical testing programs should take into consideration both the local tolerance effects at the site of administration and the potential systemic effects following absorption.

In order to be able to link toxicity with exposure in studies with dermal application, it is obviously important to be able to measure the exposure, however the low blood plasma drug levels that are often achieved in these studies do present challenges. It is important that one should develop, validate, and execute a LC-MS/MS method with a lower limit of quantification (LLOQ) in the low picogram per milliliter range. Without this, it would in many cases be impossible to demonstrate exposure. In addition, the analytical methodology should focus on possible metabolites of the parent drug, endogenous substances that might interfere with the assay methodology, and cross-contamination (where one is dealing with substances that are present in minute amounts, it is extremely important that the samples should not become contaminated with the parent drug, thus giving false results—therefore strict handling precautions from the pharmacy through the animal facility and into the analytical laboratory are mandatory). Where one is working with measurement of drug in the skin itself, we would recommend using radiolabeled compounds (3H or 14C), because recovery and measurement are relatively straightforward and enable us to address factors such as excess amount on skin, in different skin layers, serum, and so on. Working with radiolabeled compounds, the analysis is relatively fast and cheap (total radioactivity counting in scintillator). If using radiolabeled materials is not possible, then a set-up using "cold" formulation can be used; however, these require additional extraction procedures before LC-MS/MS, meaning that they are more time consuming and expensive.

PRACTICAL CONSIDERATIONS

When designing the animal studies for pre-clinical safety testing of products intended for dermal application, there are various items to consider that are not so important when using other routes of administration. There are many reasons for this. The nature of the formulations themselves can give problems—and the volumes used tend to be extremely high. Animals that have been dosed on the skin are generally less easy to handle than other laboratory animals and scientifically the very low systemic exposures (particularly in relation to the amounts of drug used) need to be fully understood in data interpretation.

The nature of the products to be applied is very variable, for example creams, gels, ointments, or some other form of liquid delivery system. More recently, patches, micropumps, and other devices have also been developed for dermal drug delivery. However, the basic fundamental rule in animal studies, where the objective is to test possible adverse effects of the product, is that the product should as much as possible be identical to that which is intended to be used in humans. This is not always possible, but it makes the results of the nonclinical studies easier to interpret. Generally dermal products, in addition to the active (drug) ingredient, contain a wide range of other constituents that might, for example, enhance absorption, or act as preservatives, which means that the actions and effects of the drug substance itself could be dependent on the concentrations and proportions of these other constituents. This might be intentional as a result of the design of the formulation or it might be an unintentional consequence. In the former case, the outcomes might be more predictable than in the latter. Therefore, as an example, if the proposed human formulation is 1% of the drug substance in a gel, data obtained from testing a 5% concentration could be expected to be different because the balance of ingredients would be altered, leading to possible differences in local effect, absorption, systemic exposure, and toxicity. In addition, if the higher drug concentration has an effect on the skin that would not be seen at the lower level, this effect in itself might cause differences at the site of application that make any other results from the study difficult to interpret. However, where the human use is proposed to be a range of concentrations of the drug, then testing of the range in animals is certainly very appropriate, and testing of high concentrations could give useful information on safety.

Based on our experience with nonclinical studies in animals, two frequently asked questions are: how much drug substance can we administer, and what should be the size of the dosing area? The answers to these two questions are linked, but when considering them we need to go back to basic toxicological principles and think carefully about what we are doing in our animal studies. The purpose of non-clinical studies for any pharmaceutical product, regardless of dose route, is to provide information on the likely toxic (adverse) effects of the drug and to establish a dosage relationship so that the findings can be used to provide a guide to selection of safe doses in humans. In an oral study, for instance, one can simply give higher dose volumes or volumes with increased concentrations in order to increase dose levels. As mentioned above, the option of increasing the dose concentration is often not appropriate in dermal studies so that the most common way of varying the dose will be either by varying the amount applied or by varying the area to which it is applied. In general terms, it is not advisable to vary both parameters (area and volume) in the same study, because this makes interpretation of results difficult.

The question of the size of the dosing area is interesting and there is in fact not much in the way of helpful guidance in the regulatory documents. In humans, particularly in the clinical situation, it might in fact be necessary to apply the treatment over significant areas of the body. In animal studies, this is normally impractical, and some standardization has to be applied. The best one can find is that the guidelines in the Organisation for Economic Cooperation and Development (OECD) series[6] for testing of chemicals refer to 10% of the animal's surface area as being the maximum one should use, and we normally follow this recommendation. The amount of material that can be applied to an animal varies depending on the nature of the material, but as a rule of thumb a practical maximum will be approximately 1 g per kilogram bodyweight of the formulated product, assuming one is using the maximum dose area (10% of the surface area). Regardless of what the recommended human dose is, we find that for practical reasons it is much easier to dose as gram per kilogram of bodyweight than to express doses as, for instance, milliliters per square centimeter. The nature of the formulation has a great influence on how much can be applied. Gels are normally rapidly absorbed and are easy to apply and the maximum amounts can be given in this form. Ointments tend to be thick and poorly absorbed and while they can be applied in large amounts as quite thick layers, the poor absorption means that in effect putting on a thick layer makes no sense because most of the applied material never comes into contact with the animal. Watery liquids are the most difficult to apply as they tend to run off, and care and patience are required in their application to ensure that the material is dosed evenly over the dosing area.

We find that by far and away the most common method used in selection of dose levels in regulatory toxicology studies in order to achieve the aim of getting a series of doses is to keep the dosing area constant and to vary the volume of material applied to that area. Clearly, though, this is only practical up to a point—there is a limit to how much material can be applied to a defined area, and there is a limit to the area that can be used, and therefore for pragmatic reasons one might be driven to use a higher concentration of active substance in order to get the maximum effect.

In summary, in a dermal toxicology study there is a need to administer high enough doses of the test compound to induce clear local or systemic toxicity. This can be achieved by either increasing the treated skin area, the volume of test article applied, or the concentration of the active compound in the formulation. The three parameters should be balanced against each other, keeping the biological and thermodynamic principles of transdermal drug delivery and the chemical/pharmaceutical properties of the formulation in mind. The treatment of the animals should mimic the clinical situation as closely as possible.

Among the other questions frequently asked when designing studies is whether the application site should be occluded or not during the exposure period. Clearly, if the human exposure would include occlusion, then this should be mimicked in the animal model. In other cases (i.e., where the human exposure does not necessarily require an occlusion) we always recommend some form of light covering, because the alternative is that the animal could interfere with the dose site and thus render ultimate interpretation of results difficult. A solution is to cover the dose site with a light gauze bandage, simply to protect it.

From time to time the question as to whether the skin of the animals should be intact or abraded arises. Within the context of regulatory safety studies, we believe that abrasion should be avoided for the purely practical reasons that (1) abrading the skin will lead to changes that could affect the interpretation of results, or affect the rate of absorption of the test article, and so on, and (2) that in the case of animals, it is virtually impossible to abrade the skin uniformly, which also impacts adversely on the ability to interpret results. For example, if during the course of a repeat-dose study the test formulations cause a dosage-related effect at the site of application, interpretation of the significance of such effects could be hindered by the artificial damage applied to the skin. Of course, human dermal treatment in many cases involves compromised (cut, burned, broken, etc.) skin, however in the animal safety studies this is difficult to recreate. In animal models of disease where products are tested for efficacy, the situation is different, and there are available models of wounded or broken skin, that are essential to demonstrate such aspects of the product, but in safety testing, it is more usual to use "normal" animals.

SUGGESTIONS FOR A STANDARD TESTING PROGRAM FOR AN NCE OR EXCIPIENT INTENDED FOR DERMAL APPLICATION

From the foregoing, it is clear that there is some potential flexibility in the design of a nonclinical testing strategy for an NCE or novel excipient. Therefore in the concluding section of this chapter, we offer our opinion of a suitable strategy. One should of course take into consideration the proposed duration of the clinical use of the product, and that it is not possible to give a "one-size-fits-all" guidance, but we have tried to present the key points that should be considered. The proposed program (see Tables 13.1–13.4) is based on the assumption that treatment in the Phase II clinical trial will be 4–13 weeks, Phase III clinical trials may exceed 13 weeks, and that the marketed product may be used by the patients repeatedly for longer periods of time (chronic or chronic intermittent use).

REFERENCES

1. International Conference on Harmonisation. ICH M3(R2): Guidance on Non-Clinical Safety Studies for the Conduct of Human Clinical Trials and Marketing Authorization for Pharmaceuticals. Available at: http://www.ich.org/products/guidelines.html.
2. International Conference on Harmonisation. ICH S1A: Guideline on the Need for Carcinogenicity Studies of Pharmaceuticals. Available at: http://www.ich.org/products/guidelines.html.
3. International Conference on Harmonisation. ICH S1B: Testing for Carcinogenicity of Pharmaceuticals. Available at: http://www.ich.org/products/guidelines.html.
4. International Conference on Harmonisation. ICH S1C(R2): Dose Selection for Carcinogenicity Studies of Pharmaceuticals. Available at: http://www.ich.org/products/guidelines.html.
5. International Conference on Harmonisation. ICH S2A: Guidance on Specific Aspects of Regulatory Genotoxicity Tests for Pharmaceuticals. Available at: http://www.ich.org/products/guidelines.html.
6. International Conference on Harmonisation. ICH S2B: Genotoxicity: A Standard Battery for Genotoxicity Testing for Pharmaceuticals. Available at: http://www.ich.org/products/guidelines.html.
7. International Conference on Harmonisation. ICH S3A: Note for Guidance on Toxicokinetics: The Assessment of Systemic Exposure in Toxicity Studies. Available at: http://www.ich.org/products/guidelines.html.
8. International Conference on Harmonisation. ICH S3B: Pharmacokinetics: Guidance for Repeated Dose Tissue Distribution Studies. Available at: http://www.ich.org/products/guidelines.html.
9. International Conference on Harmonisation. ICH S4: Duration of Chronic Toxicity Testing in Animals (Rodent and Non-Rodent Toxicity Testing). Available at: http://www.ich.org/products/guidelines.html.
10. International Conference on Harmonisation. ICH S5(R2): Detection of Toxicity to Reproduction for Medicinal Products & Toxicity to Male Fertility. Available at: http://www.ich.org/products/guidelines.html.
11. International Conference on Harmonisation. ICH S7A: Safety Pharmacology Studies for Human Pharmaceuticals. Available at: http://www.ich.org/products/guidelines.html.
12. International Conference on Harmonisation. ICH S7B: The Nonclinical Evaluation of the Potential for Delayed Ventricular Repolarization (QT Interval Prolongation) By Human Pharmaceuticals. Available at: http://www.ich.org/products/guidelines.html.
13. FDA/CDER. FDA/CDER Pharm/Tox Guidelines. Available at: http://www.fda.gov/Drugs/GuidanceComplianceRegulatoryInformation/Guidances/default.htm.
14. EMEA/CHMP. EMEA/CHMP Nonclinical Guidelines. Available at: http://www.emea.europa.eu/htms/human/humanguidelines/nonclinical.htm.
15. CANON RE. The Tg.AC mouse model passes test by failing to respond. *Toxicological Sciences* 2003; 74: 233–234.
16. THOMSON KL, SISTARE FD. Selection of drugs to test the specificity of the Tg.AC assay by screening for induction of the gadd153 promoter *in vitro*. *Toxicological Sciences* 2003; 74: 260–270.
17. THOMPSON KL, ROSENZWEIG BA, WEAVER JL, ZHANG J, LIN KK, SISTARE FD. Evaluation of the Tg.AC assay: Specificity testing with three noncarcinogenic pharmaceuticals that induce selected stress gene promoters *in vitro* and the inhibitory effects of solvent components. *Toxicological Sciences* 2003; 74: 271–278.

18. EMEA/CHMP. EMEA/CHMP Guideline: Non-Clinical Local Tolerance Testing of Medicinal Products. Available at: http://www.emea.europa.eu/htms/human/humanguidelines/nonclinical.htm.
19. OECD. OECD Guideline No. 431: *In Vitro* Skin Corrosion: Human Skin Model Test. Available at: http://www.oecd-ilibrary.org/environment/oecd-guidelines-for-the-testing-of-chemicals-section-4-health-effects_20745788.
20. OECD. OECD Guideline No. 437: Bovine Corneal Opacity and Permeability Test Method for Identifying Ocular Corrosives and Severe Irritants. Available at: http://www.oecd-ilibrary.org/environment/oecd-guidelines-for-the-testing-of-chemicals-section-4-health-effects_20745788.
21. OECD. OECD Guideline No. 406: Skin Sensitisation. Available at: http://www.oecd-ilibrary.org/environment/oecd-guidelines-for-the-testing-of-chemicals-section-4-health-effects_20745788.
22. OECD. OECD Guideline No. 429: Skin Sensitisation: Local Lymph Node Assay. Available at: http://www.oecd-ilibrary.org/environment/oecd-guidelines-for-the-testing-of-chemicals-section-4-health-effects_20745788.
23. FDA/CDER. FDA/CDER Guidance: Photosafety Testing (May 2003). Available at: http://www.fda.gov/Drugs/GuidanceComplianceRegulatoryInformation/Guidances/default.htm.
24. EMEA/CHMP. EMEA/CHMP Note for Guidance on Photosafety Testing (December 2003). Available at: http://www.emea.europa.eu/htms/human/humanguidelines/nonclinical.htm.
25. OECD. OECD Test Guideline No. 432: *In Vitro* 3T3 NRU Phototoxicity Test. Available at: http://www.oecd-ilibrary.org/environment/oecd-guidelines-for-the-testing-of-chemicals-section-4-health effects_20745788.
26. SAMBUCO CP, FORBES DP, LEARN DB, ELDRIDGE S, HOBERMAN AM. Biomarkers provide important phototoxicity data but are not sufficient for photocarcinogenic risk assessment. *The Toxicologist* 2009; 296: (poster abstract PS1429).
27. FDA/CDER. FDA/CDER Guidance: Nonclinical Studies for the Safety Evaluation of Pharmaceutical Excipients (May 2005). Available at: http://www.fda.gov/Drugs/GuidanceComplianceRegulatoryInformation/Guidances/default.htm.
28. FDA/CDER. FDA/CDER Guidance: Nonclinical Safety Evaluation of Reformulated Drug Products and Products Intended for Administration by an Alternate Route (Draft, March 2008). Available at: http://www.fda.gov/Drugs/GuidanceComplianceRegulatoryInformation/Guidances/default.htm.
29. FDA/CDER. FDA/CDER guidance: Nonclinical Safety Evaluation of Drug or Biologic Combinations (March 2006). Available at: http://www.fda.gov/Drugs/GuidanceComplianceRegulatoryInformation/Guidances/default.htm.
30. EMEA/CHMP. EMEA/CHMP guideline on the non-clinical development of fixed combinations of medicinal products (August 2008). Available at: http://www.emea.europa.eu/htms/human/humanguidelines/nonclinical.htm.
31. SWINDLE M, SMITH AC. Comparative anatomy and physiology of the pig. *Scandinavian Journal of Laboratory Animal Science* 1998; 25(Suppl. 1): 11–21.
32. MORTENSEN JT, BRINCK P, LICHTENBERG J. The minipig in dermal toxicology. A literature review. *Scandinavian Journal of Laboratory Animal Science* 1998; 25(Suppl. 1): 77–83.
33. QVIST MH, HOECK U, KREILGAARD B, MADSEN F, FROKJAER S. Evaluation of Göttingen Minipig Skin for Transdermal *in vitro* Permeation Studies. *European Journal of Pharmaceutical Sciences* 2000; 11: 59–68.
34. SVENDSEN O. The minipig in toxicology. *Experimental and Toxicologic Pathology* 2006; 57: 335–339.

Chapter 14

Topical Product Formulation Development

Marc B. Brown, Robert Turner, and Sian T. Lim

THE PHILOSOPHY OF TOPICAL FORMULATION DEVELOPMENT

When a formulation scientist starts the long and often painful process of developing a topical formulation for the treatment of a certain skin disease there are a plethora of issues that need to be considered, some of which are detailed in Figure 14.1. It should always be remembered that it is not a drug that you give to a patient but a drug product, that is, a medicine, and the pharmaceutical history is littered with examples of drugs that could have been the next "magic bullet" or turned into the next blockbuster if only a formulation could have been developed that delivered the molecules safely and efficaciously to their pathological site in a cost-effective manner. Such problems are exacerbated even further in dermal drug delivery in that patients care what they apply to the skin and often have a choice. As such, the consumer or patient should always be at the forefront of the thoughts of a formulation scientist. The dermal products developed hundreds of years ago that were greasy, with poor odor, and that stained clothes are no longer acceptable; the cosmetics and aesthetics of the final product are *almost* as important (some brand managers would argue that this should read *more*) as the product's efficacy. A good example of this is the recent development of topical foam products, which may add no real benefit in terms of drug delivery but provide the consumer or patient with an alternative that is easy to apply cosmetically and is just "different" from the classic semisolids such as creams and ointments that the consumer is used to.

An overview of the entire formulation development process beginning from pre-formulation development up to identification of the final lead formulation candidate is summarized in the flowchart shown in Figure 14.2. With this in mind, this chapter provides an overview of some of the various steps and hurdles that a

Transdermal and Topical Drug Delivery: Principles and Practice, First Edition. Edited by Heather A.E. Benson, Adam C. Watkinson.

255

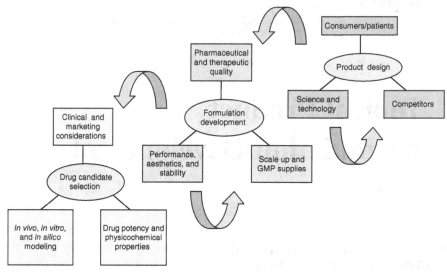

Figure 14.1   The ethos of topical formulation development.

formulation scientist should work through to develop a product that will be optimized for the drug, formulation, and consumer.

DRUG CANDIDATE SELECTION

The developments in combinatorial chemistry and high throughput screening have led to a rapid increase in drug design and discovery and ultimately the production of many potential molecules that require evaluation. For example, it is now reported that it takes 10,000 candidate molecules to produce one approved drug.[1] As such, the use of empirical or traditional screening methods such as *in vivo* and *in vitro* testing is often restricted due to the time and cost involved. Thus, modern drug selection requires rapid and cost-effective methods applicable to a large number of samples, one example being the use of mathematical models.

Over the last 25 years there has been much interest in the use of mathematical models and numerical methods to predict dermal absorption *in silico*. Formulation scientists have been tempted, especially in the pharmaceutical arena, to find the most promising compounds, by investigating the relationship between percutaneous permeation and molecular parameters such as lipophilicity (most commonly expressed as log P, the logarithm of the octanol–water partition coefficient), hydrogen bonding, molecular weight (or size), and melting point. QSPR (quantitative structure-property activity relationships) studies have meant that, if a correlation is found, it is possible to screen any number of compounds, including those that have not been yet synthesized, for the selection of those structures with the required properties for the desired delivery.

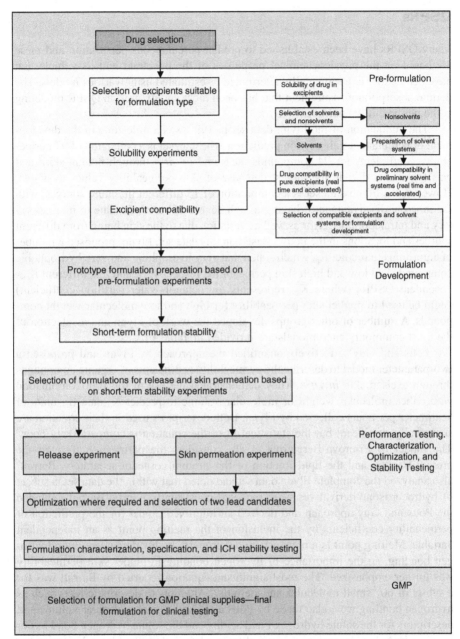

Figure 14.2   Flowchart summarizing key events of a typical topical semisolid formulation development program.

QSPRs

Many QSPRs have been established to predict percutaneous penetration and these are based on the physicochemical properties of the penetrant and its vehicle that have been either experimentally determined or estimated using various models. The dermal absorption measurement that has been most widely used in QSPR modeling is the permeability coefficient (K_p).

The publication of the Flynn data set in 1990 was a milestone in the development of percutaneous absorption prediction. The data set is a collection of 97 permeability coefficients for 94 compounds measured *in vitro* through human skin[2] and was for over a decade the largest database of skin permeability values available. However, the Flynn data set is a compilation of 15 different literature sources, with the inherent disadvantage of having a high degree of variability due to interlaboratory and intralaboratory error as well as variation due to the skin being from different sources and locations in the body.[3] Based on this data set, Flynn[2] proposed a number of algorithms to predict K_p, which stated that very hydrophilic and very hydrophobic compounds had low and high skin permeability, respectively, and that different K_{ow}-dependent QSPRs (where K_{ow} represents the octanol–water partition coefficient) could be used to predict skin permeability for high and low molecular weight compounds. A number of other groups developed the work of Flynn and a selection of the most commonly cited models are provided in Table 14.1.

Potts and Guy[4] effectively quantified the approach by Flynn and proposed a two-parameter model to describe the permeability coefficients of organic compounds through excised skin *in vitro*. They demonstrated the use of log P in combination with either molecular weight or molecular volume to predict K_p data (in units of centimeter per hour) collected by Flynn. Both descriptors used in their equation are statistically significant but the statistical fit of the equation is comparatively poor.[3] The model of Fiserova-Bergerova et al.[5] considers the permeation through the protein fraction and the lipid fraction of the stratum corneum separately. Barratt[6] also analyzed the complete Flynn data set and noted that within the data set, a subset of hydrocortisone derivatives were modeled consistently poorly. Barratt extended the Potts and Guy approach and derived an improved model for the prediction of permeability coefficients by the inclusion of the melting point as an independent variable. Melting point is a physiochemical property highly dependent upon hydrogen bonding, so the importance of hydrogen bonding to model skin permeability was further emphasized. The most significant equation reported by Barratt was for a subset of 60 "small molecules and steroids." Attempts to describe effects such as hydrogen bonding were also made by Potts and Guy,[7] where molecular volume and descriptors for the solute hydrogen bond acidity and the solute hydrogen bond basicity were included. According to the Robinson–Wilschut model, the influence of the molecular weight on the permeability coefficient is considered separately for the lipid and protein fraction of the stratum corneum and the watery layer of the epidermis, which is located beneath the stratum corneum. Pugh et al.[8] also addressed the issue of hydrogen bonding and molecular size in skin permeation. According to the model in Pugh et al.,[8] diffusion across the stratum corneum depends on H-bonding

Table 14.1 Summary of QSPRs for the Prediction of Dermal Absorption

Reference	Model	Development
4	$\mathrm{Log}\,K_p(\mathrm{cm\,sec^{-1}}) = -6.3 + 0.71\,\mathrm{log}\,K_{o/w} - 0.0061\,MW$	Quantified approach by Flynn
5	$Fl = (c_{sat}/15)\,(0.038 + 0.153P)e^{-0.016\,MW}$	Considers protein permeation
6	$\mathrm{Log}\,K_p = 0.82\,\mathrm{log}\,K_{o/w} - 0.0093\,MW - 0.039\,MPt - 2.36$	Included melting point and focused on small molecules
7	$\mathrm{Log}\,K_p = 0.0256MW - 1.72\Sigma\alpha_2^H - 3.93\Sigma\beta_2^H - 4.85$	Inclusion of molecular volume and hydrogen bonding properties
58	$K_p\;(\mathrm{cm/h}) = \dfrac{1}{\dfrac{1}{K_{psc} + K_{pol}} + \dfrac{1}{K_{aq}}}$ $\mathrm{Log}\,K_{psc} = -1.326 + 0.6097 \times \mathrm{log}\,P_{oct} - 0.1786 \times M_W^{0.5}$ $K_{pol} = \dfrac{0.0001519}{\sqrt{M_w}};$ $K_{aq} = \dfrac{2.5}{\sqrt{M_w}}$	Considered protein and lipid fractions separately
8	$\mathrm{Log}(D/h) = -1.03 - 1.25\alpha - 2.53\beta - 0.00326\,MW$	Considered retardation effects of H bonding groups
9, reanalyzed in 10	$\mathrm{Log}\,K_p = 0.772\,\mathrm{log}\,P_{oct} - 0.0103\,MW - 2.33$	Remodelled Potts and Guy

log $K_{o/w}$, octanol–water partition coefficient; MW, molecular weight; Fl, flux (milligrams per square centimeter per hour); c_{sat}, saturated concentration of a compound in the vehicle (milligrams per milliliter); MPt, melting point (degrees Celsius); $\Sigma_2^H\alpha$, solute hydrogen bond acidity; $\Sigma_2^H\beta$, solute hydrogen bond basicity; K_{psc}, permeation coefficient of the lipid fraction of stratum corneum; K_{pol}, permeation coefficient of the protein fraction of the stratum corneum; K_{aq}, permeation coefficient of watery epidermal layer; α, number of H-bond donors; β, number of H-bond acceptors.

groups in the penetrant and its molecular weight. The characteristic α and β values of the various chemical groups implies that each group has a characteristic retardant effect on diffusion. This was termed the retardation coefficient (RC). The RC depends on interaction of the H-bonding groups of the penetrant with those of the stratum corneum. Therefore, by knowing RC and α and β for the penetrant, the relative H-bonding can be estimated. A data set produced by Kirchner et al.[9] was subsequently reanalyzed by Cronin et al.[10] Percutaneous absorption, according to Cronin et al.,[10] across excised human skin *in vitro* is governed by hydrophobicity and molecular size as proposed previously by Potts and Guy.[4] The model obtained in this study had an improved correlation coefficient over that developed by Potts and Guy.[4]

Statistical Analysis (Linear vs. Nonlinear) Methods

For many QSPRs, regression analysis is the statistical method of choice as reviewed by Cronin and Schultz,[11] Yashimata and Hasida,[12] Farahmand and Maibach,[13] and Moss et al.[14] However, there are a number of disadvantages to using this method. First, it is a linear technique, and second, it is adversely affected by colinearity between independent variables (e.g., log K_{ow} and molecular weight). It is not clear whether regression analysis is a suitable tool for the development of QSPRs and nor is it clear whether linearity is appropriate for the modeling of highly hydrophilic and hydrophobic molecules. For example, Moss et al.[14] compared the statistical accuracy of Gaussian processes (GP), single-linear networks, and QSPRs by a range of statistical methods, and found that the nature of the data set was inherently nonlinear (i.e., the data were modeled by a function that was a nonlinear combination of the model parameters and depended on one or more independent variables), and that skin permeation (as represented by K_p) was best described, in purely statistical terms, by GP approaches.

GP modeling is a nonparametric method. It does not produce an explicit functional representation of the data, as QSPR modeling does in the form of an equation where the permeability is usually related to statistically significant physicochemical descriptors of a data set. In GP modeling it is assumed that the underlying function that produces the data, f(x), will remain unknown, but that the data are produced from a (infinite) set of functions, with a Gaussian distribution in the function space. This has been described in detail elsewhere.[14,15]

A range of nonlinear methods have been employed to improve predictions of skin absorption. Artificial neural networks (ANNs) have been investigated,[16] showing high predictive power. However, ANNs are a limited method in that they have a tendency to over-fit where large numbers of physicochemical descriptors exist, compared to the data points used. Such models are often weighted and are susceptible to overtraining.[17] GP methods do not alleviate all these issues, but minimize them,[15] reportedly providing better predictions of percutaneous absorption than existing models.[14]

In comparing different approaches for developing predictive models of percutaneous absorption, Moss et al.[14] suggested the inherently nonlinear nature of the skin data set used. As such, GP machine learning methods produce statistically more robust models than other approaches (single-layer networks [SLNs] or QSPR-based models). While this approach resulted in specific models that were statistically superior to others, it also clearly indicated the interdependence of the physico-chemical descriptors employed in this and in many other studies. This suggests that the approach of quantifying models of skin absorption by means of a simple equation may have limited mechanistic value. Such findings were supported by Lam et al.[18] and Sun et al.,[19] who showed that GP methods yielded predictive models that offered statistically significant improvements over SLN and QSPR models with regard to predictivity (where the rank order was: GP > SLN > QSPR). Feature selection analysis determined that the best GP models were those that contained log P, melting point, and the number of hydrogen bond donor groups as significant descriptors. Further statistical analysis also found that great synergy existed between certain parameters (i.e., molecular weight and melting point). Such synergy suggests that a model constructed from discrete terms in an equation may not be the most appropriate way of representing a mechanistic understanding of skin absorption.

Whatever the opinion on the best model to use or even if any are actually valid, there are a plethora of *in silico* models that exist for the formulation scientist to help identify the molecules that will be best absorbed. However, for the formulation scientist other factors need to be considered, including predicted or experimentally derived molecule stability, solubility, irritancy, toxicity, and potency before a final decision on candidate selection is made. Despite the developments in *in silico* modeling, they are yet to replace actual skin permeation testing using the type of *in vitro* models described in the later section and will probably remain as such until their reliability and correlation with real experimentally derived data can be confirmed. As often is the case, it is experience rather then theory that guides the best way forward.

PRE-FORMULATION STUDIES

Overview

Pre-formulation is a research and development stage where the drug's physico-chemical properties and desired dosage form along with the drug's mechanism of action and target disease are considered. For the development of topical semisolid drug products, pre-formulation studies typically involve solubility and compatibility studies. Such studies are conducted to identify any critical parameters which may affect the development of the final product. These parameters may include poor drug solubility and achievable drug concentration, inherent drug instability, potential excipient/drug, or excipient/excipient incompatibility, among others. In addition, another aim of pre-formulation studies is to develop and explore methodologies to improve these defined issues such that the target profile of the formulation dosage form can be achieved, thus pre-formulation studies are conducted to form the basis for the rationale of formulation design. A summary of a typical pre-formulation process is highlighted in Figure 14.2.

Initial Considerations of the Drug

Drug Physicochemical Properties

The physicochemical properties of a drug that can influence its performance and manufacturability should be identified and considered during pre-formulation work and include log P, pKa, solubility, and molecular weight. Such parameters play a key role in the inherent permeability of a drug across the skin as described in the section "Drug Candidate Selection." The Log P (partition coefficient) reflects how well a drug partitions between lipid (oil) and water while the pKa or dissociation constant is a measure of the strength of an acid or base and allows the determination of charge on a molecule at any given pH. Both measurements are useful parameters for use in understanding the solubility and diffusivity and/or partitioning across the stratum corneum. The effect of pH on skin enhancement of lignocaine was investigated by Valenta et al.[20] In the study, the authors showed that the flux of lignocaine hydrochloride increased across human epidermis with increasing pH as the basic molecule becomes less ionized at higher pH values. However, the permeability of unionized species is also dependent upon solubility as demonstrated by Valenta and Hadgraft.[21] The authors,[21,22] using predictive software and information available in literature, suggested that flux across skin for ionized ibuprofen and lignocaine is significantly higher than the unionized form as a result of the higher aqueous solubility and possible ion-pairing effect.

The selection and identification of potential drug salt forms or the use of a salt or free acid or base is critical during pre-formulation studies since these selections obviously influence drug solubility, stability, and ultimately drug absorption. In an *in vitro* permeation experiment, Minghetti et al.[23] evaluated the permeation of four diclofenac salts in various solvents across full-thickness human skin. Their findings suggested that the flux and permeability coefficient was highly dependent upon the diclofenac salt selected and by the solvent type used. Although the unionized form of a drug is generally thought to be a more suitable candidate for topical application due to its lower polarity and consequently higher partitioning into the stratum corneum, other considerations such as drug solubility and stability in the formulation have to be considered. These issues should be decided during the early development phase since changing the salt form at a later stage may force repetition of toxicological, formulation, and stability studies, thus increasing development time and cost. The introduction of a new salt form at a late stage must also be evaluated for potential impurity changes, and its bioequivalence, pharmacokinetic equivalence, and toxicity equivalence to the previous salt form may have to be proven.

Drug Pharmacology and Topical Efficacy

Given that the exact underlying cause of a lot of skin diseases may not be well defined or understood, the effective drug concentration required to reach the target area within the skin is also often not well defined. Thus, before a decision is made to take a drug into topical formulation development, several issues and questions should be considered (if they have not already been addressed in the candidate selection process):

1. Has the pharmacological activity of the drug been demonstrated or predicted and what is the IC50 or minimum concentration required to exert a therapeutic effect?
2. What are the pharmacological models used in assessing and/or predicting the pharmacological activity of the drug and are these models appropriate?
3. Is the target site known?
4. Is the drug metabolized in the skin?

For example, when targeting a drug to the epidermis, a highly potent drug with a low K_p may not necessarily be the most efficacious when compared to a less potent drug with a higher K_p as it is a combination of a drug's potency and its ability to permeate the skin that is important. Thus, such parameters should be well defined and understood during drug selection and during any pre-formulation work since such information will allow proper evaluation of dosage form type, dose/drug concentration, and the selection of excipients.

Dosage Forms

Topical dosage forms have been generally classified as liquids, semisolids, and solids, and typical examples are summarized in Figure 14.3. The most conventional and probably well-known topical dosage forms are creams, gels, and ointments, although classification of such topical dosage forms may be poorly defined and ambiguous depending on the literature referenced. For example, the European Pharmacopoeia (EP)[24] and British Pharmacopoeia (BP)[25] define ointments as "single-phase basis in which solids or liquids may be dispersed" and creams as "multiphase preparations consisting of a lipophilic phase and an aqueous phase," while the United States Pharmacopoeia (USP 28) and the USFDA (U.S. Food and Drug Administration) define ointments and creams as "a semisolid dosage form containing one or more drug substance dissolved or dispersed in a suitable base." Nevertheless, the initial selection of suitable dosage forms is most commonly dependent upon the drug's physicochemical properties, target disease type, required aesthetic and cosmetic properties, scalability, costs, and the target product profile. The brand and its continual evolution can also be a significant consideration for over-the-counter topical products.

Selection of Excipients

Regulatory Perspective

Pharmaceutical topical formulations rarely contain a single excipient, with the number varying from a few (e.g., aqueous gels or lotions) to greater than 10 (e.g.,

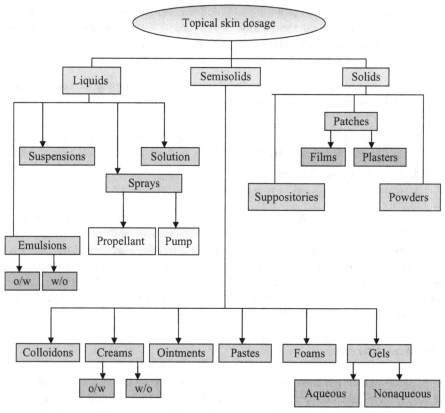

Figure 14.3   Summary of typical topical dosage forms.

emulsion systems). The simplest way to choose and utilize excipients is to select those with appropriate properties that are used in existing formulations that have received regulatory approval in the territories relevant to your product. The legislation and nature of regulatory control varies from one country to another, however, in general, acceptable pharmaceutical excipients are listed in international pharmacopoeias with extensive published safety data. Notably, the use of existing excipients requires regulatory consideration when using an established excipient for an alternative delivery route. For example, the oral consumption of an excipient that has been used in a topical dosage form may well mean that additional toxicity studies are required. Equally, a wide range of novel excipients have been developed and described in the literature. However, for the reasons highlighted above, the use of such excipients in developing a pharmaceutical product is limited, as they require supportive data similar to those required for a new drug. Although such extensive supporting data may be lessened or avoided if each excipient has extensive supportive toxicity data, previous approval for food use, oral administration or is already used cosmetically. On the other hand, regulation of cosmetic topical formulations, although controlled by legislation, has a less strict stance on excipient types, grades, and levels, thus a much wider range is available and acceptable than in the development of pharmaceutical topical formulations. With this in mind, it is obvious that the general concept of "the less the better" holds true when developing a drug product, thus it is unsurprising that dosage forms with less components such as gels are now often favored over the more traditional creams.

Role of Excipients

Excipients typically make up greater than 90% of a topical pharmaceutical product and they are included to perform a variety of functional roles in such formulations. For the purpose of a semisolid topical dosage form, such functional roles may include:

- Improvement of solubility to allow incorporation of the drug at the target concentration
- Controlling drug release and permeation
- Improving general aesthetics of the product to increase patient compliance
- Improve drug skin permeability and/or deposition
- Improve drug and formulation stability
- Prevention of microbial growth and contamination

For aqueous-based preparations such as aqueous gels and oil/water (o/w) emulsions, water is often the main drug solvent although various water-miscible solvents such as polyols (e.g., polyethylene glycol [PEG] and propylene glycol) and alcohols (e.g., ethanol, isopropyl alcohol, benzyl alcohol) can be included to improve drug solubility. Humectants such as glycerol, triacetin, and polyols have traditionally been included into aqueous-based formulations such as gels to improve the moisturizing and occlusive effect gels lack in comparison to creams and ointments. Formulations with a high emollient content such as lipids found in creams and ointments which, when applied to the skin, protect and soften the skin, making it more supple, are often used for dry and inflammatory skin conditions such as in patients with dermatitis, psoriasis, and eczema.

The stratum corneum provides a physical barrier to the skin from the external environment and as a result, prohibits or reduces the permeation of topically applied drugs. In an attempt to reduce the barrier function of the stratum corneum, a vast range of chemical permeation enhancers has been evaluated with varying degrees of success. Some of the classes of enhancers examined include azones, pyrrolidones, fatty acids, alcohols, glycols, surfactants, and phospholipids, to name a few. An in-depth review of penetration enhancer types and uses have been provided by William and Barry.[26] Among these, fatty acids, alcohols, glycols, and surfactants usually have a dual role as a solubilizer in addition to their potential enhancing capabilities. The choice and selection of enhancers depend upon the formulation type and nature of the drug, however, consideration should also be given to the enhancers' potential pharmacological activity, toxicity, duration of action, enhancing mechanism (and reversibility), stability, and cosmetic acceptability.

Many drugs in aqueous solutions are susceptible to oxidative degradation, therefore topical products that contain such drugs may require the addition of an antioxidant. The use of antioxidants can sometimes be avoided by reducing the amount of oxygen dissolved in the solution or present in the container, especially for single-use or sterile products. The inclusion of certain excipients such as fixed oils, fats, and diethyl ether-based compounds such as Transcutol P, which may contain low-level peroxides, can also accelerate drug oxidation and should be avoided for drugs prone to oxidation. Antioxidants are also occasionally included to inhibit rancidity in formulations containing unsaturated oils and fats which are common in emulsion-based systems. Examples of commonly used antioxidants may include alkyl gallates, butylated hydroxyanisole, butylated hydroxytoluene, and tocopherols, where most exhibit synergistic effects when used in combination or in the presence of metal chelators such as edetic acid. Apart from oxidation, the stability of drugs can also be affected by pH. For example, the stability of thiotepa (an alkylating agent) in acetate buffer has been shown to be highly pH dependent where rapid degradation was observed at lower pH values[27]; thus, buffers in topical formulations in general have been used to maintain pH of a formulation throughout its shelf life. Other than drugs, the behavior of certain excipients is also affected by pH. Most carbomers have a pKa of around 6 and as such require a certain pH to hydrate and form a gel. Therefore, the viscosity of a gel formulation comprising of a carbomer as a gelling agent may be affected if significant changes in formulation pH occur over storage. Another class of excipient that plays a significant role in the stability of a formulation are emulsifiers, which prevent coalescence of dispersed droplets in emulsified systems by formation of a barrier at the interface. Examples of emulsifiers may include anionic and nonionic surfactants, polysaccharides, and glycerides. Photolabile drugs, which are susceptible to photodegradation on exposure to ultraviolet (UV) or visible light such as benzodiazepines[28] and certain vitamins,[29] could potentially be stabilized by addition of photostability agents; however, the use of such chemicals have less significance in topical products since photostability can be overcome by using appropriate packaging materials.

Antimicrobials are usually included in formulations containing water such as aqueous gels and creams to prevent contamination and growth of microorganisms. In nonaqueous systems such as ointments, it is uncommon to include antimicrobial preservatives since microorganisms, while they may survive, would rarely proliferate under such conditions. A preservative should be active against a wide spectrum of microorganisms and its selection should be based on several factors such as compatibility with the formulation, toxicity, irritancy potential, and the site at which the formulation is to be applied. The actual concentration of preservative required should also be taken into consideration, since other excipients within the formulation may have some antimicrobial activity. Examples of some commonly used preservatives include alcohols (e.g., benzyl alcohol, ethanol, and phenoxyethanol), hydroxybenzoates (all salts), phenols (e.g., chlorocresol), and quaternary ammonium compounds (e.g., benzalkonium chloride and cetrimide).

Product "In Use" Considerations

During product use, most formulations undergo considerable physical changes once they are applied to the surface of the skin. For example, the effect of rubbing may decrease the viscosity of a formulation containing a thixotropic gelling agent such as xanthan gum, and this in turn may have an effect on drug release from the formulation and permeation across the skin. If a volatile solvent is present, evaporation of a drug solvent within a formulation may reduce the solubility of the drug and result in precipitation or physical instability of the formulation. However, this effect has also been used by many formulation scientists to increase the drug thermodynamic activity and thus increase drug release.[30-35] Oxidation reactions in products intended for multiple use may be accelerated because of potentially greater and longer exposure to oxygen after opening. In such cases, careful consideration must be given to the selection of an appropriate antioxidant and the conditions under which its efficacy are tested. Likewise, contamination from frequent use may warrant the inclusion of a preservative such that the microbial load throughout the product life remains below the recommended level.

Analytical Method

Most topical formulations contain several or more excipients with potentially low levels of drug, thus, an existing analytical method available for a drug may not be suitable to detect and quantify the drug in the presence of the other constituents of the formulation. Thus, modification of such analytical methods is usually necessary. Ultimately, the method will need to be stability indicting, such that it will be suitable for the resolution, identification, and quantification of drug impurities and related substances throughout the product shelf life. Also, when testing the performance of a formulation using *in vitro* experiments such as the measurement of skin permeation, extremely low levels of drug may need to be detected, necessitating sufficiently sensitive quantification of the drug. Such methods are often very different from those used for the identification and quantification of the drug and its impurities in the product. While "fit-for-purpose" methods may be sufficient for the initial development stage, a fully validated method as outlined by the International Conference on Harmonisation (ICH) guidelines (ICH Q2A,[36] Q2(R1),[37] and Q2B[38]) must be implemented for the drug and its related impurities during characterization and stability testing of the final lead formulations prior to clinical studies.

Solubility and Compatibility

Solubility

Solubility plays an essential role as part of formulation development since inadequate drug solubility in a formulation will impede the development of certain drugs if the target dose cannot be achieved. Likewise, a very soluble drug may also pose issues such as poor drug release from a system. Thus the solubility of a particular drug may necessitate the selection of a narrow range of solvents which are only suitable for specific dosage forms. For example, a highly lipophilic drug is less likely to be formulated as an aqueous gel but as a cream, ointment, or nonaqueous gel.

During pre-formulation study design, the selection of solvents is based on the initial dosage form of choice using a library of topically acceptable excipients. Some of the approaches used to dissolve drugs for topical formulation development include the use of cosolvents, pH adjustment, complexation, surfactants, and a combination thereof. Of these approaches, the use of cosolvents is probably the most practical and commonly used method to solubilize poorly soluble compounds in aqueous systems. When sufficient solubility cannot be achieved in a single solvent (most likely aqueous), cosolvents are used as an alternative option to increase drug solubility. A variety of solvents can be used and it is important that the selection of cosolvents is based on the miscibility of each solvent to avoid phase separation. In addition, solvents and nonsolvents are also used in cosolvent systems to increase the thermodynamic activity of highly soluble drugs at the desired drug concentration. pH is an effective method to increase drug solubility since most drugs are weakly ionizable acids or bases, and with a consideration of the pH of the solution and the pKa value of the drug, solubility can be optimized. In addition, it should be emphasized that the pH of the final formulation should be in the region of 5–7, although slightly more acidic pH values (>pH 4) may still be acceptable for topical formulations depending on the application site, frequency, and area. Surfactant systems have also been successfully used in the form of emulsions, microemulsions,[39] and nanoemulsions[40,41] to improve solubilization of poorly aqueous soluble drugs while other methods such as the use of cyclodextrins to complex hydrophobic molecules have also been used extensively to improve drug solubility.[42–44]

For the development of topical semisolids, typically up to 20 solvents would be selected for solubility screening during an initial pre-formulation stage. The suitability and range of such solvents are initially selected based on the physicochemical properties of the drug and the desired dosage form or product profile to be developed. The completion of this initial investigation will determine if a wider range of alternative solvents have to be investigated or if the target dose can be achieved. If the latter is achievable, cosolvent systems would be developed and together with the drug, these systems would be tested for drug/excipient and excipient/excipient compatibility.

Compatibility

Excipients are the components of a formulation that in combination produce a "successful" pharmaceutical product. Although the drug or active is of primary importance since it is responsible for the treatment of the disease, in order to "present and deliver" the drug, excipients play an equally important role. While traditionally excipients have been used as "inert" material such as bulking agents in dosage forms such as tablets, the more recent development of drug delivery systems has used the benefit of excipient–drug interaction to produce formulations with specific properties and performance specifications. Thus any interaction between excipients and the drug substance must be well understood and is fundamental in developing any drug product.

Excipient/drug or excipient/excipient compatibility can be classified as physical, chemical, or physiological and such interactions may have implications for drug stability, product manufacture, drug release, product efficacy, therapeutic activity, and side effect profiles. There are several approaches to conduct excipient compatibility screening and these can be dependent upon the dosage form; however, the main approach is based on accelerated temperature studies. In this case, an experiment is designed to investigate the effect on compatibility of the drug and excipient under real-time (25°C) and accelerated conditions (e.g., 40 or 50°C). Usually, such experiments are designed using excipients comprising of solutions of the drug in pure solvent to investigate experimental "extremes." Higher accelerated temperature conditions may be investigated, but such experiments must be based on the assumption that any reaction rate is proportional to temperature and this is often not the case. For example, based on an approximation of the Arrhenius equation (and assuming first-order kinetics), a study performed at 40°C over a month would approximately equate to approximately 4 months at 25°C. Although the majority of initial excipient compatibility for topical dosage forms are performed on solvents and excipients existing as liquids at room temperature, consideration has to be taken for certain semisolids with low melting points. For example, semisolids such as fatty acids with low melting points employed as thickeners may have enhanced potential for interaction if the product is stored at elevated temperatures. Likewise, crystallization of poorly soluble excipients at lower temperatures should also be investigated; thus, the key objective of an excipient compatibility screen is to eliminate or mitigate any risks of incompatibility at an early product development stage for a particular drug or active substance.

FORMULATION DEVELOPMENT

Although the specifics of a target product profile for a topical formulation will vary depending on its ultimate purpose, there are key aspects of most target profiles that are the same for most formulations. The most basic of these is the use of approved excipients, where the type and concentration of excipient used should be acceptable from a regulatory perspective (as discussed earlier). It is also always the case that the excipients utilized must be suitable for use in the disease state for which the formulation is designed. In addition, the extent and rate of release of drug from a formulation should be well understood. *In vitro* release rates are a useful assessment of this parameter and can also serve as a valuable quality control (QC) release tool in monitoring formulation changes on storage. Clearly it should also be demonstrated that the formulation should deliver the drug into the skin at the required concentration and to the required site of action. The cosmetic elegance and patient acceptability of any product is also of importance, while the physical and chemical stability of the drug/formulation must yield adequate shelf life. It is also important to ensure that the developed formulation can be manufactured at commercial scales.

Lastly, the cost of goods for the product must satisfy the demands of its particular market. Ultimately, it is always important to remember a general rule that the simpler a formulation is, the less things there are to go wrong.

Semisolid Topical Formulations

The three most commonly encountered semisolid topical formulations are ointments, creams, and gels. For chronic dermatological disorders such as eczema, psoriasis, and dermatitis, occlusive formulations such as ointments or anhydrous systems are often preferred since these preparations have protective properties. However, such anhydrous mixtures are also usually very tacky and greasy and have poor aesthetic properties. Although such formulation types are extremely useful as emollients due to their occlusive properties, their value as topical products is limited by their poor drug solubility. In such cases, drug solubility can only be enhanced by formulation with hydrocarbon-miscible solvents such as isopropyl myristate or propylene glycol. Anhydrous systems may also comprise of pure PEG systems or triglyceride derivatives in addition to the traditional hydrocarbon systems containing white soft paraffin and petrolatum. Alternatively, silicone-based formulations may also be used; however, the regulatory status of silicones for topical use is currently limited, even though an extensive positive safety profile is emerging.

Alternative monophasic systems to ointments are aqueous gel formulations. Such systems usually contain water-based or alcohol-based cosolvent systems with a thickening agent based on cellulose derivatives, polysaccharide polymers, or acrylate polymers. Although these systems are more aesthetically pleasing than anhydrous systems or ointments, they do not have the occlusive properties of the former systems and as such are usually used for the application of anti-inflammatories, anti-infectives, or antihistamines, or where facial application is required such as acne and rosacea, where occlusive properties are not needed and such gels are less likely to leave a greasy "residue." To improve the occlusive properties of gels, "emugels" have been developed. Emugels, or emulsified gels, are essentially biphasic systems containing an aqueous gel dispersed with a lipid phase, closely relating to a cream.

Creams are dispersed systems comprising of an outer (e.g., water) continuous phase and an inner (e.g., oil) immiscible dispersed phase. Such systems are also known as o/w emulsions. Where the phases are reversed, the system is known as a w/o emulsion. The indication for which the product will be used is an important consideration in the choice of emulsion type. o/w emulsions are significantly more common compared to w/o, given the availability of a wider range of regulatory acceptable emulsifying agents such as surfactants suitable for stabilizing o/w emulsions when compared to w/o emulsions. From a cosmetic acceptability point of view, o/w emulsions are generally less "greasy" and thus more acceptable. The development of multiple emulsions, for example, an oil in water in oil (o/w/o), would allow compartmentalization of incompatible excipients/drugs with similar physicochemical properties in this multiple-phase system. As with all multiple-phase systems, their effect on drug release should always be considered.

Liposomes have often been investigated in pharmaceuticals and cosmetics to enhance poorly soluble drugs, for drug targeting, and to improve formulation aesthetics. These colloidal systems often consist of vesicle-forming unilamellar or multilamellar phospholipids enclosing an aqueous core. Although liposomes have been investigated to improve drug localization and solubility,[45] their importance in topical pharmaceutical products has yet to be realized due to their expense, the elevated costs to produce such formulations, and their poor stability.[46] However, more recently, due to intense investigation, such disadvantages have been overcome to a certain extent.[47]

More recently, the use of emulsifier-free approaches has intensified in the development of pharmaceutical and cosmetic products. Creams or emulsion-based systems usually comprise of one or more traditional emulsifiers such as surfactants to stabilize the formulation. However, due to the irritancy potential of such surfactants,[48] polymeric emulsifiers such as carbomers, celluloses, and polyacrylates have been successfully used to stabilize emulsions and replace them.[49] The high molecular weight of such polymeric emulsifiers means that they are less likely to penetrate the stratum corneum, thus minimizing any of the unwanted effects often observed. In addition, surfactants like detergents and soaps have a tendency to emulsify and remove natural lipids within the skin, leaving a "dry-skin" feel, a drawback not observed with polymeric emulsifiers.

Development Approach

The outcome of pre-formulation work will give an indication as to whether the target drug concentration is achievable and if any potential stability concerns are likely to arise during formulation development. In consideration of all the data from the pre-formulation work and if the initial aim to develop a particular formulation type is feasible, then formulations can be developed as summarized in Figure 14.4. However, if potential incompatibility becomes obvious, alternative formulation types may have to be considered, and therefore an alternative approach such as that described in Figure 14.5 may be necessary. For the purpose of this chapter, both approaches have been confined to the development of semisolid topical formulations and three hypothetical case studies have been presented as examples. These examples are obviously not exhaustive since the development of formulations should be tailored toward the needs of the drug, disease, and target product profile. However, the principles of topical formulation development reflected in these examples are widely applicable.

Case Study 1

Aim

- To develop a topical gel formulation for the application to the facial area.

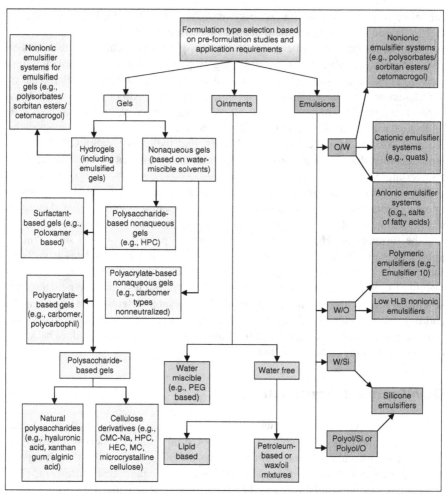

Figure 14.4 Formulation development decision tree based on formulation type. HEC, hydroxyethylcellulose; O/W, oil/water; W/O, water/oil; W/Si, water/silicone; Polyol/Si, polyol/silicone; Polyol/O, polyol/oil; HLB, hydrophilic lipophilic balance; MC, microcrystalline cellulose.

Technical Challenges

- The product is intended for application to the facial area, therefore the formulation should have minimal residue and tackiness and allow quick application when required.
- Drug is highly soluble in a wide range of solvents but a low target concentration is required, thus the combination of nonsolvents may be required to maintain a high thermodynamic activity.

Development Approach Pre-formulation studies showed that the drug was highly soluble in a wide range of solvents, thus limiting the choice of nonsolvents

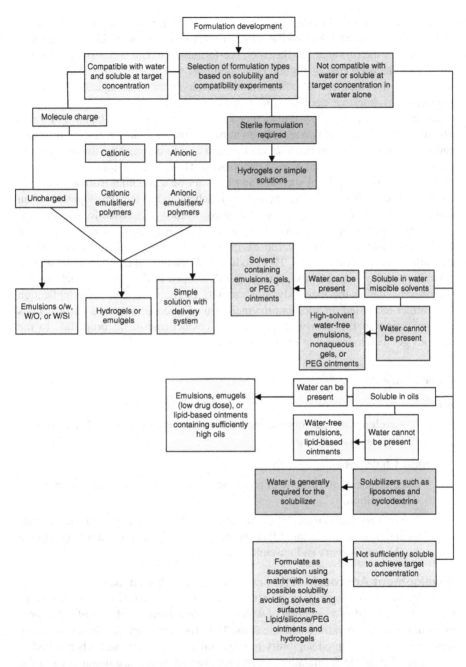

Figure 14.5   Formulation development decision tree based on drug physicochemical properties.

that could be employed to develop a monophasic gel formulation. In addition, the lack of nonsolvents also limited the scope in optimizing the thermodynamic activity of the drug in the formulation. Based on pre-formulation data and aesthetic requirements, the decision tree in Figure 14.4 highlights two feasible approaches during formulation development. The first was the development of an aqueous gel with a humectant to improve aesthetics/moisturization on application to the skin. The remainder of the cosolvent system included a volatile component, ethanol, and water. Ethanol was included for two reasons: to minimize the formulation residue on application, thus improving the in use aesthetics, and also to increase the thermodynamic activity of the drug in formulation on evaporation, However, consideration was taken to include ethanol at a level such that it would not be a potential irritant especially when applied to the face. The second approach included the development of an emulsified gel based on the best performing cosolvent system used for the aqueous gel. Using a surfactant suitable for incorporation into an aqueous-based gel, a topical pharmaceutically approved volatile excipient was included as a nonsolvent and emulsified into the formulation. This produced an opaque gel that had lower overall solubility for the drug than the aqueous gel developed in the first approach. As the silicone is volatile, the thermodynamic activity of the drug following application was further increased. In addition, the inclusion of silicone improved the aesthetics on application to the skin with comparable cosmetic/aesthetic properties to the aqueous gel developed using the first approach.

Case Study 2

Aim

- To develop a topical formulation for the treatment of hyperproliferative skin diseases such as psoriasis.

Technical Challenges

- Good cosmetic and emollient properties to manage the dry and inflammatory skin condition.
- A relatively high target drug concentration (1% w/w) was required and pre-formulation data indicated that the drug was only soluble in a very limited number of solvents and unstable in alcohols.

Development Approach Pref-ormulation studies showed the drug to have low solubility in a wide range of excipients, which included water. However, good solubility was observed in a selection of water-miscible solvents such as PEG and some oils, but it was incompatible with alcohols. Therefore, although the drug was poorly soluble in water, the good solubility in water-miscible solvents and oils resulted in a number of possible formulation approaches, two of which are highlighted in the decision tree summarized in Figure 14.5.

The first approach involved the development of a gel formulation containing water-miscible solvents. Since water-free formulations tend to give a greasy feel and as water could be present in the formulation, it was included to improve the formulation aesthetics. A cosolvent system comprising water as a nonsolvent, glycerol as a humectant, and PEG as the main solvent was developed. Suitable gelling agents were then selected based on their compatibility with high solvent content gels. The second approach was to develop an o/w emulsion. The same solvent system used for the gel was employed for incorporation into the emulsion. However, the overall solubility of the drug in the formulation on comparison to the gel was reduced due to the limited amount of solvent that could be incorporated within the oil phase to produce a stable emulsion. Since good drug solubility was observed in some oils, a medium chain triglyceride was included in the oil phase of the emulsion to increase solubility of the drug to enable the target drug concentration to be achieved.

Case Study 3

Aims

- Development of a formulation incorporating a nonsteroidal anti-inflammatory drug (NSAID) for topical application.
- The target region for the drug was regional delivery to tissues such as joints and muscles below the site of application.

Technical Challenges

- The formulation was required to be nongreasy.
- Inclusion of a sensory component to improve consumer acceptance and compliance

Development Work   The pre-formulation studies showed a good selection of both solvents and nonsolvents based on the solubility experiments where the drug was mostly soluble in water-miscible solvents; however, the compatibility experiments showed very poor stability in the presence of water. As such, formulation types that could be developed were limited to water-free emulsions, nonaqueous gels, or a suspension as shown in Figure 14.5. As a suspension formulation was undesirable (from an aesthetic and physical stability perspective), preliminary development was based on water-free emulsions and nonaqueous gels. Initial development of o/w emulsions using only water-miscible solvents in the absence of water showed the formulations to be incompatible when the drug was included. The development of nonaqueous gels was successful but limited to using a hydrophobic gelling agent such as hydroxypropylcellulose (HPC). The solvent systems incorporated a penetration enhancer for improved skin penetration and a volatile solvent to increase the thermodynamic activity of the drug in the formulation upon evaporation. In addition, a combination of volatile and nonvolatile silicone fluid to reduce the greasy skin feel and increase thermodynamic activity of the drug in the formulation on application was also included successfully with sensory components such as essential oils.

FORMULATION PERFORMANCE TESTING, OPTIMIZATION, AND SELECTION

The performance of a topical formulation can be assessed using a range of methods depending on factors such as formulation type, target disease, aesthetic requirements, and application site. However, three parameters that form a key role as part of a formulation development program are the formulation stability and the release and skin permeation characteristics of the drug from the formulation. Ultimately, a formulation optimized for drug release and permeation is often more efficacious and may require a lower concentration of drug, which may reduce the cost of the final product, drug irritation potential, and also maximize clinical efficacy.

Stability Testing

Once a series of prototype formulations are produced from the excipients evaluated at the pre-formulation stage they are placed on short-term, real-time, and accelerated stability, for example, 25 and 40°C (60% and 75% relative humidity [RH], respectively), in order to determine if there are likely to be any stability issues for the formulation over the long term. Such work is another part of the selection criteria of the lead formulation. At each time point, examples of the tests to be performed include drug content, pH, and physical appearance (microscopic and macroscopic). At this stage the validation of recovery of the drug from the formulation may not have been performed, thus both drug recovery from a generic extraction solvent and percent peak purity will be used in combination to assess for any stability trends. Ultimately, the duration of this initial stability study will dependent upon time available for product development; however, typically, a short-term study over 1–2 months may suffice at this stage to act as a screen for potential prototypes to be selected for further *in vitro* drug release and permeation testing.

In Vitro Drug Release Studies

Absorption of drugs into or through the skin depends upon a number of factors, including composition of the formulation, type and condition of the skin, and factors such as temperature, humidity, and occlusion. However, one factor that has a major influence on the rate or extent of percutaneous absorption is the thermodynamic activity of the drug in the formulation on the skin surface. This is obviously strongly influenced by the physicochemical properties of the drug and ultimately by its solubility in the solvents it is formulated with.

Synthetic membranes have been investigated as a readily available and easy-to-use tool to study the *in vitro* release profiles of drugs from topical formulations in order to ascertain batch-to-batch uniformity. Examples of artificial membranes used include silicone, polycarbonate, and cellulose. Such membranes can provide additional information contributing to the understanding of mechanistic aspects of skin permeability. For example, the thermodynamic effects of drug solubility, partition coefficient, pH, and drug–excipient interactions, and so on can sometimes be better understood by using synthetic membranes. When a formulation is applied to the skin, the drug must first diffuse across the formulation and the thermodynamic activity must then be sufficient for the drug to be released and partition into the stratum corneum. As such, this method is routinely used in order to optimize formulations for drug release.

Like classical tablet dissolution testing, *in vitro* release testing has also been employed to demonstrate "sameness" under certain scale-up and postapproval changes for semisolid products,[50] and it is assumed that *in vitro* release testing can be used to characterize performance characteristics of a finished topical dosage form, that is, semisolids such as creams, gels, and ointments. Important changes in the characteristics of a drug product formula or the thermodynamic properties of the drug(s) it contains should show a difference in drug release.

A typical *in vitro* release method for topical dosage forms is based on an open chamber diffusion cell system such as a Franz cell system, fitted usually with a synthetic membrane (Fig. 14.6). The test product is placed on the upper side of the membrane in the open donor chamber of the diffusion cell and a sampling fluid is placed on the other side of the membrane in a receptor cell. Diffusion of drug from the topical product across the membrane is monitored by assay of sequentially collected samples from the receptor fluid. Aliquots removed from the receptor phase can be analyzed for drug content by high-pressure liquid chromatography (HPLC) or other analytical methodology as appropriate. A plot of the amount of drug released per unit area (micrograms per square centimeter) against the square root of time yields a straight line, the slope of which is representative of the release rate.

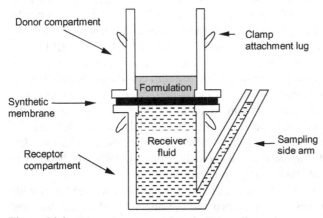

Figure 14.6   Schematic representation of a Franz cell.

In Vitro Skin Permeation Studies

Human or animal skin has also been widely used in *in vitro* studies of topical products. Sources of human skin utilized in this way have included cadaver skin, skin excised during cosmetic surgery, and diseased skin. *In vitro* studies based on cadaver skin may be useful but can exhibit substantial variability and, owing to the nonviable state of the preparation, do not take into account certain skin processes such as metabolism that may impact on drug permeation into the skin. Despite these limitations, *in vitro* experiments conducted using human skin have yielded valuable information on permeation of topically applied drugs.[51-53] This approach has been used to screen formulations in product development and potentially could be used to assess *in vivo* performance (see Chapter 9 of this volume). Such models have also been used to screen for drug candidates suitable for topical delivery and used as an alternative to *in silico* models or as a means to confirm *in silico* predictions.

However, a validated, reliable, and reproducible test procedure defining the use of human or animal skin is essential for meaningful interpretation of drug permeability. As such, extensive guidelines on conducting skin permeation experiments have been made available by the Organisation for Economic Cooperation and Development (OECD) (Guidance Document for the Conduct of Skin Absorption Studies—OECD Series on Testing and Assessment 28) and the European Commission (Guidance Document on Dermal Absorption, rev 7, 2004).

As with *in vitro* drug release experiments, *in vitro* skin permeation experiments involve the use of a diffusion cell designed to mimic the physiological and anatomical conditions of skin *in situ* (see Chapter 9 for a detailed discussion on this subject). An example of the model used is the Franz diffusion cell as described in Figure 14.6. However, full-thickness skin, epidermal membrane, or stratum corneum instead of a synthetic membrane is positioned between the two halves, with the stratum corneum facing the donor compartment. A finite dose (1–10 mg/cm^2) of formulation is applied to the surface of the skin membrane. The receptor compartment of the Franz cells is filled with a suitable receiver fluid to maintain sink conditions and the cells fixed in a water bath maintained at 37°C. The receptor chamber content is continuously agitated by small magnetic followers and at regular time intervals, samples of receiver fluid are taken from the receptor compartment, replaced with fresh receiver medium, and assayed by a suitable assay method such as HPLC.

Upon completion of the skin permeation study, quantification of the residual drug on the surface of the membrane, within the stratum corneum, epidermal membrane, and/or dermis (full mass balance) can be performed. This technique can involve removal of the stratum corneum by tape stripping and separation of the epidermis and dermal layer where the active can be recovered by a suitable analytical method. From these models and applying similar principles, various other models utilizing diseased skin to mimic the clinical setting more closely can be used to assess for drug permeation during product development.

Although *in vitro* systems to determine drug release and skin permeation provide useful data, each system has to be validated and optimized based on the drug and dosage form to be tested in order to obtain meaningful data. For example, in a drug release experiment, the drug physicochemical properties would have to be considered when selecting an artificial membrane of choice such that the rate of drug release should be influenced by the formulation characteristics and not restricted by poor partitioning and diffusion of the drug across the synthetic membrane used. Occlusion of the donor compartment is often used to prevent evaporation of the formulation to be tested over; however, such practice may not be appropriate for all formulation types. For example, the performance of a topical dosage form containing a volatile solvent would be affected since the rate of evaporation of the volatile component from such a formulation would most probably affect drug solubility, the thermodynamic activity of the drug, and therefore drug release and permeation.

Formulation Optimization

Formulation optimization is a continuous process and several approaches can be used to optimize a product during the development stage; examples include using factorial design, single-factor approach, and a systematic approach.

Factorial designs are commonly used during product development, particularly when different formulation components (e.g., excipient/excipient and/or drug/excipient) are thought to interact significantly. Since the identification of key contributing factors such as parameter type, level, and range is often difficult, the risk of potentially omitting a real parameter often exists. In addition, where key contributing factors cannot be identified, such designs could potentially lead to a large number of repetitions for each variable in order to ascertain data validity, and interpretation of responses may not always be straightforward. As the name suggests, a single-factor approach involves varying each factor in series and such an approach is normally restricted to single-parameter responses and is mostly unsuitable for the development of topical formulations that typically contain multiple variable parameters. A systematic approach is more often used by experienced formulators, and in such an approach, key contributing factors are systematically determined. An example of such an approach is highlighted in the flowchart described in Figure 14.2 where the development process involves a series of pre-formulation tests prior to development and testing of formulation prototypes to identify lead candidates. Throughout this process, the prototype formulations developed are "optimized" according to the outcome from the series of experiments performed in relation to the set out aims. Under most circumstances, optimization would usually involve larger changes during initial prototype development while smaller changes would normally be performed following completion of *in vitro* testing of formulation prototypes and it is at this stage where optimization of a formulation is mostly referred to.

The completion of stability studies, *in vitro* release, and skin permeation studies, depending on the outcome, may result in the need for a significant change to the formulation and thus iterations of the performance tests described above. For example, drug recovery from the epidermal layer following a mass balance study, if found to be below the target concentration, may be a result of several factors:

1. *Poor or No Drug Release from the Formulation.* Likely reasons for this may be drug binding to excipients or simply low drug thermodynamic activity. Such a phenomenon would be obvious when an *in vitro* drug release experiment is performed.

2. *Poor Inherent Drug Permeability.* The suitability of a drug candidate to permeate across the skin can usually be predicted by assessing its physicochemical properties. For example, hydrophilic drugs with unfavorably high molecular weight (>600 Da) would be less likely to partition across the stratum corneum compared to a more lipophilic drug with low molecular weight. In some cases, the inclusion of penetration enhancers can remedy poor drug physicochemical characteristics, but this approach is not a panacea for all such situations.

3. *Insufficient Dose or Drug Concentration.* Such risks are usually mitigated by performing a dose-ranging study to cover a sufficiently wide range of drug concentration. In some cases, alteration of drug concentration may result in significant redevelopment work.

4. *Drug Metabolism.* Although the metabolism of a drug is less significant when using excised skin, some degree of metabolism, depending on the skin storage condition, may still be present and this parameter should at least be considered.

Formulation Selection

Along with formulation stability, drug release, and skin permeation testing, other performance assessments can include aesthetic and cosmetic acceptability, perhaps by a consumer panel, the use of pre-clinical disease models, and early-stage toxicity assessment if required. In addition, stability in various packaging materials may be determined. Ultimately the objective is to test the performance of the developed candidate formulations in order to mitigate the risk of failure during clinical investigation. However, once all such assessments and formulation optimization has been completed, one lead and preferably at least one back-up formulation should be selected for full characterization and stability testing.

FORMULATION CHARACTERIZATION AND ICH STABILITY

Detailed characterization of a formulation is usually performed once the lead candidate(s) formulation has been defined. Formulation characterization is performed to define a provisional product specification and methods of measurement for these parameters such that that the capability or performance of a product can be monitored during ICH stability tests and to ensure that they remain within the set specifications throughout its shelf life. For topical semisolids, some examples of typical parameters determined are described in the subsequent text.

Formulation Characterization

Macroscopic/Microscopic Appearance and Odor

Macroscopic or product visual appearance may include color changes, absence of particulates, and/or formulation appearance (e.g., phase separation of semisolid formulations on storage), where such observations provide first-hand information on the stability of the drug product. Microscopic appearance to observe for the formation of drug particulates could be determined using optical microscopy or more sophisticated instruments such as X-ray diffraction. Development of odor over time could be a stability indication for formulations containing triglycerides, for example, which are prone to hydrolysis or microbial contamination.

Drug Content and Uniformity, Related Substances, and Degradation Products

A validated analytical method capable of measuring drug content and impurities at the required levels should have been established by this stage of the development program. Although the specifications for drug content of a topical product would typically range between 95% and 105% for semisolids, the levels of impurities would be dependent upon the drug in question and thus will have to be justified and characterized according to the analytical method and drug product. Extensive guidance on the testing of drug products and related substances/impurities and new dosage forms is available in the form of ICH guidelines and from the EMA.[54] The determination of formulation uniformity is especially important for biphasic systems such as emulsions. For example, a lipophilic drug may be preferably distributed within the oil phase of an o/w emulsion, therefore it is important to demonstrate that the drug is uniformly distributed within the formulation. Uniformity is usually determined by analysis of the drug content from sampling of the top, middle, and bottom of a bulk sample.

Preservative Content

For products containing preservatives, part of the product specification should be to ensure that the specified level of preservative is present. In addition, preservative effectiveness must be monitored as part of the final ongoing stability program and this can be accomplished through analysis for the level of preservative previously shown to be effective and/or through preservative efficacy testing.

pH

The skin has a pH between 5 and 6.5[55] and as discussed previously, the pH of a product can influence not only the solubility and stability of a drug in the formulation, but may also affect its potential to cause skin irritation, therefore, many topical products are formulated to be in that pH range. Although development of products with lower pH values (up to pH 3.5) may be adequate, such products would require considerable justification from a formulation development point of view and such potentially irritable pH values may be acceptable depending on the product use and frequency as well as application site.

Rheology and Viscosity

Testing for rheological or flow properties of a drug product is normally performed for formulations with bioadhesive or mucoadhesive properties where the rheological property and residence time would have an impact on the performance or release of the drug product. Thus for most semisolids applied to the skin, viscosity/rheology is normally employed to monitor or assess the "thickness" or rheological behavior of a product type, respectively, where changes in viscosity or rheological behavior of a product can be indicative of changes in physical stability or performance of a product. For example, a loss in viscosity over time from a gel formulation could indicate a possible breakdown in molecular weight of the polymer as a result of microbial contamination, which is common with polysaccharide-based polymers and may therefore affect the overall physical stability of the formulation. Therefore it is important that batches comprising of similar molecular weight range are used to ensure consistency between product batches. Such observations have previously been reported in the literature,[56] where seven Carbomer 934 lots were studied and the rheological behavior in aqueous dispersion was found to differ significantly, possibly due to differences in mean molecular weight. The authors also found that such differences in viscosity significantly affected the release rate of theophylline and chlorthiazide.

Microbial Quality or Microbial Limit Test (MLT) and Preservative Efficacy Test (PET)

The inclusion of an MLT for a drug product is dependent upon the dosage form and therefore typically used only for nonsterile products which contain sufficient water to support the growth of microorganisms. Therefore, semisolid dosage forms such as ointments and other nonaqueous systems such as nonaqueous gels with little or no water sufficient to support microorganism growth would not be routinely tested unless an excipient or the drug within the product is susceptible to microbial contamination.

Most multidose products for topical application would contain a preservative or combination of preservatives. A PET is performed usually on aqueous-based semisolids to determine the minimum effective concentration of one or more preservatives required for adequate control of contamination, thus products are considered satisfactorily preserved if they meet the requirements set out by the pharmacopoeia. The appropriate preservative system for a particular drug product should be demonstrated to be effective below its target concentration (typically between 70% and 95% of target concentration), where the antimicrobial efficacy of the preservative in the final product should be assessed during product development, particularly during stability studies and at the end of the proposed shelf life using a test outlined by a pharmacopoeia.

Sterility

Sterile semisolid formulations to be applied to the skin are mostly aimed for wound or burn indications, single-use products, and comprise of topical gels or solutions. Since the method of sterilization is dependent upon the formulation type, composition, and also packaging, such factors should be taken into consideration even during pre-formulation stage, and sterility testing should be performed in the final packaging such that container closure integrity can also be assessed. It is also important that the relevant sterility test is performed according to requirement since the sterility test outlined within the USP has several significant differences from the EP while the JP is identical to that of the EP.

ICH Stability

Once characterized, the formulation(s) are placed on long-term accelerated and real-time stability studies performed at ICH conditions 25°C/60% RH, 30°C/65% RH, and 40°C/75% RH (ICH Q1A(R2)).[57] Such a study may span over a period of at least 2 years and typical time points may include t = 0, 1, 3, 6, 9, 12, 18, and 24 months where all characterized parameters described in the section "Formulation Characterization" are tested to monitor the performance of the product over its shelf life. At the same time, the primary packaging materials may also be selected and investigated with the formulation as a final product.

CONCLUSIONS

The development of any product is unique to the particular drug and dosage form where various issues have to be identified and considered during the development process. This chapter has provided a general overview from drug selection to formulation selection for good manufacturing practice (GMP) scale-up and pre-clinical and clinical evaluation. The performance of such a development program is complex and drug/disease specific with influences from marketing, regulatory, and scientific perspectives, and this chapter discusses some of these aspects and summarizes general approaches with specific examples that will serve as a useful guide for the development of any topical product.

REFERENCES

1. BOWN MB. The lost science of formulation. *Drug Delivery Technology* 2005; 10: 1405–1407.
2. FLYNN GL. Physicochemical determinants of skin absorption. In: Gerrity TR, Henry CJ, eds. *Principles of Route-to-Route Extrapolation for Risk Assessment.* Elsevier, New York, 1990; 93–127.

3. Moss GP, Cronin MTD. Quantitative structure-permeatibility relationships (QSPRs) for percutaneous absorption: Re-analysis of steroid data. *International Journal of Pharmaceutics* 2002; 238: 105–109.

4. Potts RO, Guy RH. Predicting skin permeability. *Pharmaceutical Research* 1992; 12: 663–669.

5. Fiserova-Bergerova V, Pierce JT, Droz PO. Dermal absorption of industrial chemicals: criteria for skin notation. *A. J. Ind.* 1990; 17: 617–635.

6. Barratt MD. Quantitative structure-activity relationships for skin permeability. *Toxicology in Vitro* 1995; 9: 27–37.

7. Potts, RO, Guy, RHA. Predictive algorithm for skin permeability: The effects of molecular size and hydrogen bond activity. *Pharm Res* 1995; 12: 1628–1633.

8. Pugh WJ, Roberts M, Hadgraft J. Epidermal permeability—penetrant structure relationships: 3. The effect of hydrogen bonding interactions and molecular size on diffusion across the *stratum corneum*. *International Journal of Pharmaceutics* 1996; 138: 149–165.

9. Kirchner LA, Moody RP, Doyle E, Bose R, Jeffery J, Chu I. The prediction of skin permeability by using physicochemical data. *Alternatives to Laboratory Animals* 1997; 25: 359–370.

10. Cronin MTD, Dearden JC, Moss GP, Murray-Dickson G. Investigation of the mechanism of flux across human skin *in vitro* by quantitative structure-permeability relationships. *European Journal of Pharmacy and Pharmacology* 1999; 7: 325–330.

11. Cronin MTD, Schultz TW. Development of quantitative structure-activity relationships for the toxicity of aromatic compounds to Tetrahymena pyriformis: Comparative assessment of the methodologies. *Chem. Res. Toxicol.* 2001; 14: 1284–1295.

12. Yamashita Y, Hashida M. Mechaniostic and empirical modelling of skin permeation of drugs. *Advanced Drug Delivery Reviews* 2003; 55: 1185–1199.

13. Farahmand F, Maibach HI. Estimating skin permeability from physicochemical characteristics of drugs: A comparison between conventional models and an *in vivo* based approach. *International Journal of Pharmaceutics* 2009; 375: 41–47.

14. Moss GP, Sun Y, Prapopoulou M, Davey N, Adams R, Pugh WJ, Brown MB. The application of Gaussian processes in the prediction of percutaneous absorption. *Journal of Pharmacy and Pharmacology* 2009; 61: 1147–1153.

15. Rasmussen CE, Williams CKI. *Gaussian Processes for Machine Learning*. Massachusetts Institute of Technology, Cambridge, MA, 2006.

16. Degim IT, Hadgraft J, Ilbasmis S, Ozkan Y. Prediction of skin penetration using artificial neural network (ANN) modelling. *Journal of Pharmaceutical Sciences* 2003; 92: 656–664.

17. Neumann D, Kohlbacher O, Merkwirth C, Lengauer T. A fully computational model for predicting percutaneous drug absorption. *Journal of Chemical Information and Modelling* 2006; 46: 424–429.

18. Lam LT, Sun Yi, Davey N, Adams R, Prapopoulou M, Brown MB, Moss GP. The application of feature selection to the development of Gaussian process models for percutaneous absorption. *J. Pharm. Pharmacol.* 2010; 62(6): 738–749.

19. Sun Y, Brown MB, Propapopolou M, Davey N, Adams R, Moss GP. The applications of stochastic machine learning methods in the prediction of skin penetration. *Applied Soft Computing* 2011; 11: 2367–2375.

20. Valenta US, Kratzel, M, Hadgraft, J. The dermal delivery of lignocaine: Influence of ion pairing. *Int. J. Pharm.* 2000; 197(1–2): 77–85.

21. Valenta C, Hadgraft J. pH, pKa and dermal delivery. *International Journal of Pharmaceutics* 2000; 200: 243–247.

22. Watkinson AC, Brain KR, Walters KA. The penetration of ibuprofen through human skin *in vitro*: Vehicle, enhancer and pH effects. In: Brain KR, James VJ, Walters KA, eds. *Prediction of Percutaneous Penetration*. STS Publishing, Cardiff, UK, 1993; 335–341.

23. Minghetti, P, Cilurzo F, Casiraghi A, Montanari, L, Fini A. Ex vivo study of transdermal permeation of four diclofenac salts from different vehicles. *J. Pharm. Sci.* 2007; 96: 814–822.

24. European Pharmacopoeia 6.3. Monographs on dosage forms, Semi-Solid Preparations for Cutaneous Application, Ointments and Creams, p. 3980.

25. British Pharmacopoeia, General Monographs, 2009, *Topical Semi-solid Preparations of the British Pharmacopoeia*, Vol. 111, p. 2253.
26. WILLIAM AC, BARRY BW. Penetration enhancers. *Advanced Drug Delivery* 2004; 56: 603–618.
27. COHEN BE, EGORIN MJ, BALACHANDRAN NAYAR MS, GUTIERREZ PL. Effects of pH and temperature on the stability and decomposition of *N,N'N"-triethylenethiophosphoramide* in urine and buffer. *Cancer Research* 1984; 44: 4312–4316.
28. CORNELISSEN PJG, BEIJERSBERGEN VHGMJ, GERRITSMA KW. Photochemical decomposition of 1,4-benzodiazepines. *International Journal of Pharmaceutics* 1978; 1: 173–181.
29. GASPAR LR, MAIA CAMPOS PMBG. Photostability and efficacy studies of topical formulations containing UV-filters combination and vitamins A, C and E. *International Journal of Pharmaceutics* 2007; 343: 181–189.
30. REID ML, JONES SA, BROWN MB. An investigation into solvent-membrane interactions when assessing drug release from organic vehicles using regenerated cellulose membranes. *Journal of Pharmaceutics and Pharmacology* 2008; 60: 1139–1147.
31. BROWN MB. The next generation in topical drug delivery. *Drug Delivery Report* 2008; Winter: 24–26.
32. JONES SA, REID ML, BROWN MB. Transient supersaturation using a topically applied metered dose aerosol to enhance drug delivery of corticosteroids. *Journal of Pharmaceutical Science* 2009; 2: 543–553.
33. REID ML, JONES SA, BROWN MB. Determining the degree of saturation after application of transiently supersaturated metered dose aerosols for topical delivery of corticosteroids. *Journal of Pharmaceutical Science* 2009; 98: 543–554.
34. REID ML, JONES SA, BROWN MB. An investigation into the effects of transient drug supersaturation kinetics on the release of beclomethasone dipropionate from rapidly drying films. *International Journal of Pharmaceutics* 2009; 371: 114–119.
35. REID ML, BROWN MB, JONES SA. Manipulation of corticosteroid release from a transiently supersaturated topical metered dose aerosol using a residual miscible co-solvent. *Pharmaceutical Research* 2008; 25: 2573–2580.
36. ICH. Q2A: Text on validation of analytical procedures: Definitions and terminology. Proceedings of the International Conference on Harmonisation. US FDA Federal Register. 1995.
37. ICH. Q2(R1): Validation of analytical procedures: Methodology. Proceedings of the International Conference on Harmonisation. US FDA Federal Register. 1996.
38. ICH. Q2B: Validation of analytical procedures: Methodology. Proceedings of the International Conference on Harmonisation. US FDA Federal Register. 1996.
39. LI CJ, OBATA Y, HIGASHIYAMA K, NAGAI T, TAKAYAMA K. Effect of 1-0-ethyl-3-butylcyclohexanol on the skin permeation of drugs with different physicochemical characteristics. *International Journal of Pharmaceutics* 2003; 259: 193–198.
40. WU HL, RAMACHANDRAN C, WEINER ND, ROESSLER BJ. Topical transport of hydrophilic compounds using water-in-oil nanoemulsions. *International Journal of Pharmaceutics* 2001; 220: 63–75.
41. HOELLER S, SPERGER A, VALENTA C. Lecithin based nanoemulsions: A comparative study of the influence of non-ionic surfactants and the cationic phytosphingosine on physicochemical behaviour and skin permeation. *International Journal of Pharmaceutics* 2009; 370: 181–186.
42. MASSON M, LOFTSSON T, SIGURDSSON HH, MAGNUSSON P, GOFFIC FL. Cyclodextrins as co-enhancers in dermal and transdermal drug delivery. *Pharmazie* 1998; 53: 137–139.
43. VENTURA CA, TAMMASINI S, FALCONE A, GIANNONE I, PAULINO D, SDARAFKAKIS V, MONDELLO MR, PUGLISI G. Influence of modified cyclodextrins on solubility and percutaneous absorption of celecoxib through human skin. *International Journal of Pharmaceuticals* 2006; 314: 37–45.
44. MANNILA J, JARVINEN K, HOLAPPA J, MATILAINEN L, AURIOLA S, JARHO P. Cyclodextrins and chitosan derivatives in sublingual delivery of low solubility peptides: A study using cyclosporine A, α-cyclodextrin and quaternary chitosan *N*-betainate. *International Journal of Pharmaceuticals* 2009; 381: 19–24.
45. SCHMID MH, KORTING HC. Therapeutic progress with topical liposome drugs for skin disease. *Advanced Drug Delivery Review* 1996; 18: 335–342.

46. GREGORIADIS G. Liposomes in drug delivery: Present and future. In: Braun-Falco O, Korting HC, Maibach HI, eds. *Liposome Dermatics*. Springer, Heidelberg, Germany, 1992; 346–352.
47. CHEN C, HAN D, CAI C, TANG X. An overview of liposome lyopholisation and its future potential. *Journal of Controlled Release* 2010; 142: 299–311.
48. WILHELM K-P, CUA AB, WOLFF HH, MAIBACH HI. Surfactant-induced *Stratum Corneum* hydration *in vivo*: Prediction of the irritation potential of anionic surfactants. *Journal of Investigative Dermatology* 1993; 101: 310–315.
49. BOBIN MF, MICHEL V, JOURNET E, MARTINI MC. Study of formulation and stability of emulsions with polymeric emulsifiers. *Colloid and Surfaces* 1999; 152: 53–58.
50. FDA. Guidance for Industry. Nonsterile Semisolid Dosage Forms. Scale-Up and Postapproval Changes: Chemistry, Manufacturing, and Controls; *In Vitro* Release Testing and *In Vivo* Bioequivalence Documentation. U.S. Department of Health and Human Services, FDA, CDER, May, 1997, SUPAC-SS, CMC 7.
51. HOTCHKISS SAM, HEWITT P, CALDWELL J, CHEN WL, ROWE RR. Percutaneous absorption of nicotinic acid, phenol, benzoic acid and tricllopyrbutoxyethyl ester through rat and human skin *in vitro*: Further validation of an *in vitro* model by comparison with *in vivo* data. *Food and Chemical Toxicology* 1992; 20(10): 891–899.
52. LODEN M, AKERSTROM U, LINDAHL K, BERNE B. Bioequivalence determination of topical ketoprofen using a dermatopharmacokinetic approach and excised skin penetration. *International Journal of Pharmaceutics* 2004; 284: 23–30.
53. TROTTEL L, OWEN H, HOLME P, HEYLINGS J, COLLIN IP, BREEN AP. Are all acyclovir cream formulations bioequivalent? *International Journal of Pharmaceutics* 2005; 304: 63–71.
54. EMEA. ICH Topic Q 3 B (R2) Impurities in New Drug Products. CPMP/ICH/2738/99, 2006.
55. BEHRENDT H, GREEN M. *Patterns of Skin pH from Birth through Adolescence: With a Synopsis on Skin Growth*. Charles C. Thomas, Springfield, IL, 1971; 1–115.
56. PEREZ-MARCOS B, MARITNEZ-PACHECO R, GOMEZ-AMOZA JL, SOUTO C, CONCHEIRO A, ROWE RC. Interlot variability of Carbomer 934. *International Journal of Pharmaceutics* 1993; 100: 207–212.
57. ICH. Q1A(R2): Stability testing of New Drug Substances and Products. Proceedings of the International Conference on Harmonisation. US FDA Federal Register. 2003.
58. WILSCHUT A, TENBERGE WF, ROBINSON PJ. Estimating skin permeation—The validation of 5 mathematical skin permeation models. *Chemosphere* 1995; 30(7): 1275–1296.

Chapter 15

Transdermal Product Formulation Development

Kenneth J. Miller

OVERVIEW

"Transdermal" means through the skin. Consequently, a transdermal product is applied to the skin for the purpose of delivering a drug to the bloodstream. This is in contrast to a topical product, which is intended to deliver drug *to* the skin rather than *through* the skin.

There are three basic types of transdermal products: aerosol sprays, semisolids, and (self-adhesive) patches.

Transdermal sprays and semisolids tend to be hormone products (estrogens and androgens) that are sprayed on, or rubbed into, the skin. The greatest advantage of these products is that they are invisible. It is virtually impossible to identify the user of a transdermal spray or semisolid. Unfortunately, this can also be a disadvantage since the drug can be unintentionally and unknowingly transferred from the skin of the patient to pets and other people.[1,2] Since transdermal sprays are still relatively new and transdermal semisolids are closely related to topical products, this chapter focuses on transdermal patches.

Self-adhesive transdermal patches are unit-dose products with defined surface areas, dosages, and potencies. Many of the product development concepts in this chapter are broadly applicable to all transdermal products, but the self-adhesive transdermal patch has the greatest number of distinct design elements and is the least like any other dosage form.

There are two basic types of transdermal patches: liquid/gel reservoir and solid matrix patches.

Liquid/gel reservoir (also known as form-fill-seal) patches sequester a drug-containing fluid or semisolid within a cavity formed between an impermeable backing film and a permeable film (usually by heat-sealing the periphery). The

Transdermal and Topical Drug Delivery: Principles and Practice, First Edition. Edited by Heather A.E. Benson, Adam C. Watkinson.

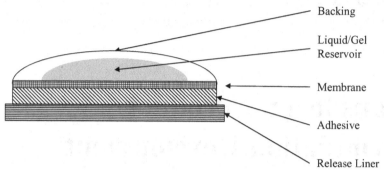

Figure 15.1   Schematic of liquid/gel reservoir transdermal patch.

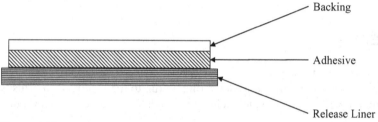

Figure 15.2   Schematic of solid matrix transdermal patch.

reservoir is either covered or surrounded by the adhesive that attaches the patch to the skin. Figure 15.1 illustrates the basic structure of a liquid/gel reservoir patch. The advantage of this design is the ability to somewhat decouple the drug delivery function from the skin adhesion function. The disadvantage is the reliance on sophisticated manufacturing processes to assure that the reservoir compartment is properly formed and well sealed. Liquid/gel reservoir patches have recently amassed unwanted attention due to the potential for the reservoir to rupture or leak. Most notably, the original Duragesic® patch and the generic competitors of similar design face increasing scrutiny due to manufacturing defects and the resulting leakage of the powerful narcotic (fentanyl) that can result.[3]

In a solid matrix patch, the adhesive and drug are mixed in the same layer to simultaneously deliver drug and affix the patch to the skin. Because of the different performance criteria for the matrix (pressure-sensitive adhesive and drug delivery medium), solid matrix patches are more complex to develop than liquid/gel reservoir patches. The advantage over liquid/gel reservoir patches is a cheaper, more robust manufacturing process. Typically, the solid matrix is coated in a continuous film on a substrate and patches are die-cut from the resulting laminate in very large batches. In addition to an adhesive film, a liquid/gel reservoir patch also requires that the gel be sealed within a semipermeable membrane. If the seal fails, the reservoir can leak and the patch will not function as intended.* Figure 15.2 shows the different layers of a simple solid matrix patch.

* There is no seal in a matrix patch, so this can't happen.

This chapter focuses on the interplay of the materials and performance criteria that go into developing solid matrix transdermal patches. The development of this type of product is particularly challenging because it requires the optimization of multiple disparate performance criteria. The exercise is made even more challenging by the interplay between the constituent materials and the performance criteria in this deceptively simple dosage form. Most of the concepts apply to both types of systems (even aerosol and semisolid transdermals), but examples and references are exclusively of the solid matrix variety because they provide the most complete view of the commercial transdermal product development landscape.

HISTORY*

The age of the modern transdermal patch began on December 31, 1979, when Alza's Transderm Scōp® was approved by the U.S. Food and Drug Administration (FDA). Barely a year later, the United States' (and Alza's) second transdermal patch (Transderm Nitro®) was approved. Although Key Pharmaceutical's Nito-Dur®[4] debuted later that same year, Alza clearly dominated the field with its Catapres-TTS® (1984), Estraderm® (1986), Durogesic® (1990), and Nicoderm® (1991) patches.

In fact, it wasn't until a decade after approval of Alza's Transderm Scōp that any other companies entered the field (Pharmatrix with Habitrol®[5] in 1991 and Elan with Prostep® in 1992).

In 1993, Alza struck again with Testoderm® before the relative frenzy of "me-too" product approvals ensued. Between 1994 and 1998, 14 different branded transdermal patches were approved by the FDA, but only one new drug.[†] The lack of new compounds gave many the impression that the heady days of transdermals were over. While some companies like Alza and 3M focused their attention on newer drug delivery technologies (pulmonary delivery, extended-release oral products, etc.), others like Noven and Theratech/Watson continued the search for new compounds to deliver through the skin. Even a few new companies like Hisamitsu and Teikoku began the hunt.

For three years, no new products were approved, but in 2001, Ciba-Geigy's Ortho Evra® contraceptive patch made transdermal products "sexy" (in more ways than one). For the first time, a transdermal patch was developed and marketed to hip, healthy, vibrant (female) individuals. When worn on a visible surface, Ortho Evra provided assurance to a potential partner that at least some of the risks of a physical encounter were mitigated: transdermal delivery was "cool" again.

Although recent years have not witnessed a flood of transdermal products like the mid-1990s, there has been a steady stream of new transdermal product approvals: TheraTech's Oxytrol®; 3M's Climara Pro® and Menostar®; Mylan Technologies' EMSAM®; Noven's Daytrana®; LTS' Neupro®, Exelon®, and BuTrans®; and Strakan's Sancuso®.

---

* Unless otherwise noted, commercial product information was obtained from Drugs @ FDA (http://www.accessdata.fda.gov/scripts/cder/drugsatfda/index.cfm) and/or the US Patent and Trademark Office (http://patft.uspto.gov).

† Norethindrone acetate in Noven's CombiPatch®.

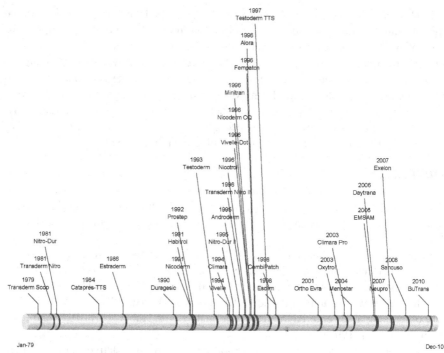

Figure 15.3   FDA-approved branded transdermal patches.

Today the field of transdermal patches has grown large enough to attract generic competitors. Sano/Elan, Mylan Technologies, Corium, Aveva, Lavipharm, and Watson are among the companies that have marketed and/or developed generic versions of nicotine, nitroglycerin, fentanyl, estradiol, and clonidine patches (Fig. 15.3).

PHILOSOPHY OF PRODUCT DEVELOPMENT

The philosophy of product development (transdermal or otherwise) is not a concept often discussed within the walls of universities. The formal education system is designed to teach skills for solving defined problems, one at a time. Commercial product development, by contrast, typically requires using less than cutting-edge science to solve a host of poorly defined, interrelated problems simultaneously—it's rather like herding cats.

Successful product development is absolutely dependent on the fundamentals learned in traditional academic environments. A solid background in chemistry, physics, biology/anatomy, mathematics, and engineering is necessary, but not sufficient to the commercial product development scientist. Many bright, talented, and successful researchers struggle (and sometimes fail) to transition from the university laboratory to the industrial laboratory. It is my hope that this chapter provides a glimpse into commercial product development and illustrates how this vocation is a departure from the highly focused science with which all classroom students are familiar.

Constrained Optimization

Transdermal products must meet a variety of performance criteria and it is rare, indeed, that a scientist has the luxury of optimizing one variable without sacrificing another. Therefore, it is most often a matter of achieving *acceptable* performance of all criteria rather than achieving *exceptional* performance in any one dimension.

Serendipity and Synergy

Precisely because commercial product development is a *commercial* endeavor, the ultimate goal is to fulfill the various aspects of the potential product's profile in as little time and at as little cost as possible. Although never a formal part of any development plan, serendipity plays a role more often than expected. The key to using serendipity in product development is to recognize it when it occurs. That is, to recognize the potential of an otherwise unfortunate result.

EXAMPLE: During the development of the Mylan Fentanyl Transdermal System, crystals of fentanyl spontaneously appeared after drying the adhesive blend. After multiple attempts to prevent crystallization proved inadequate, the suspended crystals were incorporated into the design and became the basis for the rate-controlling mechanism in the commercial product.

Synergy refers to the conscious manipulation of variables to achieve more than one goal. In a sense, this is the ultimate quest of product development because it shortens a more time-consuming iterative optimization process.

EXAMPLE: Silicone medical fluid is used as a dispersant for fentanyl and a nonvolatile tackifier for the adhesive matrix in Mylan's Fentanyl Transdermal System.

Function over Form/Time = Money/Research versus Development

One of the hardest concepts for any commercial product development scientist to embrace is the notion that there will always be questions without answers. It is often the case that the development scientist knows that certain combinations of materials are incompatible even though he or she will never know exactly why. Despite the fact that we are scientists, we must accept that we are not compensated to contribute to the collective scientific knowledge base of our species. We remain gainfully employed for rapidly and economically developing widgets that patients, physicians, pharmacies, and hospitals will choose to buy from our sponsors.

This concept is a cornerstone of commercial product development and is difficult for some people to embrace. Therefore, a career in commercial product development may not be a viable option for everyone.

CONSIDERATIONS IN FORMULATION DESIGN

Performance Criteria (DEWSI)

DEWSI is an acronym and mnemonic device that I use to remind myself of the key performance parameters necessary to a transdermal product. The order of these performance parameters is immaterial since all are equally important and must be achieved.* They represent **D**elivery, **E**xcipients, **W**ear, **S**tability, and **I**rritation.

Drug Delivery

In order to be a feasible transdermal project, the active pharmaceutical ingredient (API) must have a combination of sufficient permeability and potency such that an adequate number of molecules are delivered systemically to produce a pharmacological effect. That means that we must be conscious of not only the fundamental ability of the compound to diffuse through the stratum corneum, but also how much of it needs to be delivered. Table 15.1 illustrates this relationship by juxtaposing five commercial transdermal products with their respective delivery rates, dose ranges, and patch sizes.[6–10]

Table 15.1   Transdermal Product Examples

	Drug (product, manufacturer)	Approximate transdermal flux (μg/cm^2/h)	Therapeutic dose range	Patch size (cm^2)
Example 1	Estradiol (Vivelle-DOT®, Noven)	0.4	0.025–0.1 mg/day	2.5–10
Example 2	Clonidine (Catatpres-TTS®, Boehringer Ingelheim)	1.2	0.1–0.3 mg/day	3.5–10.5
Example 3	Fentanyl (FTS, Mylan)	4	25–100 μg/hr	6.25–25
Example 4	Nitroglycerin (NTS, Mylan)	28	0.1–0.6 mg/hr	3.5–21
Example 5	Nicotine (Nicoderm CQ, Glaxo SmithKline)	40	7–21 mg/day	7.3–22

---

* Besides, most other acronyms are unpronounceable.

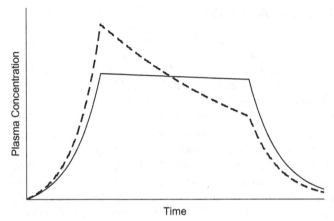

Figure 15.4 Idealized PK profiles.

Rate and Extent In order to have an effect, sufficient drug must pass through the skin and enter the circulatory system to reach a therapeutic concentration. On the other hand, if the systemic concentration rises too high, there is a risk of toxicity, adverse effects, or even death.

The rate and extent of drug delivery is usually characterized in pharmacokinetic studies as C_{max} and AUC (area under the curve).[11] C_{max} refers to the maximum concentration recorded during dosing, and AUC refers to the total systemic exposure to the drug from a single dose or during a single treatment cycle (in the case of a multidose study). The AUC can also be used to determine the average plasma concentration (AUC/dosing period). If the average plasma concentration during treatment is much less than the C_{max}, the delivery profile (Fig. 15.4, dashed line) will have a pronounced peak, whereas a constant rate of delivery will produce a relatively flat profile (Fig. 15.4, solid line) without a sharp C_{max}, even though the AUC for both curves in Figure 15.4 is the same.

Efficiency Efficiency in this context simply means that the finished transdermal product has neither too much nor too little drug. Achieving this goal is not as simple as it sounds even though the benefits of efficiency are readily apparent. Ideally, the goal is to deliver all of the drug in the patch. However, this is not practical since, at some point, the rate of delivery will depend on the concentration in the matrix.

To a first approximation, the delivery rate from a patch is proportional to its degree of saturation or thermodynamic activity (relative to the solid drug). This means that the rate of delivery will decrease as drug leaves the patch unless there is some other mechanism to replenish it. The amount of drug that must remain in a "spent" transdermal system depends on the width of the therapeutic window* since the rate of delivery must fall between these limits in order to be safe and effective.[12]

---

* The range between the minimum and maximum therapeutic plasma concentrations.

Excipient Compatibility and Acceptability

Excipient compatibility and acceptability goes beyond the obvious notion that one should not combine chemicals that are fundamentally incompatible. This is a very broad, nebulous goal that is too often neglected until very late (and very expensive to rectify). A laboratory developer sometimes give little thought to the source of the materials in their formulary and may use what is close to hand rather than seeking commercially available, pharmaceutical-grade, or unexpired materials.

A healthy respect for how different grades or sources of excipients can affect a formulation is gained through experience. Although this concept applies to the development of all products, it is particularly applicable to topical or transdermal products. Common formulary excipients (e.g., polymers, metal oxides, fatty acids, alcohols, plant extracts, etc.) may or may not have standard monographs (United States Pharmacopeia/National Formulary, British Pharmacopeia/European Pharmacopeia, Japanese Pharmacopeia, etc.) but even if they do, the monographs rarely have anything to do with performance in a transdermal product. Failure to consider the potential effects of supplier variability (quality, source, purification/purity) early in the development process can lead to some nasty surprises during scale-up or commercialization.

Wear

Obviously, a transdermal product must have adequate and appropriate wear properties.[13] Less obvious is exactly what that means. A transdermal product delivers its active ingredient(s) at a rate proportional to its surface area.* If the patch does not remain fully attached over its entire area, the drug delivery rate will be less than intended. There are a number of ways a patch can lose contact with the skin: the most obvious is to have the patch completely fall off before the wear period expires. A partial loss of surface contact is difficult to quantify and can result from edge lift, center lift, folding, or puckering.

The type of adhesion failure depends on the patch (adhesive, backing, size, wear period, etc.).

Edge lift is the easiest to comprehend and refers to the loss of adhesion at the edge of the patch. Sometimes this occurs along a portion of the edge and creates a flap that can catch on clothing or other surfaces in the environment (bed linens, furniture, etc.) and get progressively worse until the patch ultimately pulls free of the skin. Sometimes, the entire edge lifts (i.e., all the way around) and leaves only the center attached.

Center lift usually occurs for relatively large patches, patches that have a separate peripheral adhesive or liquid/semisolid reservoir systems. In these instances, the center of the patch detaches from the skin, but the edge does not. This may not affect delivery if there is sufficient moisture trapped at the skin surface to provide an uninterrupted diffusion path, in which case drug delivery continues more or less normally, but this is still something to be avoided if possible.

---

* A quick review will show that nearly all multidose commercial transdermal systems have delivery areas directly proportional to their labeled doses.

A third type of failure occurs when the patch fails by puckering and adhering to itself and can occur either before (mishandling the patch after removal of the release liner), during application to the skin, or after application to the skin (e.g., a consequence of lift during wear).

Regardless of the mechanism of patch dishesion, the measurement is usually captured as the fraction of the total contact area. Conceptually, this is straightforward, but in practice much more difficult and subjective. The relevance of this measurement corresponds, to a first approximation, to the decrease in drug delivery since drug delivery is proportional to treatment area.

There are other aspects of wear that are less directly associated with delivery. A very soft adhesive will have a tendency to spread beyond the edge of the backing film. This does not usually increase the rate of delivery because the total increase in area is usually negligible* and the backing does not occlude the added area. However, the exposed adhesive will tend to collect dead skin cells, clothing fibers, and other flotsam to form a black ring around the patch. The longer the wear period, the worse the ring will become. Although largely a cosmetic issue, it is nonetheless something to be avoided.

Lastly, in some rare cases, a patch may adhere too aggressively. This is most likely when a patch is designed to be worn for a very short time period (less than a day) or if it is intended to be worn on skin that is abnormal for some reason. It is easy to forget when striving for "more, more, more" that one can develop a product that adheres so aggressively that the act of peeling the patch off the patient coincides with peeling the patient off the ceiling.

Stability

The mention of stability usually brings to mind thoughts of dropping potency or the rise of related compounds, but transdermal products must also be physically stable. In fact, it is probably more useful to consider stability of a transdermal product as the ability to maintain the other critical parameters over the shelf life (drug delivery, excipient acceptability, wear, and irritation).

There is one aspect of transdermal patch (in)stability that can only be detected over time: cold flow. Cold flow is the spontaneous movement or flow of the adhesive. Patches that are subject to cold flow will develop a ring of adhesive around the patch over time and this ring can grow large enough to adhere the patch to the inside of its package. If the adhesive remains in the package when the patch is removed, the potency of the patch will be reduced.

Irritation and Sensitization

Irritation includes erythema (redness), edema (swelling), or erosion (blisters, fissures, exudate, scabbing, bleeding, etc.) and is a response to direct cell injury or an immunological response.[14,15] Irritation is most typically assessed on a scale of redness

---

* A 1-mm ring around a 10-cm^2 patch would only increase delivery by 12%.

and swelling (on a scale of 0–7) augmented by "other effects" which include glazing, lesions, scabbing, paticchei, exudate, and so on.[14]

Sensitization (sometimes referred to as delayed-contact sensitization or delayed-contact hypersensitivity) is an immunological phenomenon manifested as an inflammatory response at a naïve site only *after* a patient has been exposed at a different site.[15] By contrast, there are a variety of potential causes of primary irritation because the nature of the assault of a product on the same site after repeated applications can be chemical, mechanical, or immunological.

Chemical irritation (as its name implies) is a chemical interaction of the product or an excipient of the product with the skin that causes irritation. This irritation could be caustic or corrosive (pH driven), oxidative, and so on, such that the skin sustains injury sufficient to cause an inflammatory response.

Mechanical irritation can be caused by any sharp edges (chafing) or a particularly aggressive adhesive that removes a considerable quantity of the stratum corneum upon removal. This repeated removal of stratum corneum can lead to irritation at the site that is independent of the chemical constituents of the product.

Similar to sensitization, the product can also trigger an immunological response during repeated application of the product (before reaching the challenge phase of the sensitization study).

Excipients

First off, let us define "excipients," although conventions vary; here, an excipient refers to everything except the drug itself. Therefore, excipients include not only the inactive constituents of the adhesive matrix (including the adhesive), but also the backing and protective release liner films. All commercial transdermal systems have at least one *pressure-sensitive adhesive*, a *backing film*, and a *release liner*. Other common excipients are *adhesive modifiers* and *permeation enhancers*.

Adhesives

The adhesive is the primary material responsible for creating a bond between the skin and the product. There are a variety of polymeric, medical-grade, commercial, pressure-sensitive adhesives available to the formulation scientist.[16–18] These adhesives are most often available from suppliers as organic solvent solutions, aqueous emulsions, or bulk solids. The solvent-borne or aqueous adhesives are usually combined with other excipients before drying to create the adhesive matrix. Bulk-solid adhesives can either be solvated in the formulation process, melted, or extruded with the other components of the adhesive matrix.

The choice of adhesive impacts all performance criteria and is (essentially by definition) the primary component in a transdermal product adhesive matrix.[19] In terms of chemistry, there are three basic types of pressure-sensitive adhesive polymers used in contemporary transdermal products: acrylic copolymers, silicone polymers, and rubber.[20]

Acrylic pressure-sensitive adhesives are generally copolymers (two or more monomers) in proprietary combinations. The monomers contain at least one vinyl group (C=C) that allows them to polymerize. The various monomers and ratios in which they are combined provide different physical properties and some are engineered to cross-link on drying. Advantages of acrylic copolymer adhesives are their seemingly infinite "tenability" (by varying monomers, ratios, and cross-linking), excellent affinity for drugs and other excipients, and relatively low cost. The primary disadvantage tends to be the unavoidable presence of unreacted monomers, some of which are toxic in sufficient quantity.[21]

Silicone polymer adhesives are produced through a condensation reaction of a silanol end-blocked polydimethylsiloxane (PDMS) with a silicate resin.[22] Advantages of silicone adhesives are low irritation, high delivery, and very low reactivity. Disadvantages tend to be high cost and low solubility/miscibility with drugs and other excipients.[23]

Rubber adhesives consist of a variety of covalently cross-linked polymers of either natural (i.e., derived from the latex of a plant) or synthetic origin. Although once widely used, natural rubber use has decreased due to the potential for severe allergic reactions which increases with repeated exposure (up to 10% of operating room personnel may have developed antibodies to latex proteins).[24] Far more common now are synthetic, cross-linked polymers such as polyisobutene and styrene-butadiene copolymers. Advantages of rubber adhesives are their chemical inertness and low cost. Disadvantages tend to be poor affinity for drugs or other excipients and low solubility in solvents.[25]

Backing Films

The backing film provides protection for the adhesive matrix during storage and during use as well as a physical structure and support for the adhesive matrix. The requisite properties of a backing film are (in no particular order): robust and permanent adhesion to the matrix, chemically inert with respect to the matrix contents, nonirritating, appropriate occlusivity/permeability, comfortable to wear, and aesthetically acceptable.[26]

> *Adhesion to the Matrix.* The bond between the adhesive matrix and the backing is intended to be permanent. Failure of this bond (delamination) can occur under two different circumstances. First, the adhesive can delaminate from the backing when the patient attempts to remove the release liner, making the patch unusable. Second, the adhesive can delaminate from the backing after the patch has been adhered to the skin. This can be anything from a nuisance to a potential overdose if the matrix continues to deliver drug and a new system is applied elsewhere.

> *Nonreactive.* Although chemical interaction of a polymer backing with the contents of the adhesive matrix is unusual, it cannot be completely ruled out. Absorption of drug or permeation enhancer into a backing film, on the other hand, is all too common[26] and some suppliers design their backing films to

limit the potential for absorption or chemical interaction.[27] Polyester (poly-ethylene terephthalate [PET]) films tend to be chemically inert, highly occlu-sive, and possess a very low tendency for absorption.[27] However, PET is often combined with a softer film for comfort and aesthetic purposes.[27] These softer films, or the adhesives used to adhere them to the PET substrate, sometime absorb measurable amounts of the drug or excipients in the adhe-sive matrix.[27] For this reason, it is advisable to proactively evaluate the tendency for a candidate backing film to absorb the constituents of the adhe-sive matrix. Little can be done to prevent absorption by a given film, so the approach is to evaluate the potential impact of absorption (i.e., can the product tolerate it?) and choose appropriately.

Nonirritating. The plethora of commercial backing films available may all be considered nonirritating. However, any potential for irritation (from the adhesive, reservoir, drug, etc.) will be amplified by a highly occlusive backing film.

Appropriate Occlusivity/Permeability. Regarding transdermal systems, occlu-sivity generally refers to the backing's tendency to trap water at the skin surface and increase the level of hydration of the stratum corneum. As the level of hydration increases, the permeability of the skin to most substances increases. In this way, the backing can contribute directly to the rate of absorption in a transdermal system. As indicated above, however, there are positive and negative aspects of highly occlusive backings. Not only is a highly occlusive backing more likely to increase any potential for irritation, maintaining a moist environment at the skin surface for an extended period of time can also lead to bacterial proliferation and skin breakdown/maceration. Another consideration is the permeability of adhesive matrix components through the backing.* In extreme situations, a metalized film is incorporated to further decrease the permeability of the backing film (which is synony-mous with maximizing its occlusivity).[†]

Comfortable and Aesthetically Acceptable. Whether a backing film should be thick, thin, compliant, or more rigid in order to be comfortable depends on the size of the patch, anatomical area of application, and duration of wear. Generally, however, it is preferable to have a soft, matte backing that simulates the feel of skin.[27] Polyurethanes are well suited to this as well as certain polyolefin and EVA (ethylene-vinyl acetate mixture) films. Regarding pigment, less is more. In other words, it is usually preferable to use a translucent film to allow the natural color of the skin to show through and make the patch as unobtrusive as possible. Under some circumstances,

---

* This is distinguished from absorption in that a film may lack sufficient mass (volume) to absorb a significant quantity of drug or excipient, but still allow the passage of a significant amount through the film and into the environment or package to either limit stability or decrease delivery during wear.

† This is less popular now due to concerns about the metalized film interacting with the magnetic field in magnetic resonance imaging (MRI), causing burns or image artifacts.

however, a pigmented film may be preferred. If a metalized film is required, a pigmented outer layer is needed to hide the shiny metal layer. If treatment causes noticeable redness, one may wish to downplay this by selecting a pigmented film. Lastly, if the adhesive matrix is light sensitive, opaque, or colored, a pigmented film provides a consistent and, arguably, more natural appearance.*

Release Liners

The disposable release liner provides protection for the adhesive matrix during storage, but is removed and discarded by the patient prior to use. Typically, the release liner is a polymer film with a low-energy coating bonded to the surface in contact with the adhesive. This low-energy coating assures that the release liner will adhere lightly to the adhesive matrix during storage, but peel away easily to expose the adhesive before use. Failure of the release liner to cleanly or easily peel away from the matrix is sometimes known as blocking or lock-up.

Most commercial transdermal product release liners are clear polyester films with a low surface energy coating, although they can also be made of paper or polypropylene.[27,28] The surface energy of the coating must be high enough to allow the adhesive blend to uniformly coat the surface without beading or leaving dry spots. On the other hand, the surface energy must be low enough to prevent the adhesive from forming a permanent bond. As with backing films, a variety of commercial release liners are available and the suppliers are the best sources for determining the appropriate release liner for a given application. In general, the release agents are either silicone polymers (for use with nonsilicone adhesives) or fluorocarbon or fluorosilicone polymers (for general use, including silicone adhesives).[27–29]

Adhesive Modifiers

Adhesive modifiers are compounds intended to improve the adhesive performance by restoring the proper combination of viscous and elastic properties. Although there are now commercially available adhesives designed to withstand or be compatible with permeation enhancers and drugs, historically, adhesive modifiers have been necessary to restore pressure-sensitive adhesive properties to drug- and enhancer-loaded matrices. Necessary modifications tend to fall into two very broad categories: hardening and softening.

Shear builders or fillers are added to counter the effects of enhancers or drugs that plasticize the adhesive. These materials are generally insoluble solids (polymers, metal oxides) that retard or prevent viscous flow of the adhesive matrix through simple mechanical reinforcement (like the steel rebar in concrete) or as a high-energy surface on which immiscible matrix excipients can adsorb.[30]

---

* A consequence of developing transdermal patches for a large market is that "flesh tone" is a misnomer. As evidence of this, consider the trend toward translucent adhesive bandages.

Plasticizers or tackifiers are generally liquids or semisolid polymers added to the matrix to counter the effects of suspended solid materials (sort of the opposite of a filler) or when the adhesive is simply too stiff or hard to effectively bond with the skin.[31]

Permeation Enhancers

Permeation or penetration enhancers are chemical compounds intended to increase the rate or extent of delivery. Chapter 2 of this book is devoted to this topic, so there is no need to discuss it here except to stress that the addition of "permeation enhancers" can have effects on the formulation other than permeation enhancement.

INTERACTION AND EXAMPLES

In a sense, the sections "Performance Criteria (DEWSI)" and "Excipients" introduce the performance criteria and the physical constituents of solid matrix transdermal patches, respectively. In this section, the permutations of the criteria and constituents illustrate some of the multidimensional aspects of product design and optimization. The interrelationship among the performance criteria is one of, if not *the* most important take-home concept in this chapter. Table 15.2 summarizes some of the potential interactions and can be used as a quick, future reference.

Delivery versus . . .

Simply put, the delivery rate of the API through the skin depends on thermodynamics (activity or driving force) and kinetics (diffusivity or mobility). Any excipient in a transdermal patch has the potential to influence delivery.

Drug. The transdermal delivery of a drug is, of course, dependent on the drug you choose. The diffusivity of the drug will depend on the size (molecular weight) as well as the structure (polarity, reactive groups). Moreover, whether or not one can achieve a therapeutic level of delivery depends on how potent the drug is.

Adhesive. Because different adhesives have different affinities for a given drug, the solubility of that compound will also vary. Therefore, changes to the adhesive can have profound effects on the delivery of the drug through the skin.

The Mylan and Apotex Fentanyl Transdermal Systems both deliver fentanyl through the skin at the same rate, both contain the same amount of fentanyl, and neither contains a permeation enhancer. But the poly isobutylene (PIB) adhesive matrix of the Apotex system is more than three times the size of the silicone adhesive matrix of the Mylan patch.[8,32]

Backing Film. As discussed earlier, the backing film can significantly influence drug delivery through the skin by controlling the hydration level of the skin

Table 15.2 Examples of Interactions between Performance Parameters and System Components

	Delivery	Excipient compatibility and acceptability	Wear	Stability	Irritation/ sensitization
Drug	Molecular weight Structure Physiological potency	Reactivity Solubility/ miscibility	Solid/liquid/ suspension Solubility/ miscibility	Reactivity Solid/liquid/ suspension Solubility/ miscibility	pK/pH Irritant Sensitizer
Adhesive	Solubility Density Occlusivity	Reactivity Solubility/ miscibility	Chemistry Duration Excipient tolerance	Reactivity Cold flow Excipient tolerance	N/A[a]
Backing film	Occlusivity Absorption/ transmission	Reactivity Absorption/ transmission	Composition Thickness/ compliance	Reactivity Absorption/ transmission	Thickness/ compliance
Release liner	Lock-up Absorption/ transmission	Lock-Up Absorption/ transmission	Lock-up	Lock-up Absorption/ transmission	N/A[b]
Adhesive modifiers	Concentration Surface energy of dispersed solid	Reactivity Solubility/ miscibility	Concentration Surface energy Stiffening of the matrix	Reactivity Cold flow	Irritant Sensitizer
Permeation enhancer	Lipid barrier disruption Solubility/ miscibility	Reactivity Solubility/ miscibility	Plasticization of the matrix Solubility/ miscibility	Reactivity Cold flow	Irritant Sensitizer

[a] Commercially available medical adhesives are tested and verified as nonirritating to the skin.
[b] The release liner is not part of the system during wear.

under the patch. As the backing film becomes more occlusive, it traps more water, making the skin more permeable.

Relatively obvious, but rare, is the situation where absorption of material into the backing film or transmission through the backing film has a measurable effect on delivery. If this occurs, the effect will become more pronounced as the patch ages.

Release Liner. Although perhaps indicative of a greater problem, the release liner can affect delivery if it cannot be removed from the adhesive matrix (in which case the delivery is reduced to zero since the patient cannot wear it). The Daytrana product has been recalled multiple times for difficulty or inability of the patient to remove the release liner.[33]

It is possible in theory (although unlikely) that a PET film or its low surface energy coating can absorb enough drug or matrix excipient to influence delivery. If so, this would most likely occur in a patch containing a very small amount of drug.

Adhesive Modifiers. The diffusivity of drugs within a polymer matrix depends on the polymer. Similarly, the addition of materials to the polymer matrix can influence drug diffusion by changing the density of the matrix, providing a thermodynamically favorable (or unfavorable) surface for drug diffusion or creating an immiscible phase within the continuous matrix.

Permeation Enhancers. The purpose for including a permeation enhancer in a transdermal patch is to improve the rate or extent of delivery. There is little to say about the relationship between drug delivery and permeation enhancers that is not obvious; however, permeation enhancers can sometimes have the opposite effect.

Consider a patch containing a drug and a pressure-sensitive adhesive. A permeation enhancer could be added to decrease the barrier of the skin. But if the drug is soluble in the permeation enhancer, the thermodynamic activity of the drug in the matrix will decrease. This decreases the driving force for diffusion (offsetting the decrease in the skin barrier).

Excipient Compatibility

Not all excipients play well together. The fundamental requirements for excipient compatibility are lack of reactivity among the excipients and physical compatibility (solubility, miscibility). In addition, the backing film and release liner should be impermeable to, and absorb little or no drug.

Drug. The active ingredient is often the most chemically delicate component of a finished pharmaceutical product (transdermal or otherwise). Chemical structure is the basis of drug pharmacological activity and any uncontrolled change to its chemical structure or conformation will almost certainly be devastating to the finished product.

Many drugs contain amine groups that can accept a proton in acidic environments to become positively charged ions. This not only affects the solubility of the drug in the matrix (and, hence, its activity), but also its ability to partition into the skin. Therefore, any other excipient capable of changing pH needs to be carefully screened.

Some drugs are susceptible to oxidation by free radicals, so adhesives or adhesive modifiers created by free radical polymerization need to be carefully screened for the effects of residual initiator.

Some drugs are susceptible to hydrolysis or dimerization, so the presence of water, alcohol fatty acids, ethers, and esters could be problematic.

The intent here is not to create an exhaustive list of potential interactions, but rather to illustrate that there are many opportunities for matrix excipients to interact with the drug.

Somewhat different is the case of a drug that is light sensitive. Although the product will probably experience very little or no light exposure inside its package, it may not be able to tolerate exposure to sunlight during use. Therefore, the product would require an opaque backing or be worn on an area of the body that is not exposed to light in order to prevent degradation during wear.

Adhesive. The most common problem choosing adhesives is basic physical incompatibility with the other excipients in the matrix.

If the adhesive is immiscible with a liquid permeation enhancer or liquid drug, the liquid will eventually collect at an interface. If the liquid collects at the release liner/matrix surface, the bond between the liner and the matrix can approach zero (the liner spontaneously falls off) or infinity (the liner becomes permanently bonded to the matrix). If the liquid collects the backing film/matrix surface, the adhesive may delaminate from the backing film or the liquid could be prevented from reaching the skin surface.

Excessive amounts of solid material in the adhesive matrix (crystalline drug, for example) can stiffen the adhesive to the point where it loses its pressure-sensitive adhesive qualities.

Backing Film. There are three main considerations when choosing a backing film: the adhesive bond with the matrix must be strong and robust, drug absorption potential is negligible, and drug transmission (diffusion of drug through the backing) is negligible. Although chemical reactions between the backing film and the solid matrix components are possible, they are rare.

Release Liner. Release liners generally come in two categories: silicone-coated liners for use with nonsilicone adhesives and fluorocarbon- or fluorosilicone-coated liners for general use. Choosing an inappropriate release liner can result in lock-up (permanent bonding to the adhesive matrix). Since release liner lock-up can take months or years, it is important to monitor the force required to remove the release liner over time as part of the development process.

Adhesive Modifiers. Adhesive modifiers such as tackifying resins, metal oxides, or plasticizers are generally inert, but physical incompatibility (with the adhesive, for example) could lead to pooling, cold flow, or other changes over time (see the "Adhesive" discussion above).

Permeation Enhancers. Permeation enhancers tend to have one or more polar groups while some adhesive polymers are nonpolar. Consequently, the solubility or miscibility in these systems can be limited. This can lead to unintended emulsification and phase separation.

Some permeation enhancers also have the potential to disrupt or prevent the cross-linking (curing) in some acrylic adhesives, leaving the matrix unexpectedly soft and subject to cold flow.

Wear versus . . .

Drug. Often, the drug itself can affect the physical properties of the adhesive and, thus, wear properties. The potential effects depend on drug concentration, whether the drug is a solid or liquid, and whether the drug is dissolved or suspended/immiscible in the matrix.[34-36]

Adhesive. Different adhesives wear differently. As the primary component of the matrix, the adhesive is a critical element for achieving adequate wear on the skin.

Backing Film. A backing film must be compliant enough to move with the skin, but not so soft that it permanently deforms during normal wear. The appropriate amount of "give" depends on both the location and duration of wear.

Release Liner. The only ways in which the release liner can affect wear are if the release liner cannot be removed or the adhesive matrix is physically deformed in the process of removing the release liner, or if there is a transfer of the release coating from the liner to the adhesive such that its ability to adhere is compromised.

Adhesive Modifiers. The purpose of including adhesive modifiers is to improve the physical properties of the adhesive matrix. Although the adhesive matrix has to have sufficient structural integrity to resist cold flow during storage, any other intentional modification of the physical properties should be to improve wear. Therefore, wear and adhesive modifiers are not usually at odds with one another.

Permeation Enhancers. Permeation enhancers can soften the adhesive matrix to the point that the patch exhibits cold flow or slides around on the skin during wear.

Stability versus . . .

A stable transdermal product has no meaningful chemical degradation of the drug or any other excipient, no meaningful change in assay, no meaningful change in physical properties, and no meaningful change in appearance.

Drug. The chemical stability of a drug product is almost always related to the stability of the drug itself. Consequently, the more delicate the drug is, the more challenging it will be to develop a stable product.*

As noted earlier, transdermal patches must also be physically stable and the drug can have a profound influence on the physical stability of the product. This usually occurs when the concentration is relatively high, the drug is in suspension, or the drug is a liquid at room temperature. The most

---

* Most transdermals contain the un-ionized form of the drug (free base or free acid) and these forms are often less stable than the corresponding salts typically found in oral products.

common manifestation of physical (in)stability is cold flow, although changes in shear, peel, and tack may be measurable too.*

Adhesive. Instability issues associated with the adhesive tend to be physical rather than chemical and, as noted above, can appear as cold flow on stability or changes in shear, peel, and tack.

Backing Film. Absorption of drug or enhancer by the backing film may not appear as a stability problem if the assay method can still extract the drug from the backing, but this could still affect the performance of the product over time. A drug release test (similar to a dissolution test for a solid oral product) is generally a more sensitive measurement of the availability of the drug in the product and whether it is changing.

Release Liner. If the release liner absorbs drug or enhancer, the potency or enhancer assay of the patch will fall over time (perhaps reaching an equilibrium value). Fortunately, the potential for the release liner to absorb a meaningful amount of drug is low, so the most common stability issue is the increasing effort necessary to remove the release liner as the product ages.

Adhesive Modifiers and Permeation Enhancers. If a low molecular weight adhesive modifier or permeation enhancer is only marginally compatible with the adhesive, there could be a drift in the physical properties (changes in tack, peel, and shear) or changes in appearance (e.g., blooming).

A solid adhesive modifier can affect the physical stability of a patch if adsorption at its surface is very slow. In other words, a solid adhesive modifier can lead to a progressive loss of plasticizer from the bulk adhesive matrix.

Irritation/Sensitization versus . . .

Drug. Some drugs are primary irritants or sensitizers. If so, there is no way to prevent contact between the skin and the drug. However, if the potential for irritation/sensitization is moderate and dose dependent, there is still potential for success. Clonidine is an example of a drug that has successfully been formulated into transdermal products despite being a sensitizer.

Adhesive. Medical-grade, pressure-sensitive adhesives are not irritating per se, but some adhesives can harbor bacteria or trap moisture better than others. Also, as mentioned earlier, a particularly aggressive adhesive can cause mechanical irritation upon removal. Lastly, the natural protein in latex (rubber) adhesives is a known sensitizer.

Backing Film. An overly occlusive backing film, worn for an extended period of time, can lead to excessive hydration and breakdown of the skin. If the

---

* Shear, tack, and peel tests were originally developed and standardized for the pressure-sensitive tape industry, but are widely used to test self-adhesive transdermal patches. Examples of how these tests are used for patches can be found in Wokovich et al.[26]

skin reaches a point where its mechanical integrity is lost, almost any assault can cause irritation, including normal skin flora or the physical stress of removing the patch. Also, a backing film with sharp edges can cause mechanical irritation (chafing) at the patch periphery.

Release Liner. Since the release liner is removed prior to application of the patch, it doesn't really influence irritation or sensitization. A hypothetical possibility would be an irritating or sensitizing coating that is transferred to the adhesive from the release liner prior to application.

Adhesive Modifiers. Probably the greatest likelihood of irritation due to an adhesive modifier is a gritty or rough surface. This can be attenuated by keeping both the level and particle size to a minimum. Another possibility would be the use of a natural plant resin (like latex) which could be a sensitizer.

Permeation Enhancers. By their nature, permeation enhancers are supposed to interact with the skin. If this interaction is sufficiently invasive, irritation may result. After all, the purpose of the skin is to isolate the interior of the body from the hazards of the environment. Sufficiently compromising this barrier is sufficient cause for the body to take corrective action in the form of an inflammatory response.

CONCLUSIONS

If you can conduct hundreds of experiments in a week; interpret, organize, and archive the data in real time; cope with not being able to answer every question; juggle a dozen variables in each of a dozen projects that wax and wane in importance on any given day; and accept cost as the penultimate metric . . . you will be a successful transdermal product development scientist.

REFERENCES

1. Medication Guide AndroGel®. Available at: http://www.fda.gov/downloads/Drugs/DrugSafety/UCM188474.pdf (accessed September 8, 2010).
2. FDA Drug Safety Communication. Ongoing safety review of Evamist (estradiol transdermal spray) and unintended exposure of children and pets to topical estrogen. Available at: http://www.fda.gov/Drugs/DrugSafety/PostmarketDrugSafetyInformationforPatientsandProviders/ucm220185.htm (accessed September 8, 2010).
3. FDA Patient Safety News, Show #74, April 2008. Available at: http://www.accessdata.fda.gov/scripts/cdrh/cfdocs/psn/transcript.cfm?show=74 (accessed September 8, 2010).
4. GONZALEZ M, et al. Personal communication. August 30, 2010.
5. BAKER RW, et al., inventors; Pharmetrix Corporation, assignee. Novel transdermal nicotine patch. US Patent 4,839,174, June 13, 1989.
6. Vivelle-Dot® Prescribing Information. Available at: http://vivelledot.com/documents/vivelle-dot-prescribing-information.pdf (accessed August 16, 2011).
7. Catapres-TTS® Prescribing Information. Available at: http://bidocs.boehringer-ingelheim.com/BIWebAccess/ViewServlet.ser?docBase=renetnt&folderPath=/Prescribing+Information/PIs/Catapres+TTS/CatapresTTS.pdf (accessed September 7, 2010).

8. Mylan Fentanyl Transdermal System Prescribing Information. Available at: http://mylantech. com/ transdermal_technology/~/media/mylan-tech/content-pdfs/FTS_R17.pdf (accessed August 16, 2011).

9. Mylan Nitroglycerin Transdermal System Prescribing Information. Available at: http://mylantech.com/ transdermal_technology/~/media/mylan-tech/content-pdfs/NTG_R13.pdf (accessed August 16, 2011).

10. VENKATRAMAN S, et al. An overview of controlled release systems. In: Wise DL, ed. *Handbook of Pharmaceutical Controlled Release Technology*. Marcell Dekker, New York, 2000; 448.

11. Code of Federal Regulations, Title 21, Chapter 1, Subchapter D, Part 320 2009 [21CFR320].

12. Guideline for the format and content of the clinical and statistical sections of an application. Center for Drug Evaluation and Research, Food and Drug Administration, Department of Health and Human Services, July 1988. Available at: http://www.fda.gov/downloads/Drugs/ GuidanceComplianceRegulatoryInformation/Guidances/UCM071665.pdf.

13. WICK KA, et al. Adhesion-to-skin performance of a new transdermal nitroglycerin adhesive patch. *Clinical Therapeutics* 1989; 11: 417–424.

14. BERGER RS, BOWMAN JP. A reappraisal of the 21-day cumulative irritation test in man. *Journal of Toxicology, Cutaneous and Ocular Toxicology* 1982; 1: 109–115.

15. GOLDSMITH LA. *Physiology, Biochemistry, and Molecular Biology of the Skin*, 2nd ed. Oxford University Press, Inc., New York, 1991; 1458.

16. Pressure Sensitive Adhesives—Medical. Available at: http://cytec.com/specialty-chemicals/ psa-medical.htm (accessed August 16, 2011).

17. Products: Healthcare (Medical). Available at: http://www.dowcorning.com/applications/search/ default.aspx?Ne=4294965941&N=4294965921&DCCD=PRODUCT&WT.svl=1&DCCT= PRODUCT (accessed August 16, 2011).

18. Henkel International—Brands & Solutions. Available at: http://www.henkel.com/cps/rde/xchg/ henkel_com/hs.xsl/markets-2707.htm?iname=Transdermal+Adhesives+&countryCode=com&BU= industrial&parentredDotUID=0000000H0K,00000002LA,000000XOGT&redDotUID= 0000011ZUX&noCrawl=true (accessed August 16, 2011).

19. BUSHKIRK GA et al. Scale-up of adhesive transdermal drug delivery systems. *Pharmaceutical Research* 1997; 14: 848–852.

20. SACHAN NK et al. Transdermal approaches in drug delivery. *Der Pharmacia Lettre* 2009; 1: 34–47.

21. KRAELING ME, BRONAUGH RL. *In Vitro* Percutaneous Absorption of Acrylamide and Styrene in Human Skin From Cosmetic Vehicles. 2004 FDA Science Forum, 2004. Available at: http:// www.accessdata.fda.gov/ScienceForums/forum04/D-20.htm (accessed August 16, 2011).

22. DOW CORNING® BIO-PSA Standard Silicone Adhesives Product Information. Ref. No. 52-1052A-01, 2008. Available at: http://www2.dowcorning.com/Datafiles/090007c8801ca2a1.pdf (accessed May 27, 2010).

23. BARNES K. 2005. in-Pharma Technologist: Silicone solutions. Available at: http://www.in-pharmatechnologist.com/Materials-Formulation/Silicone-solutions (accessed May 27, 2010).

24. WEISS ME. Latex allergy. *Canadian Journal of Anaesthesia* 1992; 39: 528–532.

25. TAN HS, PFISTER WR. Pressure-sensitive adhesives for transdermal drug delivery systems. *Pharmaceutical Science & Technology Today* 1999; 2: 60–69.

26. WOKOVICH AM, et al. Transdermal drug delivery system (TDDS) adhesion as a critical safety, efficacy and quality attribute. *European Journal of Pharmaceutics and Biopharmaceutics* 2006; 64: 1–8.

27. M Transdermal Components-3M Drug Delivery Systems. Available at: http://solutions.3m.com/wps/ portal/3M/en_WW/DrugDeliverySystems/DDSD/technology-solutions/transdermal-technologies/ components/ (accessed August 31, 2010).

28. Mylan Technologies Inc. (MTI). MEDIRELEASE®. Available at: http://mylantech.com/component_ materials/standard/mediRelease.aspx. (accessed September 2, 2010).

29. Flexvue, performance films for specialty applications. Available at: http://flexvuefilms.com/en/ Specialty-Films.aspx (accessed September 2, 2010).

30. SHCHERBINA Y, et al. Physical properties of gum karaya-starch-essential oil patches. *AAPS PharmSciTech* 2010; 11: 1276–1286.

31. MINGHETTI P et al. Design of a new water-soluble pressure-sensitive adhesive for patch preparation. *AAPS PharmSciTech* 2003; 4: 1–9.
32. A-Z Product List: F-Apotex Products: United States. Available at: http://www.apotex.com/us/en/products/search.asp?qt=A2Z&qs=F&t=Search (accessed September 2, 2010).
33. Recalls, Market Withdrawals, & Safety Alerts. Available at: http://www.fda.gov/Safety/Recalls/default.htm (accessed September 10, 2010).
34. GOVIL SK, WEIMANN LJ, inventors; Mylan Technologies, Inc., assignee. Adhesive mixture for transdermal delivery of highly plasticizing drugs. US patent 7,070,808, July 4, 2006.
35. MULLER W, inventor; LTS Lohmann Therapie-Systeme, AG, assignee. Topical plaster with non-steroidal antirheumatic agents with an acid group. US patent 6,676,962, January 13, 2004.
36. TSURUDA K, IKEURA Y, inventors; Hisamitsu Pharmaceuticals Co., Inc., assignee. Adhesive preparations. US patent 7,250,546, July 31, 2007.

Chapter 16

Sensitivity and Irritation Testing

Belum Viswanath Reddy, Geetanjali Sethi, and Howard I. Maibach

INTRODUCTION

The discovery, manufacture, and use of newer topical medications, cosmetics, and industrial or agricultural chemicals is growing. In each of these cases, chemicals with little or no potential for producing skin or systemic injury must be identified. Consumers, workers at production facilities and industrial sites, and patients using topical medications derived from these chemicals are at constant risk. Hence, adverse cutaneous reactions triggered by repetitive low-dose exposure to such chemicals mandate accurate prediction. This situation has driven the need to develop newer models and assays that attempt to categorize chemicals according to their irritation/sensitization potential.

There is much variability among the rules of regulatory bodies, both within the United States and worldwide for the testing of chemicals that are to be applied to the skin. U.S. regulatory bodies such as the Consumer Product Safety Commission (CPSC), Department of Transportation (DOT), Food and Drug Administration (FDA), and international organizations such as the Organisation for Economic Cooperation and Development (OECD) and the European Economic Community (EEC) have variable requirements for the evaluation of such chemicals. This chapter discusses the rationale and methodology of tests and assays used for predicting the irritation and sensitizing potential of topically applied substances.

HISTORICAL PERSPECTIVE

In 1867, Paul Langerhans described a nonpigmentary dendritic cell in the skin.[1] In 1891, Koch and Jadassohn described skin reactions in humans whose development was delayed and could not be explained to be due to an irritant etiology.[2]

Transdermal and Topical Drug Delivery: Principles and Practice, First Edition. Edited by Heather A.E. Benson, Adam C. Watkinson.
© 2012 John Wiley & Sons, Inc. Published 2012 by John Wiley & Sons, Inc.

The first investigator to use a patch test for contact allergy in humans was Jadassohn (1895).[3] In 1906, Von Pirquet defined allergy as a change of reactivity of an organism to toxic substances or infective agents.[4] Frey and Wenk demonstrated in guinea pig studies that the draining lymph node is important during the induction phase of the development of contact sensitivity.[5,6] Another important step in the understanding of the mechanism of contact allergy was the proof by Inge Silberberg of the relationship between the epidermal Langerhans cell and the contact dermatitis (CD).[7] Later, Pollack summarized many developmental steps for the mechanism of CD and described the different stages of contact sensitivity, such as the preparation phase, the antigen recognition phase, the proliferative phase, and the propagative phase.[2]

Almost 50 years after the first patch test (based on studies done in cellular immunology), the first predictive studies in animals and man were elucidated by Draize et al. (1944), Schwartz and Peck (1944), and Shelanski and Shelanski (1953).[8–10] Studies were mainly done in guinea pigs by Landsteiner and Chase (1937, 1941, 1942), Landsteiner and Jacobs (1935, 1936), Draize (using a modified protocol in 1959), Buehler (1965), and Magnusson and Kligman (1969).[11–18]

New predictive assays in man were described by Kligman (1966), Marzulli and Maibach (1974), and Stotts (1980).[19–21] Based on practical experience, it has been shown that the guinea pig models have been quite successful in protecting humans from allergic contact dermatitis (ACD).

A number of the many experimental models developed over the years have been included in regulatory guidelines. These include the Magnusson and Kligman maximization test, Draize test (DT), Freund's complete adjuvant test (FCAT), Maurer optimization test, Buehler's test (BT), open epicutaneous test (OET), and split adjuvant test (SAT). The Test Method B6 of the European Community (EEC, 1984) and the subdivision F of the pesticide assessment guidelines (US-EPA/FIFRA, 1984) both accepted the above seven methods of testing except that the latter organization omitted the DT and included the footpad technique instead.[22,23]

Protocols involving mice (local lymph node assay, LLNA) have been standardized and accepted by many regulatory bodies for hazard identification. This measures induction (amount of chemical necessary to cause induce sensitization) but not elicitation potency (amount of chemical required to elicit a discernible allergic reaction in a previously sensitized subject).

DERMATOPHARMACOKINETICS

Proper understanding of cutaneous pharmacokinetics is necessary to exploit the potential for transdermal drug delivery development. Presently, this assumes even greater significance as there has been a surge in efforts worldwide to develop newer methods and cosmetic products aimed at delivering drugs transdermally.

The fate of any topically applied compound is determined by numerous factors. The skin's ability to absorb, retain, and permit diffusion/penetration, besides the concentration and type of vehicle, all play a major role (Table 16.1).[24] *In vitro* and

Table 16.1   Factors Affecting Percutaneous Absorption

Release from vehicle (varies with):
   Solubility in vehicle
   Concentration
   pH
Kinetics of skin permeation (influenced by):
   Anatomical site
   Degree of occlusion
   Intrinsic skin conditions
   Animal age
   Concentration of dosing solution
   Surface area dosed
   Frequency of dosing
Tissue distribution
Excretion kinetics
Substantivity to the skin
Volatility
Wash and rub resistance
Binding to skin components
Cutaneous metabolism
Anatomic pathways
Lateral spread

Source: Adapted from Wester and Maibach.[24]

in vivo assays permitting the estimation of absorption through the skin have been devised. While existing models and assays need to be streamlined, efforts to develop better, ideal, and more humane methodologies should continue.

Animal and human models have been developed to predict the irritation and sensitization potential of compounds; the resulting tests are described in Table 16.2.

TESTS FOR PREDICTING SENSITIZATION POTENTIAL

Guinea Pig Sensitization Tests

These predictive tests conducted on the guinea pig help determine the potential of substances to induce delayed-type hypersensitivity in humans.[25-27] The tests share many common features, however each has its own advantages and disadvantages.

Young (1–3-month old or weighing 250–550 g), randomly bred albino guinea pigs, housed in facilities with ambient temperatures ($20 \pm 1°C$) and relative humidity (40%–50%, 12-hour automatic light cycle), are utilized. This helps reduce the possibility of seasonal variability during a reaction. In addition, food

Table 16.2   Tests to Predict the Irritation and Sensitization
Potential of Compounds

Tests for predicting sensitization potential

Guinea pig sensitization tests
1. The Draize test (DT)
2. Open epicutaneous test (OET)
3. Buehler's test (BT)
4. Freund's complete adjuvant test (FCAT)
5. Optimization test (OT)
6. Split adjuvant test (SAT)
7. Guinea pig maximization test (GPMT)
Sensitization tests in mice
1. LLNA
2. MEST
3. VAET
Human sensitization assays
1. S-P tests (and modifications)
2. RIPT
3. Human maximization test
4. Modified Draize human sensitization test
In vitro assays for ACD
Tests for predicting irritation potential
Irritation tests in animals
1. Draize rabbit model
2. Cumulative Irritation assays
3. Immersion assay
4. Mouse ear model
5. Other methods
Irritation tests in humans
1. Single-application patch tests
2. Cumulative irritation test
3. The chamber scarification test
4. Immersion tests
5. Bioengineering devices in irritancy evaluations
In vitro assays of skin irritation and corrosion

---

and water are made available at all times. The guinea pigs also receive vitamin C
supplementation.

Skin over the test sites is epilated using electric clippers or by a chemical depila-
tor. Descriptive scales for erythema and edema are used to grade the response
(production of visible dermatitis). The assays listed under this category (DT, OET,
BT, FCAT, optimization test [OT], SAT, and guinea pig maximization test [GPMT])
differ with regard to the following: sex of the group, route of exposure, adjuvant
use, induction interval, and number of exposures.

The Draize Test

This is the oldest predictive test devised and is still in use.[16,28,29] The materials comprise of 20 guinea pigs, 1% solution of the test material in saline and paraffin oil or polyethylene glycol (PEG). The test is conducted in three stages, namely induction, challenge, and evaluation.

Induction   On day 0, one flank of all the 20 guinea pigs is shaved for injection of the 0.05 mL of the 1% test solution into the anterior aspect. This is followed by injection of 1.1 mL of the test solution into a new site every time, on the same flank from day 1 through day 20.

Challenge   After a 2-week "rest" period, the opposite untreated flank of each guinea pig is shaved and challenged (injected) with 0.05 mL of the test solution. Twenty previously untreated guinea pigs, injected at the same time, serve as controls.

Evaluation   At 24 and 46 hours after the challenge, test sites are visually inspected and the intensity of the reaction is noted. A larger and intense erythematous response in test subjects vis-à-vis controls is recorded as a positive test result, and expressed as the *percentage of animals positive* or as the *ratio of positive animals tested.*

OET

Test material is topically applied to replicate conditions of human use. The purpose of the assay is to ascertain the dose required to induce sensitization and elicit a response in sensitized animals.[29–31]

For evaluation of the *irritancy profile*, different concentrations (usually undiluted—30%, 10%, 3%, 1%) of the test material (in ethanol, acetone, water, PEG, or petrolatum) are used. Six to eight guinea pigs are chosen for application of 0.025 mL of dosing solutions to 2 cm^2 areas of a shaved flank. Solubility in the vehicle and usage characteristics is taken into account when test concentrations are decided. After 24 hours, the test sites are visually examined for the presence/absence of erythema. The minimum irritant concentration (MIC; dose causing a reaction in 25% of animals) and maximum nonirritant concentration (MNIC; dose not causing a reaction in any animal) are determined.

Induction Phase   An 8 cm^2 area of flank skin in six to eight guinea pigs is shaved and 0.10 mL of test solution is applied. This is done either daily for 3 weeks, or five times a week for 4 weeks. While six groups of guinea pigs are treated with different concentrations, the control group is treated only with the vehicle. The MIC is usually the highest dose tested. Lower doses are also tested and are based on usage concentrations or a graded reduction (e.g., 30%, 10%, 3%, 1%). The test solutions are applied to the same site every day unless an inflammatory response develops.

Challenge Phase   Twenty-four to 72 hours after the last induction treatment, a 2 cm^2 area of the previously untreated flank of each animal is treated with 0.05 mL of the MIC, MNIC, and five solutions of lower concentrations.

Evaluation   At 24, 48, and 72 hours postapplication in the challenge phase, the results are noted (on an all-or-none basis). The maximum nonirritating concentration in the control group (vehicle treated) is estimated. Guinea pigs displaying inflammatory responses to lower concentrations in the test groups are considered sensitized.

Although the OET is time consuming and laborious, it provides suitable information on irritation, dose response, and sensitization.

BT (Occlusion Only)

This test also involves the application of test materials topically. The materials used include 0.4 mL of test substance saturating an absorbent patch (2 × 2 cm Webril®, Covidien, Mansfield, MA), Blenderm™ tape (3M, St. Paul, MN) to secure the patch, a test group (10–20 guinea pigs with shaved flanks), and a control group (10–20 guinea pigs).[17,32,33]

Induction Phase   Different concentrations of the test patches (from undiluted to usage strengths) are applied over 6-hour periods. Based on an irritancy screen (conducted in other animals), an optimum concentration that produces slight erythema is selected. The animal is then wrapped with an occlusive wrapping and placed in a special restrainer fitted with a rubber dam to maintain even pressure. The control group is patch tested with only the vehicle. The same steps are repeated at 7 and 14 days after initial exposure.

Challenge Phase   This is performed 2 weeks after the last induction patch, wherein the animals are patched on both flanks with a nonirritating concentration of test material and the vehicle (if other than water or acetone), in a manner similar to induction. Six hours later, the patch is removed and the skin is depilated.

Evaluation   This is performed 24–48 hours after patch removal. The guinea pigs that develop an erythematous response are considered sensitized, provided the irritant controls do not respond.

The number of positive reactions and the average intensity of the response are estimated.

FCAT

This test is accomplished by means of injecting the test material intradermally, in a 1:1 mixture of Freund's complete adjuvant (FCA) and distilled water. This test has witnessed many modifications; the most recent published method is summarized below.[29,31]

Induction Phase   The procedure involves shaving a 6×2 cm area across the shoulders of two groups of 10–20 guinea pigs which would be used as injection sites. The first group is injected with 0.1 mL of a 5% solution of the test material (in FCA/water). A total of three injections are given at an interval of 4 days. The second group (control) is injected only with FCA/water. Using the OET, the minimum irritating and maximum nonirritating concentrations are determined following topical application of 0.025 mL solutions to a 2 cm^2 area of skin in at least four naïve guinea pigs.

Challenge Phase   Twenty-one days following the first induction injection, 0.025 mL of the MIC, MNIC, and two lower concentrations are applied to 2 cm^2 areas of the shaved flanks. At this time the test sites are left open.

Evaluation   The test sites are examined at 24, 46, and 72 hours postapplication for the presence of any erythema. The minimum, nonirritating concentration in FCA-/water-treated controls is determined. The guinea pigs injected with the test material during induction that respond to lower doses are considered sensitized. The threshold of concentration for elicitation of response and the incidence of sensitization can be calculated.

Optimization Test

This test involves the use of both intradermal and topical routes, and incorporates the use of an adjuvant in some injections for induction.[29,31,34] It resembles the DT in many aspects.

Induction Phase   A total of 10 injections of 0.1 mL of test material (0.1% concentration) in 0.9% saline or in 1:1 FCA: saline are given to 20 test animals over 3 weeks. In the first week (day 1), a shaved flank and dorsal skin area are injected. On days 2 and 4, a new dorsal area is injected. During the first week, the test material is administered after dilution in saline. Twenty control animals are injected with the saline. In the second and third weeks, on every other day, test material (diluted in FCA/saline) is injected into the shaved area of a shoulder. Controls are administered as FCA/saline.

Evaluation   The two largest diameters (mm) of an erythematous reaction over the injection site are measured, and skin thickness is recorded with the help of calipers. The "reaction volume" (fold thickness × the two largest diameters) is calculated as the intensity of a 24-hour response during week 1 and is expressed in microliters. The mean reaction volume of each animal during the first week (in a saline vehicle) is also estimated.

Challenge Phase   This phase involves two steps. Initial challenge is done 35 days after the first injection. The guinea pigs are administered 0.1 mL of 0.1% test material in saline, while control animals are injected with plain saline.

Evaluation   During the challenge phase, the reaction volume for each guinea pig is calculated and compared to the mean reaction volume of the same animal. An animal developing a reaction volume greater than the mean + 1 SD (standard deviation) during induction is considered sensitized.

The second challenge is done 45 days after the first injection. A 0.05 mL of nonirritating concentration of test material (in a suitable vehicle) is applied to a 1 cm^2 area of flank skin, away from the previous injection sites. The area is occluded with a 2 × 2 cm piece of paper backed by an occlusive dressing for 24 hours. Control guinea pigs are patched with only the vehicle.

Evaluation   The 4-point *Draize primary erythema scale* is used to visually evaluate the reaction. Fischer's exact test is used to statistically compare the number of positive test results in the test group to the positives in controls. The comparison between dermal and epicutaneous challenge is done separately and a p value of ≤ 0.01 is considered significant.

This assay has been useful in classifying materials into strong, moderate, weak, or nonsensitizers. Based on the results of this a test, a classification scheme has been devised. (Table 16.3)

SAT

This test involves application of test material topically, and utilizes skin damage and FCA as adjuvants.[29,36,37]

Induction Phase   This involves shaving the skin (just behind the scapula) of 10–20 guinea pigs, and then treating with dry ice for 5–10 seconds. The area is then covered with a layer of loose-meshed gauze dressing and stretch adhesive, leaving a 2 cm opening over the shaved area, which in turn is secured by an adhesive tape. This dressing stays in place throughout induction. On day 1, creams/solid test material (approximately 0.2 mL) or liquid (0.1 mL) is spread over the test site and covered with filter paper (two layers) backed by occlusive tape, and attached to the dressing by adhesive tape. The concentration tested is decided by the irritancy potential, use conditions, and so on. After 2 days, the test material is reapplied to

Table 16.3   Optimization Test: Classification Scheme

Interdermal-positive animals (%)	Epidermal-positive animals (%)	Classification
NS, 0–30	NS, 0	Nonsensitizer
S, 30–50	NS, 0–30	Weak sensitizer
S, 50–75	S, 30–50	Moderate sensitizer
S, >50	S, >75	Strong sensitizer

S, statistically significant; NS, not statistically significant (by exact Fisher's test).
Source: Adapted from *Principles and Methods of Toxicology* (2007).[35]

the same area by lifting and replacing the filter paper. On day 4, two doses of 0.075 mL FCA are injected into the edges of the same test site. On day 7, the test material is reapplied and on day 9 the dressing is removed.

Challenge Phase   The challenge phase is carried out 22 days after the initial treatment. The test material (0.5 mL) is applied topically over a 2×2 cm area of shaved mid-back of the guinea pig. The test site is occluded by filter paper, which is held in place by adhesive tape and reinforced elastic adhesive bandage around the animal. A control group of 10–20 guinea pigs are treated similarly.

Evaluation   A day later, the dressing is removed and the test site is examined at 24, 48, and 72 hours, using a 7-point descriptive visual scale. Individual animals are considered sensitized if they show significantly stronger reactions than control animals.

GPMT

This test combines the FCA test, irritancy, an intradermal injection and a topical application.[18,29,38]

Induction Phase   The shoulder regions of two groups of 20–25 guinea pigs are shaved. The animals are injected with two identical sets of injections of 0.1 mL (50:50) FCA: water, test material in water, paraffin oil, or propylene glycol; the same dose of the test material in FCA/vehicle are placed in a 2×4 cm area. On day 6, if the test material is found nonirritating, the test site is treated with 10% sodium lauryl sulfate (SLS) to provoke an irritant reaction. On day 7, the test article is placed on filter paper over the injection site and occluded with approximately 4×8 cm surgical tape, which in turn is secured in place with an elastic bandage wrapped around the animal. The filter is saturated with the solution, if a vehicle other than petrolatum is used for topical application. Control guinea pigs are patched with only the vehicle. The dressing is removed 48 hours after application.

Challenge Phase   In this phase, the test and control animals are patched on the shaved flank with the highest nonirritating concentration, with approximately one-half of the highest nonirritating concentration and with the vehicle. The test solutions are applied to 1×1 cm pieces of filter paper and secured in place, for a period of 24 hours.

Evaluation   Evaluation is done 24 and 48 hours after removal of the patch, but the challenged area may be shaved 3 hours prior if required. A comparison between the intensity of responses to test material and vehicle in the test group and controls is done. A reaction is considered positive when the response is more intense as compared to controls. The test materials are then judged incrementally from weak to extreme sensitizers, based on the number of positives in the test group (Table 16.4).

Table 16.4   GPMT: Classification of Materials

Sensitization rate (% responding at challenge)	Grade	Classification
0–8	I	Weak
9–28	II	Mild
29–64	III	Moderate
65–80	IV	Strong
81–100	V	Extreme

Source: Adapted from *Principles and Methods of Toxicology* (2007).[35]

SENSITIZATION TESTS IN MICE

The classical guinea pig sensitization assays, even though very popular, are fraught with difficulties. They are expensive, time consuming, use subjective end points posing difficulties in data interpretation, and may cause a significant amount of stress during their manipulation, in order to alter the normal physiological function. Hence, in the last 10 years, there has been an increased interest in developing and standardizing predictive assays in mice.[39–41]

Sensitization tests in laboratory animals such as mice have made it possible to study delayed hypersensitivity reactions in lesser time, especially with the development of new techniques. Less subjective methods for evaluating the allergic response such as changes in the water content of challenged ears,[42] measurement of ear thickness with a micrometer,[43,44] and response of lymphocytes[43,45–47] have been proposed.

There have been many suggestions over the years toward developing standardized assays in mice. The most interesting of these involve use of the mouse ear and are:

1. Mouse ear swelling test (MEST)
2. LLNA
3. Vitamin A enhancement test (VAET)

The first two methods have now been developed sufficiently and will be discussed in some detail below.

MEST

Preliminary work done on the MEST lead to the incorporation of many findings in the main protocol elaborated below.[48,49]

1. The MEST involves both topical and injection exposures for induction and a topical challenge of the pinnae (the outer visible part of the ear).

2. Visual evaluation is replaced by measurement of ear thickness with a micrometer.

3. Albino mice (BALB/c, CF-1 or SW strains) are a better choice, as they favor the study of immune responses generated due to allergic sensitization.

4. Females, due to their less aggressive behavior, were chosen to allow group housing and minimal damage to the ears.

5. It was noted that responses of mice aged less than 5 weeks or more than 13 weeks were weaker than mice 6–10 weeks of age.

6. Induction doses administered to the animal's stomach region yielded a higher rate of sensitization than the back.

7. Tape stripping and preinjection of the test site with FCA was found to increase the efficacy of the induction method marginally.

8. Patch test by occlusion did not lead to increased sensitivity of the assay. In contrast, the response was found to be diminished due to the same.

Induction Phase CF-1, BALB/c, or SW female mice (6–8 weeks old) are gang housed and quarantined in direct bedding cages for a period of 5–7 days. Around 10–15 test animals and five controls with healthy pinnae are utilized (animals with damaged pinnae are excluded). The fur over the abdomen is shaved with electric clippers and stripped with a surgical adhesive tape (Dermaclear, GB Skincare, Montrose, CA) until a sheen appears on the skin.

FCA (0.05 mL) is injected intradermally in divided doses, using a tuberculin syringe attached to a 30-gauge needle, into two sites within the shaved area along the borders. This is followed by application of 100 µL of vehicle containing the test material/vehicle alone (controls) to the center of the shaved area. The mouse is then returned to the cage once the abdomen dries.

This process of tape stripping and application of test material to the abdomen is repeated from day 1 through day 3.

The dose selection is based on "*dermal irritation toxicity range finding* studies," which are conducted before testing each compound. Four groups of two mice each are subjected to the same induction procedure, followed by exposure of the ears to at least four different concentrations of challenge doses. The minimum irritating and nonirritating concentrations are then selected for induction.

The choice of vehicle depends on solubility and chemical compatibility with the test substance. Acetone, methyl ethyl ketone, or 70%, 80%, and 95% ethanol in water have been demonstrated to be acceptable vehicles in contrast to mixed ethanol/olive oil.

Challenge Phase Seven days after the last topical induction application, 20 µL of the test material in vehicle is applied to one ear of each animal (test and control) and 10 µL of the vehicle to the opposite ear. The ear thickness is measured with a micrometer before and 24–48 hours after application of the challenge. The thickness of both ears is measured and the animals are lightly anesthetized for the same.

Evaluation   A two- to threefold increase in thickness of the test ear compared to the vehicle-treated control ear is considered a positive test. The thickness of the control ear must not be more than 10% the original for the test to be considered valid. The study should be repeated with lower doses if the control group shows a greater than 10% increase in thickness.

The "degree of ear swelling" can be estimated by dividing the thickness of the ear tested by the thickness of the ear (control) treated with the vehicle. The percentage of respondents can also be calculated.

It has been proposed that the results produced by MEST (and classical guinea pig assays) could also be used to calculate the "potency index of sensitization." A comparison of MEST and various guinea pig techniques have been conducted in various studies.[50]

LLNA

LLNA is a unique test that involves topical induction, followed by measurement of the mitotic activity of the draining lymph node (efferent phase of the response).[51,52] T cell hyperplasia has been observed in the auricular lymph nodes upon exposing the dorsum of the pinnae to a sensitizer. Measuring lymphocyte proliferation has been proposed as an alternative approach to visual evaluations or measurement of edema of the mouse ear.[53-56]

BALB/c mice strains were found to be more sensitive than other strains for this test.[54] It was observed in preliminary studies that a test dose, when divided into three exposures over 3 days, leads to a more intense response than the same dose delivered in one exposure.[57] Cultures of excised lymph node cells labeled with ^{3}H-thymidine with or without exogenous interleukin (IL)-2 used in initial studies have been replaced by exposing proliferating cells to ^{3}H-thymidine *in situ* by intravenous injection.[54,55]

Materials Required   A minimum of three groups of four CBA/ca mice aged 8–12 weeks are used. They may be of either sex, however only a single sex may be used for each assay. Solubility and viscosity of the test solution and suspension guide the choice of vehicle and test concentration. A nontoxic dose should be chosen. The vehicles admissible are 4:1 acetone/olive, methyl ethyl ketone, dimethyl formamide, propylene glycol, dimethyl sulfoxide, and 2.5% hydroxypropyl cellulose in methanol.

Procedure   From a series of concentrations (100%, 50%, 25%, 10%, 5%, 2.5%, 1%, 0.5%, 0.25%, 0.05%, 0.001%), three consecutive concentrations are chosen for testing. Twenty-five microliters of the test solution is applied to the dorsal surface of the pinnae every day for three consecutive days. The vehicle alone is applied onto the controls. On day 5, after the first exposure, 250 mL of phosphate-buffered saline (PBS) containing 20 μL methyl thymidine is injected into the tail vein of each animal. Five hours later, the animals are euthanized by carbon dioxide asphyxiation.

The respective auricular lymph nodes are excised and grouped with the nodes from other animals from the same group. A cell suspension is now obtained from each lymph node and subjected to a series of biochemical steps in order to obtain the amount of ^{3}H–thymidine incorporation into the test group and the control. Subsequently, a ratio between the test and control group is calculated for each dose. The material is considered a sensitizer if the ratio for any test dose is two to three times greater than the control group.

Many variations of the LLNA and comparisons with other guinea pig assays exist. Usage of a lesser number of animals, lower cost, and lesser time required to conduct the assay are the advantages. The results are similar to the Buehler and guinea pig maximization assays (in validation studies); however, there has been no attempt to study the clinical relevance (e.g., relation between LLNA data and frequency of ACD in humans) of LLNA data or the benchmarks used. Many new reviews on LLNA have been published recently.[58–60]

VAET

The VAET is not considered a standard test by many laboratories, even though it has been used to evaluate the ingredients in many consumer products. This test works on the principle that the administration of a diet high in vitamin A intensifies the immune system reactivity for a preconditioning period and throughout induction and challenge. This in turn enables the dose of strong sensitizers to be decreased during the test.[61–65]

The doses used during induction and challenge are determined by dose–response studies in different groups of mice. Accordingly, the MIC is used for induction and the MNIC is used for challenge. Nonirritancy and solubility of the test substance guide the choice of vehicle.

The test is conducted in three phases: (1) vitamin A-rich diet for 28 days (preconditioning period); (2) six doses of the test material administered for 12 days over the shaved abdomen and thorax (induction); and (3) 4 days after induction (challenge).

Statistical comparison of the test and control groups is done. Sensitization is indicated by a 50% increase in response of the test group over the controls. The long preconditioning period and choice of micrometer were the main points of concern of this assay. This test was never submitted for formal validation.

HUMAN SENSITIZATION ASSAYS

These assays can be conducted in a limited number of human volunteers after informed consent has been obtained, only if the results of predictive tests in animals are available, the test material is a new compound, or if it contains significantly increased levels of common ingredients. Humans are usually not tested with materials that have been identified as sensitizers in animals unless the material is expected to be beneficial n some way. In the above case, the study must be reviewed by an institutional review board. Subjecting animals to higher doses of the test material imparts a certain margin of safety in potential human subjects.

Individuals should be randomly screened and the following precautions must be taken:

1. **Mastectomized Subjects.** Intact lymph nodes draining the test site are deemed important to induce sensitization. Hence, consenting subjects with unilateral mastectomies must be tested on the opposite side of the body and testing on scar tissue is unacceptable.

2. **Dermatology Patients.** Individuals with chronic and recurring skin conditions such as psoriasis and eczema are required to obtain a clearance from their dermatologist prior to enrolment. This is due to the risk of inciting koebnerization (Koebner's phenomenon, refers to the appearance of skin lesions appearing along a site of injury) following patch testing and minor trauma.

3. **Concomitant Diseases.** A history of ACD or other dermatological diseases must be solicited. Testing with known allergens, proven by diagnostic patch test in the volunteer, is usually counterproductive.

The human sensitization tests currently in use are described below:

1. Single-induction, single-challenge patch test
2. Repeated insult patch test (RIPT)
3. RIPT with continuous exposure (modified Draize)
4. Maximization test

Regulatory agencies approve of the RIPT, modified Draize, and human maximization tests. Sponsors usually use one of the above assays and define it as the "standard of the industry." All tests use standard, customized, occlusive, and semiocclusive patches such as the Webril, Hill-top chamber®, and Duhring and Finn chambers. Occlusive patches are superior to semiocclusive patches in terms of induction of sensitization.[66,67]

Most of the tests (except maximization) involve 150–200 subjects. Statistically, if no positive reactions are observed in 200 randomly selected subjects, then only 15/1000 of general population may react (95% confidence). Reducing the sample size of the test will decrease the predictive ability of adverse reactions in the general population.[68]

The FDA device group has worked on formulating many details of sensitization procedures, and has published guidelines for evaluating skin sensitization to chemicals in rubber products.[69] They recommend the modified Draize procedure. Tests for evaluating transdermal products are underway.

Schwartz–Peck Test (and Modifications)

This test was described by Schwartz and Schwartz–Peck, and is also known as the single-application, single-induction challenge patch test or the Traub–Tusing–Spoon method.[9,70,71]

The complete Schwartz–Peck (S-P) method involves a single induction patch, a usage period, and single-challenge patch test, while the incomplete S-P tests do not have a usage period.

Induction Phase   A patch impregnated with the test material (diluted/undiluted) is applied to the outer aspect of the upper arm in 200 test subjects for a period of 24–72 hours. The nature of the patch test (dose tested, duration of contact, presence or absence of occlusion) varies with the intended use. For example, cosmetics are tested by open patch or semiocclusive patches. Evaluation for erythema and edema is done 24–48 hours after removing the patch.

Usage Period   This period lasts for 4 weeks and is not a part of the incomplete S-P test.

Challenge Phase   At the end of the usage period, the same site of the upper arm is used to apply the challenge patch for 24–72 hours. For the incomplete S-P test, the second patch is applied 10–14 days following the induction patch. The test site is evaluated in the same manner as during induction. A stronger skin reaction during challenge indicates sensitization.

The S-P test initially described was the incomplete version, and was designed to study the effect of nylon garments on the skin (adverse effects, irritation, sensitization). The usage period was supposed to be performed in 1000 subjects after the challenge. This test was designed at a time when the mechanism of skin allergy was unknown. While Schwartz and Peck referred to it as the "prophetic patch test," it has now been observed that only potent haptens induce sensitization in this assay.

Some groups still use this assay, although it is inferior to all its counterparts. It has been modified in various ways by eliminating the usage test or patching completely, and placing a usage period between the induction and challenge phases.[72,73]

RIPT

Described below are the four main variations of the RIPT that are commonly used:[10,16,32,74,75]

1. The Draize human sensitization test
2. Shelanski–Shelanski test (S-S test)
3. Voss–Griffith test
4. Marzulli–Maibach modification

The RIPT was originally described by Shelanski (based on a verbal description of a method devised by Draize) and has gone through a series of modifications by Voss and Griffith. The current guidelines and protocol of the RIPT are now published by the FDA and given on their website in the medical devices section (http://www.fda.org).

1. Draize human sensitization test

    Induction Phase. Patches of test material are applied under occlusion, on the upper arm/back of a group of 200 volunteers for 24 hours and then removed. Soon after, the test site is evaluated for erythema and edema. A day after the first patch is removed, a new site is chosen for application of a second patch test. This process is repeated 10 times. A Monday–Friday schedule may be followed for simplicity so that the patient can remove the patch on Saturday on his own, thus allowing a 72-hour interval between the Friday and Monday patch applications.

    Challenge Phase. This is done 10–14 days following application of the last induction patch. The challenge patch is applied at a new site for a period of 24 hours and then evaluated for any reaction. A comparison is made between the responses obtained in early induction patches and challenge patches. The incidence of sensitization is also estimated.

2. Shelanski–Shelanski test (S-S test)

    Induction Phase. The S-S test is similar to the Draize RIPT, except that the induction cycle is repeated 15 times and the patches are applied to the same site every time. After each induction patch removal, the test site is evaluated and in the event of a reaction, a new patch is applied on the adjacent normal skin.

    Challenge Phase. This is carried out 2–3 weeks after the induction period. The challenge patch is applied for 48 hours, following which the test site is noted for any erythema/edema. The incidence of positive responses is calculated.

    Shelanski–Shelanski felt that the patch test responses during induction were due to "skin fatigue" or cumulative irritation and the time of such development (number of patches required to achieve this state) was called the "fatigue index."

3. Voss–Griffith test

    A small pilot group of 10–12 subjects are tested before conducting the test in 60–70 individuals.

    Induction Phase. Voss modified the S-S test by decreasing the number of 24-hour induction patch test cycles to nine, applied over 3 weeks.

    Challenge Phase. The challenge patch is applied 2 weeks after the last induction patch, wherein duplicate patches are placed for 24 hours at the original test site. Forty-eight and 96 hours after patch application, the sites are observed for inflammatory response.

    Many more details and modifications of the RIPT have been published by Griffith[76,77]:

    a. Testing areas drained by different lymphatic groups—four different test materials have been patched simultaneously and duplicate challenges have been applied to the induction sites as well as to the opposite arm.

    b. A new concept of rechallenge of subjects with reaction that was difficult to interpret was introduced.

c. The test group was scaled to 200 subjects and patch tests were conducted on multiple panels.

d. Detailed examples of proper interpretation of the human RIPT have been elaborated by Stotts.[21] Sensitization was defined as challenge reactions stronger than reactions early in the induction phase, by persistence of responses through delayed readings, by delayed appearance of a response, or by weak responses in a few subjects when the material has not produced irritation in the panel.

For reasons of cost-effectiveness and efficiency, many test materials are tested simultaneously. The term "Draize RIPT" is now being used by investigators for patches applied to the same site during induction, leading to blurring of the difference between the Draize and Voss–Griffith tests. However, the S-S test with over five to six induction applications has retained its identity.

4. Marzulli–Maibach modification

This modification ensures compliance of the patient in that the laboratory removes the patch (rather than the subject). The patch is applied on 3 days of the week (Monday, Wednesday, and Friday) for 3 weeks. Elicitation is for a 48-hour period and the test site is evaluated 1 hour after removal of the patches (at 49 and 96 hours), according to the International Contact Dermatitis Research Group (ICDRG) guidelines.

Human Maximization Test

This test was advanced by Kligman,[78] who found all human predictive sensitization assays in use (from 1966) to be inadequate in inducing sensitization to nine clinical allergens. He realized[19] that:

Emphasis must shift from prophecy to the more practical objective of identifying potential allergens. Once the allergenic potential is known with reasonable certainty, a judgment of risk might be ventured after examining all pertinent variables.

Kligman introduced a whole new perspective to the predictive sensitization assays. His objective was to ease the difficulties in performing and interpreting tests. Irritancy was used as an adjuvant in the maximization test.[79–81]

Induction Phase Compounds which cause irritation are patch tested at a concentration that induces moderate erythema in 48 hours. If the material is found to be nonirritating, then the test site is pretested (patched) with 5% SLS for a period of 24 hours. Moreover, the pre-treatment SLS patches may be applied prior to each patch application until a brisk erythema is produced. The test materials are dissolved in petrolatum (preferred vehicle) at a concentration at least five times higher than usage levels. Up to four dissimilar induction patches (under occlusion) are tested simultaneously and placed on the outer aspect of the arm or lower back, using custom-made Webril/Blenderm patches or Duhring chambers. To make sure that the patches are properly occluded, extra tape or bandage sprays may be used. The different sets of patches remain at the same site for 48 hours, followed by a 24-hour rest period (patches are removed). They are then reapplied.

Challenge Phase   A 2-week rest period follows the induction phase. A provocative patch of SLS is then applied to the lower back on previously untreated areas for 1 hour. The concentration of SLS to be used is determined by the season and individual response. Immediately after the SLS patch, the challenge patch is applied for 48 hours. The control area is also patched with SLS for 1 hour and then the vehicle (petrolatum) for 48 hours.

Evaluation   The tests areas are examined immediately after patch removal at 24 and 48 hours for inflammatory reactions. The number and percentage of individuals developing a positive response is calculated and a sensitization index to each test material is drawn.

The skin damage caused as a result of this test, unacceptable to most subjects, is a major drawback of this test. Nevertheless, the maximization test is the most sensitive method to detect allergenicity.

Modified Draize Human Sensitization Test

This is a modification of the RIPT procedure, wherein the subject is exposed continuously to the test material in the patch. This method is the test of choice for chemicals in natural rubber products.[69]

Induction Phase   Ten patches of the test material are applied over a 3-week period (on Monday, Wednesday, and Friday), on the outer upper arm of each subject.[20,82] After a rest period of 30 minutes, a fresh patch is applied. This short interval allows clearing of responses, occurring due to the tape, and also assists in grading the responses. The new patches are applied to the same area unless the original test site is moderately inflamed (patch is placed on adjacent, noninflamed skin). This type of patch application allows a total exposure time of 504–552 hours (216–240 hours for RIPT), with induction concentration levels much above usage levels.

Challenge Phase   The challenge patch (nonirritating concentration) is placed 2 weeks after induction onto a new area for a period of 72 hours. The sites are examined for any reaction at the time of patch removal and 24 hours later.

In Vitro Assays for ACD

Delayed hypersensitivity research at the cellular level has enabled us to understand and develop newer techniques of predicting allergenicity in humans. The *in vitro* assays are an attempt to replace diagnostic patch testing and serve as early screening predictive assays. The work done so far was mainly concentrated on measuring the effect of lymphokines (cytokines released by sensitized lymphocytes) on target cells as a marker for allergy. The current focus of *in vitro* assays on the afferent phase of antigen binding and stimulation of target cells has met with limited experimental success.

The phenomenon of "migration inhibition" of peritoneal exudate cells from capillary tubes has been described, and was found to be due to an antigen to which the guinea pigs (donors) were sensitized.[82] Later, the antigen was identified as a migration inhibition factor (MIF), which also retarded the macrophage mobility and caused their adherence to glass. This was produced by sensitized lymphocytes in the presence of a sensitizing antigen.[83,84]

Further, our understanding of MIF was refined due to experiments conducted by Rocklin et al. (who found that MIF was produced by highly purified populations of proliferating T cells), Moorehead et al. (demonstrated that MIF production is dependent on Ia-T cell subsets), and Pearmain et al. (reported that the tuberculin caused the same effect in peripheral blood leucocyte cultures from sensitized patients but not from unsensitized patients).[85–87] Phytohemagglutinin was found to initiate mitotic activity and cause blast transformation of lymphocytes.

Similar *assays in nickel-sensitive subjects* and unsensitized controls were conducted. McLeod et al. used ^{14}C thymidine uptake to confirm blast transformation and they found that more than half of the nickel-sensitive subjects tested positive for the same. The unsensitized controls did not show any blast transformation.[47,88–91]

Assays with dinitrochlorobenzene (DNCB) in guinea pigs have been conducted, with similar results by at least two investigators.[45,92] They found that lymphocyte transformation occurred to a greater degree in guinea pigs sensitized with 2,4-dinitro-1-fluorobenzene (DNCB) and incubated with DNFB (as the dinitrophenyl group would attach to protein using either material) than the unsensitized controls. The blast transformation was measured by tritiated thymidine.

Experiments conducted in human volunteers and epidermal extracts for conjugation revealed similar results. For example, leukocyte and erythrocytic membranes used for conjugation produced the same effect (Miller and Lewis).[46,93] Cytotoxicity in experimentally induced ACD has been shown to be produced by lymphotoxin.[94]

A hypothetical *in vitro* assay involving the use of Langerhans cells (LC) to predict sensitization potential was proposed, in which the binding to LC would be measured.[42]

In recent times, a lot of resources have been devoted to developing reliable *in vitro* assays with the aim of eliminating predictive testing on animals and humans.[95–97]

SKIN IRRITATION AND CORROSION

Skin irritation is a localized inflammation of the skin that is not mediated by the immune system (i.e., sensitized lymphocytes or antibodies). Chemicals can irritate the skin in a single exposure (active irritants) or on repeated applications to the same area of the skin (cumulative irritation or skin fatigue).[74] Some chemicals destroy the skin immediately on application, causing necrosis and scar formation and are labeled as corrosives.

Regulatory agencies have made it mandatory to screen various chemicals for their potential to cause skin irritation and corrosion, as there is always a chance for accidental exposure. Since it is not appropriate to conduct corrosion studies in humans, tests have been conducted in animals using standardized protocols. If animal studies establish the noncorrosive nature of the material besides a low risk of systemic toxicity, then humans may also be tested. Further efforts are in progress to replace animal studies with *in vitro*/human assays.

The mechanism of induction of skin irritation is not well known, but it is thought that chemicals destroy and disrupt cell functions and trigger the release of autocoids, which (1) increase vascular permeability, (2) cause low increases in blood flow, (3) attract white blood cells (WBCs) into the area, and (4) damage cells directly. All these result in local skin inflammation. Histamine, prostaglandins, leukotrienes, kinins, reactive oxygen species (ROS), complement, and WBC products have been implicated, as some of the mediators of irritant reactions.[98,99]

In a study conducted to understand the mechanism of acute skin irritation using open topical application of chemicals to the ear of the mouse, it was confirmed that different pathways of mediator involvement existed for skin irritation. Hence, to screen materials for skin irritation, a number of *in vitro* assays would be required, as no single assay would be adequate..[85,100,101]

There are a number of factors that affect the development of skin irritation. They have been classified into extrinsic and intrinsic factors[102–104] and have been important in designing assays for skin irritation. The various extrinsic factors are the dose and duration of contact of chemical, type of appliance, chamber and tape used for patch testing, degree of occlusion, surface temperature of the skin, which may increase with occlusion, and type of vehicle.[78,101,105]

Tests for Predicting Irritation Potential

Draize Rabbit Model

The Draize model utilizes albino rabbits and is used to test skin irritation.[8] This method has been adopted as a standard procedure by many governmental agencies, such as the U.S. Federal Hazardous Substance Act (FHSA).[101,106,107]

The hair on the dorsum of six albino rabbits is clipped (two areas of 1 in.[2] each). One site is left intact and the other abraded with a hypodermic needle. The undiluted test material (0.5 mL of liquids and 0.5 g of solids/semisolids) is then applied to both test sites. The test areas are occluded with 1 in.[2] surgical gauze and a rubberized cloth is placed on the entire trunk for a period of 24 hours. The test sites are assessed at 24 and 72 hours after patch application.

Draize utilized the visual scoring system (Table 16.5) to calculate the primary irritation index (PII), which is estimated by averaging the erythema and edema

Table 16.5   The Draize–FHSA Scoring System[101]

Erythema and eschar formation	Score
No erythema	0
Very slight erythema (barely perceptible)	1
Well-defined erythema	2
Moderate to severe erythema	3
Severe erythema (beet redness) to slight eschar formation (injuries in depth)	4

Edema formation	Score
No edema	0
Very slight edema (barely perceptible)	1
Slight edema (edges of the area well defined by definite raising	2
Moderate edema (raised >1 mm)	3
Severe edema (raised >1 mm and extending beyond the area of exposure)	4

Table 16.6   Interpretation of the PII Value

PII	Interpretation regarding the test material
<2	Nonirritating
2–5	Mildly irritating
>5	Severely irritating

scores of all sites (abraded and nonabraded). When the two averages are added together, the PII value is obtained and is interpreted as shown in Table 16.6.

The CPSC defines a value of 5 as irritant. However, it is recommended by laboratory and clinical experience that these values must not be viewed in the absolute sense or extrapolated to humans. This is because there are many substances which are irritating to the rabbit, but well tolerated by human skin.

It must be noted that vesiculation, ulceration, and severe eschar formation are not included in the Draize scoring system. Even then, all the Draize-type tests are used to evaluate corrosion and irritation. When severe reactions occur, the tests sites are observed again on days 7 and 14 or later if required.

Inability to adequately differentiate between mild and moderate irritants constitutes the main drawback of this test. However, the Draize model helps in hazard identification and even overpredicts the severity of human skin reactions and so is recommended by regulatory bodies.

Various modifications of the Draize assay have been tried in order to improve the prediction of irritation potential in humans.

Cumulative Irritation Assays

The effects of cumulative exposure to potential irritants have been studied by many researchers. Surfactant solutions have been tested with the application of test material, seven times at 10-minute intervals, over the clipped dorsum of albino mice under occlusion (with a rubber dam to prevent evaporation). The skin was then evaluated microscopically for any erosion of the epidermis.[108]

Protective creams which are used against chemical irritants such as SLS, sodium hydroxide, and toluene were tested in the guinea pig repeat irritation test (RIT).[109,110] Chemical irritants were applied on the shaved skin of the back in young guinea pigs every day for 2 weeks. Barrier creams were also applied onto the skin of the test animals, 2 hours before and immediately after exposure to the irritant. Only irritants were applied to the control guinea pigs. The test sites were examined visually (for erythema) and by bioengineering methods (using laser Doppler flowmetry and transepidermal water loss). This method of RIT has been proposed as an animal model to test the efficacy of barrier creams.

A human version of the RIT has also been proposed and developed, wherein the irritant material is applied under occlusion to the same area for 3–21 days. The types of patches vary from Draize-type gauze dressings to metal chambers; hence, a reference irritant material is added to the test to simplify analysis of the results. The sensitivity of this test may be influenced by the degree of occlusion since it affects percutaneous penetration of the test material. This test has been replicated in various other animal species, including the guinea pig and rabbit.[111,112]

RIT has also been used as an open application assay in rabbits, wherein the test substances are applied 16 times over a 3-week period.[113] The results are evaluated visually (for erythema) and by measuring the skin thickness. There is a high correlation between these two parameters of evaluation, which was demonstrated between the scores of 60 test substances in the rabbit and man. Thus, rabbit assay is a powerful tool for predicting irritation potential.

An open application procedure has also been tried in guinea pigs to classify weak irritants.[114]

Immersion Assay

The irritant potential of aqueous surfactant solutions and aqueous dilutions of agricultural chemicals were tested using this assay. The test involves 10 guinea pigs that are restrained and immersed in a 40°C test solution while keeping their head above water. This is done for 4 hours daily for 3 days. A control group is also immersed in a reference solution. Twenty-four hours after the last immersion, the animals' flanks are shaved and examined for erythema, edema, and fissures.

This utility of this study is restricted because of systemic absorption of a lethal dose of the test material. Hence, this assay is restricted to testing products with limited toxic potential, with a maximum test concentration of 10%.[115–118]

This assay has also been utilized to test the dermatotoxic effects of detergents in guinea pigs.[119]

Mouse Ear Model

The mouse ear has been used for testing shampoos.[120] The undiluted shampoo is applied to one ear of mice every day for 4 days, following which the degree of inflammation (vessel dilation, erythema ,and edema) is assessed. Ear thickness has also been used to quantify inflammation due to surfactants and other chemicals.[121] This method of evaluation allows quantification of the dose–response relationship along with comparison of chemicals.

The above mechanism was used to compare skin inflammation induced by mustard oil and capsaicin.[122] Mice were first pretreated with various receptor antagonists, such as 5-HT2, H1, and tachykinin antagonists. It was demonstrated that the tachykinin NK-1 receptor was an important mediator of inflammation induced by mustard oil. Even though mouse models help in making simple and objective measurements, their relevance in humans requires elucidation.

Other Methods

A few more assays of skin irritation in animals have been proposed. The quantity of Evans blue dye recovered from the skin after exposure to irritants has been estimated.[123] In another experiment, myeloperoxidase in polymorphonuclear leukocytes was used as a biomarker for inflammation of the skin.[124]

Human Models

Most of the skin irritation tests are species relevant. This eliminates erratic extrapolation of animal and *in vitro* results to humans. However, data from prior animal studies help in excluding particularly toxic substances and concentrations from human exposure.

Many products and concentrations can be tested and compared at the same time as the test area required is small. A reference irritant substance is included in the patch series to allow interpretation of the test substances with ease. The various assays are summarized below.

Single-Application Patch Testing

This test was outlined by the National Academy of Sciences (NAS).[26] The test material is applied onto the intrascapular region of the back or dorsal surface of the forearms and occluded for 4 hours; however, the exposure time can vary. For new or volatile materials, a relatively nonocclusive tape and a shorter time of contact (30–60 minutes) is recommended, as the severity of response increases with better occlusion. Studies have also been performed with patches applied for greater than 24 hours.

The skin is examined 30–60 minutes after removal of the patch using the Draize scale for erythema and edema (Table 16.5). However, this scale does not provide

Table 16.7 Human Patch Test Grading Scales

A. Simple patch test grading scale	
0	Negative, normal skin
+/−	Questionable erythema
1	Definite erythema
2	Erythema and induration
3	Vesiculation
4	Bullous reaction
B. Detailed human patch test grading scale	
0	No apparent cutaneous involvement
½	Faint, barely perceptible erythema or slight dryness (glazed appearance)
1	Faint but definite erythema, no eruptions or broken skin, *OR* No erythema but definite dryness; may have epidermal fissuring
1½	Well-defined erythema or faint erythema with definite dryness; may have epidermal fissuring
2	Moderate erythema, may have a few papules or deep fissures, moderate to severe erythema in cracks
2½	Moderate erythema with barely perceptible edema, *OR* Severe erythema not involving a significant portion of the patch (halo effect around the edges), may have a few papules, *OR* Moderate to severe erythema
3	Severe erythema (beet red). May have generalized papules, *OR* Moderate to severe erythema with slight edema (edges well defined by raising)
3½	Moderate to severe erythema with moderate edema (confined to patch area), *OR* Moderate to severe erythema with isolated eschar formations or vesicles
4	Generalized vesicles, *OR* Eschar formation, *OR* Moderate to severe erythema and/or edema extending beyond patch area

Source: Adapted from *Principles and Methods of Toxicology* (2007).[35]

scoring for papular, vesicular, or bullous responses. Hence, integrated scales with points ranging from 4 to 16 have been defined (Table 16.7). The test data can also be subjected to statistical analysis, to calculate (1) IT50 (time required to produce irritation in 50% of the subjects) and (2) ID50 (dose required to produce irritation in 50% of the subjects after a 24-hour exposure).[125]

Using the visual scoring for assessing erythema, a variety of irritants have been tested on Caucasians and Asians. SLS (20%) was used as a benchmark for relative ranking of irritancy. Further, the "threshold of skin irritation" in six different skin types has been studied and no significant difference was found between various skin types.[126] The threshold of skin irritation was defined as the lowest concentration of SLS that would produce skin irritation under the 4-hour occluded patch conditions.

Cumulative Irritation Testing

This assay was described by Lanman et al. and Philips et al. and is also known as the "21-day cumulative irritation assay."[111,127] The main objective of this test was to screen new formulations before their marketing. The test material (liquid/semisolid) is added to a 1 in.[2] of Webril and applied to the skin of the upper back under occlusion, for a period of 24 hours. In the case of liquids, the patch is saturated with the material, and for semisolids 0.5 g of the viscous substance is used. After 24 hours, the area is examined for any reactions and then repatched. This process is repeated for 21 days, following which the IT50 may be calculated.

The drawback of the cumulative patch test was that it could not predict the adverse reactions to the skin damaged by acne, shaving, or sensitive areas like the face.[128]

Two cumulative irritation models have been by testing skin reactions to metalworking fluids (MWFs).[129] In the first model, MWFs were applied with Finn chambers on the subject's mid-back, removed after 1 day, and then again reapplied for another 2 days. The second model used the guinea pig RIT for induction of dermatitis, 6 hours daily for 2 weeks (omitting the weekends).

Evaluation of the results was done by visual scoring, transepidermal water loss (used mainly for low irritancy materials), and chromametry. The first model, which lasted 3 days, was preferred due to its shorter duration and better discriminatory potential of irritancy.

The Chamber Scarification Test

The main objective of this assay was to test the irritant potential of materials on damaged skin.[130,131] On the volar aspect of the forearm, six to eight 1-mm scratches (four parallel and four perpendicular scratches) are made with a 30-guage needle, taking care not to cause bleeding. The test material (0.1 g of ointments, creams ,or powders) are placed on Duhring chambers and then applied onto the skin. Liquid test material (0.1 mL) is saturated on a fitted pad and placed on the skin. Chambers containing fresh test material are reapplied every day for 3 days and the test sites are examined visually 30 minutes after the removal of the final sets of patches.

A "scarification index" can be calculated when both normal and scarified skin are tested (score of scarified skin divided by the score of intact skin).

The role and relationship of this assay to routine use of substances on damaged skin has not yet been established.

Immersion Tests

These tests were developed to improve irritancy prediction by simulating consumer use and use aqueous solutions. In the first test done by Kooyman and Snyder, soap solutions (up to 3%) were prepared in troughs at a temperature of 105°F.[132] The subjects immersed one hand and forearm in each trough for 10–15 minutes, thrice daily for 5 days, or until there was development of irritation in both arms. It was found that the antecubital fossa was the first site to develop irritation, followed by the hands.[108,132] This lead to the development of antecubital wash tests and hand immersion assays.[107]

Another immersion protocol (30 min/4 days) was designed to examine the effects of temperature and anionic character, on the degree of irritation caused by detergents.[133]

The evaluation was done by assessing the stratum corneum barrier function (transepidermal water loss), skin redness (color parameter), and skin dryness (capacitance method). It was found that all three parameters (integrity of the skin, higher anionic content, and temperature) caused an increased irritant response of the detergents under consideration.

An "arm immersion model of compromised skin" was designed by Allenby et al. to study the irritant or allergic potential of substances on damaged skin.[134,135] The test involved immersion of the subject's forearm into a solution of 0.5% sodium dodecyl sulfate twice every day for 10 minutes, until an erythema reading of 1 to 1+ (degree of damage occurring in one morning's wet domestic work was reached on the visual scale). Patches of different irritants were applied onto the dorsal and volar aspects of both pretreated and untreated forearms and back. It was observed that the degree of reaction was much greater on compromised skin than on normal skin.

Bioengineering Methods in Model Development

Most of the animal and human models discussed above do not utilize the modern bioengineering methods that are now available. These new methods circumvent any imprecision which may occur due to the investigator skill and inter- or intraobserver variation. The results obtained by using these techniques are reproducible and hence increase the statistical power of the data obtained. Transepidermal water loss, capacitance, ultrasound, laser Doppler flowmetry, spectroscopy, and chromametric analysis are few of the techniques which can be used singly or in combination. These tests and techniques have been further elaborated.[107]

A comparison between the various bioengineering methods was made by Andersen and Maibach. They demonstrated that the skin reactions, which looked clinically indistinguishable, induced a significantly different change in barrier function and vascular status.[136]

In Vitro *Assays of Skin Irritation and Corrosion*

Over the past few years, a great deal of effort has gone into developing *in vitro* alternatives to the Draize-type tests for skin and eye irritation. Humane objections to animal testing, the need for a system that can deliver quantitative and reproducible results, and advances in techniques to culture human cells have been the driving forces behind their development. They are also being considered as research tools for toxicology and as aids in the formulation of milder products.

Various approaches have been used toward the development of these assays, which include[89,137-148]:

Cell toxicity

Measurement of inflammatory mediators

Effect on cell recovery and survival

Effect on cellular physiology

Cell morphology

Biochemical end points

Effect on membranes and artificial membranes

Use of metabolic activators

Use of nonmammalian cells

As of now, the *in vitro* assays for skin irritation and corrosion have not been validated. Thus, animal and human tests are the only ways of assessing any irritation potential.[149] However, many proposals for validation of these methods have been advanced, with the likelihood of being accepted in the near future. A few of the techniques in use deserve mention.

Of late, there has been a surge in the use of laboratory-cultured skin for irritation testing, with the availability of two commercial products, Skin[2] and Epi-Derm™.[150-152]

Skin[2] (Advanced Tissue Sciences, La Jolla, CA) is a 3D coculture of human fibroblasts and epidermal keratinocytes. The culture is constructed by seeding human neonatal fibroblasts onto a specially treated nylon mesh substrate. The fibroblasts adhere to the mesh and lay down a dermal collagen matrix. A proper degree of confluence is awaited, and subsequently, keratinocytes are seeded onto the fibroblast matrix-containing mesh. The epidermis is then exposed to the environment (air interfaced), following which a partially differentiated stratum corneum consisting of three to six layers is formed. This system is available and has been used for many of the cytotoxicity assays, and assays for the release of inflammatory mediators.

Epi-Derm (MatTek, Ashland, MA), also known as the reconstructed human epidermis (RHE), is a commercially marketed, 3D, human cell-derived skin tissue model that is mitotically and metabolically active. It consists of a multilayered corni-fied epithelium, with a well-differentiated stratum corneum but lacking a dermal component.[153] Implementation of this system to study skin corrosion, using the dimethyltriazoldiphenyl tetrazolium-formazan (MTT) cell viability assay, has met with limited success.[154] Efforts are ongoing to improve the sensitivity of the test protocol.

Other synthetic dermal assay systems such as the Skintex and Corrositex (both from Invitro International, Irvine, CA) are membrane barrier/protein matrices that comprise two component systems and utilize protein denaturation and changes in the arrangement of macromolecules as an end point.[5,155-157] The first compartment consists of a barrier matrix that contains an indicator dye, the release of which signals protein disruption and denaturation. The second compartment consists of a reagent system that increases in turbidity upon exposure to irritants. Spectrophotometry allows the detection of the above changes. The DOT has accepted Corrositex as a substitute to the DT for skin corrosion, and it has also been validated for limited purposes by the Interagency Coordination Committee on the Validation of Alternative Methods (ICCVAM).[158]

In Europe, excised rat and human skin have also been used to study skin corrosion by employing a change in transcutaneous electrical resistance (TER).[159-163] Full-thickness skin (including the dermis) is tied onto the top of a small tube (epidermal surface uppermost) with a rubber "O" ring. These small tubes are then suspended into a larger tube, containing an electrolyte solution in distilled water. The test material (150 µg) is applied onto the surfaces of at least three skin surface discs. At the end of 24 hours, the skin is rinsed and treated with ethanol, following which an electrolyte solution is added to the surface of the skin. Evaluation is done by measuring the TER using a commercial instrument. A value above 11–12.5 kΩ/ disc indicates corrosion of the test material. The results of this assay may vary by investigator and source of skin. This method appears to be reproducible, provided there is a judicious use of reference materials to set threshold values for classifying materials as corrosives. It is yet to receive full validation.

CONCLUSION

These descriptions provide a starting point. As in most scientific endeavors, the generation of a valid result depends to a great extent on the sophistication and experience of the investigator.

REFERENCES

1. SAKULA A. Paul Langerhans (1847–1888): A centenary tribute. *Journal of the Royal Society of Medicine* 1988; 81: 414–415.
2. POLAK L. Immunological aspects of contact sensitivity. *Monographs in allergy* 1980; 15: 1–170.
3. JADASSOHN J. Zur kenntniss der medicamentosen dermatosen. *Verhandlungen der Deutschen Dermatologischen Gesellschaft* 1895; 5: 103.
4. VON PIRQUET C. Allergie. *Annals of Allergy* 1946; 4: 388–390.
5. FREY JR, WENK P. Experimental studies on the pathogenesis of contact eczema in the guinea pig. *International Archives of Allergy and Applied Immunology* 1957; 11: 81–100.
6. FREY JR, WENK P. Function of regional lymph nodes in the development of dinitrochlorobenzol contact eczema in guinea pigs. *Dermatologica* 1958; 116: 243–259.
7. SILBERBERG I, BAER RL, ROSENTHAL SA. The role of Langerhans cells in allergic contact hypersensitivity. A review of findings in man and guinea pigs. *The Journal of Investigative Dermatology* 1976; 66: 210–217.
8. DRAIZE JH, WOODARD G, CALVERY HO. Methods for the study of irritation and toxicity of substances applied topically to the skin and mucous membranes. *The Journal of Pharmacology and Experimental Therapeutics* 1944; 82: 377–390.
9. SCHWARTZ L, PECK SM. The patch test in contact dermatitis. *Journal of the National Association of Chiropodists* 1946; 36: 7–16.
10. SHELANSKI HA, SHELANSKI MV. A new technique of human patch tests. *Proceedings of the Scientific Section of the Toilet Goods Association* 1953; 19: 46–49.

11. LANDSTEINER K, CHASE MW. Studies on the sensitization of animals with simple chemical compounds IV. Anaphylaxis induced by picryl chloride and 2:4 dinitrochlorobenzene. *The Journal of Experimental Medicine* 1937; 66: 337.

12. LANDSTEINER K, CHASE MW. Studies on the sensitization of animals with simple chemical compounds IX. Skin sensitization induced by injection of conjugates. *The Journal of Experimental Medicine* 1941; 73: 431–438.

13. LANDSTEINER K, CHASE MW. Experiments on transfer of cutaneous sensitivity to simple compounds. *Proceedings of the Society of Experimental Biology and Medicine* 1942; 49: 688–690.

14. LANDSTEINER K, JACOBS J. Studies on sensitization of animals with simple chemical compounds. II. *The Journal of Experimental Medicine* 1936; 64: 625–639.

15. LANDSTEINER K, JACOBS J. Studies on sensitization of animals with simple chemical compounds. *The Journal of Experimental Medicine* 1935; 61: 643–656.

16. DRAIZE JH. Dermal toxicity. In: *Appraisals of the Safety of Chemicals in Food, Drugs and Cosmetics*. Association of Food and Drug Officials of U.S, Texas State Department of Health, Austin, TX, 1959; 46–59.

17. BUEHLER EV. Delayed contact hypersensitivity in the guinea pig. *Archives of Dermatology* 1965; 91: 171–177.

18. MAGNUSSON B, KLIGMAN AM. The identification of contact allergens by animal assay. The guinea pig maximization test. *The Journal of Investigative Dermatology* 1969; 52: 268–276.

19. KLIGMAN AM. The identification of contact allergens by human assay. III. The maximization test: A procedure for screening and rating contact sensitizers. *The Journal of Investigative Dermatology* 1966; 47: 393–409.

20. MARZULLI FN, MAIBACH HI. The use of graded concentrations in studying skin sensitizers: Experimental contact sensitization in man. *Food and Cosmetics Toxicology* 1974; 12: 219–227.

21. STOTTS J. Planning, conduct and interpretation of human predictive sensitization patch tests. In: Drill VA, Lazar P, eds. *Current Concepts in Cutaneous Toxicity*, Vol. 41. Academic Press, New York, 1980; 41–53.

22. European Union. EEC Council Directive of 25 April 1984 amending for the 6th time Directive 67/548/EEC on the approximation of the laws, regulations and administrative provisions relating to the classification, packaging and labeling of dangerous substances (Annex V). *Official Journal of the European Communities* 1984; L251(27): 1.

23. EPA (U.S. ENVIRONMENTAL PROTECTIVE AGENCY). *Pesticide Assessment Guidelines. Subdivision F: Hazard Evaluation—Human and Domestic Animals*, rev. ed. Environmental Protection Agency, Washington, D.C., 1984. PB 86-108958, Series 81-6.

24. WESTER RC, MAIBACH HI. Cutaneous pharmacokinetics: 10 steps to percutaneous absorption. *Drug Metabolism Reviews* 1983; 14: 169–205.

25. JAPAN/MAFF. *Testing Guidelines for Evaluation of Safety of Agriculture Chemicals*. The Ministry of Agriculture, Forestry and Fisheries, Tokyo, Japan, 1985.

26. NATIONAL ACADEMY OF SCIENCES. *Principles and Procedures for Evaluating the Toxicity of Household Substances*. Committee for the Revision of NAS Publication 1138, Washington, D.C., 1977; 23–59.

27. RITZ HL, BUEHLER EV. Planning, conduct and interpretation of guinea pig sensitization patch tests. In: Drill VA, Lazar P, eds. *Current Concepts in Cutaneous Toxicity*. Academic Press, New York, 1980; 25.

28. JOHNSON AW, GOODWIN BFJ. The Draize test and modifications. In: Andersen KE, Maibach HI, eds. *Contact Allergy Predictive Tests in Guinea Pigs*. Karger, Basel, Switzerland, 1985; 31–38.

29. KLECAK G. Identification of contact allergens: Predictive tests in animals. In: Marzulli FN, Maibach HI, eds. *Dermatotoxicology*. Hemisphere, New York, 1983; 193–236.

30. KERO M, HANNUKSELA M. Guinea pig maximization test, open epicutaneous test and chamber test in induction of delayed contact hypersensitivity. *Contact Dermatitis* 1980; 6: 341–344.

31. KLECAK G. The Freund's complete adjuvant test and the open epicutaneous test. In: Andersen KE, Maibach HI, eds. *Contact Allergy Predictive Tests in Guinea Pigs*. Karger, Basel, Switzerland, 1985; 152–171.

32. Buehler EV. A new method for detecting potential sensitizers using the guinea pig. *Toxicology and Applied Pharmacology* 1964; 6: 341.

33. Buehler EV. A rationale for the selection of occlusion to induce and elicit delayed contact hypersensitivity in the guinea pig: A prospective test. In: Anderson KE, Maibach HI, eds. *Contact Allergy Predictive Tests in Guinea Pigs*. Karger, Basel, Switzerland, 1985; 38–58.

34. Maurer T, Thomann P, Weirich EG, Hess R. The optimization test in the guinea-pig. A method for the predictive evaluation of the contact allergenicity of chemicals. *Agents Actions* 1975; 5: 174–179.

35. Hayes BB, Patrick E, Maibach HI. Dermatotoxicology. In: Hayes AW, ed. *Principles and Methods of Toxicology*, 5th ed. Informa Healthcare, New York, 2007; 1359–1405.

36. Maguire H Jr. Mechanism of intensification by Freund's adjuvant of the acquisition of delayed hypersensitivity in the guinea pig. *Immunological Communications* 1972; 1: 239–246.

37. Maguire HC Jr. Proceedings: Alteration in the acquisition of delayed hypersensitivity with adjuvant in the guinea pig. *Monographs in Allergy* 1974; 8: 13–26.

38. Wahlberg JE, Boman A. Guinea pig maximization test. In: Andersen KE, Maibach HI, eds. *Contact Allergy Predictive Tests in Guinea Pigs*. Karger, Basel, Switzerland, 1985; 9–106.

39. Asherson GL, Ptak W. Contact and delayed hypersensitivity in the mouse. I. Active sensitization and passive transfer. *Immunology* 1968; 15: 405–416.

40. Crowle AJ. Delayed hypersensitivity in the mouse. *Advances in Immunology* 1975; 20: 197–264.

41. Crowle AJ, Crowle CM. Contact sensitivity in mice. *The Journal of Allergy* 1961; 32: 302–320.

42. Bos JD. A new approach to contact allergenicity screening. *Medical Hypotheses* 1984; 15: 103–108.

43. Bäck O, Larsen A. Contact sensitivity in mice evaluated by means of ear swelling and a radiometric test. *The Journal of Investigative Dermatology* 1982; 78: 309–312.

44. Van Loveren H, Kato K, Ratzlaff RE, Meade R, Ptak W, Askenase PW. Use of micrometers and calipers to measure various components of delayed-type hypersensitivity ear swelling reactions in mice. *Journal of Immunological Methods* 1984; 67: 311–319.

45. Milner JE. *In vitro* lymphocyte responses in contact hypersensitivity. *The Journal of Investigative Dermatology* 1970; 55: 34–38.

46. Milner JE. *In vitro* lymphocyte responses in contact hypersensitivity. II. *The Journal of Investigative Dermatology* 1971; 56: 349–352.

47. Pauly JL, Caron GA, Suskind RR. Blast transformation of lymphocytes from guinea pigs, rats, and rabbits induced by mercuric chloride *in vitro*. *The Journal of Cell Biology* 1969; 40: 847–850.

48. Gad SC, Dunn BJ, Dobbs DW, Reilly C, Walsh RD. Development and validation of an alternative dermal sensitization test: The mouse ear swelling test (MEST). *Toxicology and Applied Pharmacology* 1986; 84: 93–114.

49. Gad SC, Dunn BJ, Gavigan FA, Reilly C, Walsh RD. Development validation and transfer of a new test system technology in toxicology. In: Goldberg AM, ed. *New Test System in Toxicology*. Mary Ann Liebert, New York, 1987; 275–292.

50. Gad SC. A scheme for the prediction and ranking of relative potencies of dermal sensitizers based on data from several systems. *Journal of Applied Toxicology* 1988; 8: 361–368.

51. Basketter DA, Scholes EW, Kimber I, Botham PA, Hilton J, Miller K, Robbins MC, Harrison PTC, Waite SJ. Interlaboratory evaluation of the local lymph node assay with 25 chemicals and comparison with guinea pig test data. *Toxicological Methods* 1991; 1: 30–43.

52. Scholes EW, Basketter DA, Saril AE, Kimber I, Evans CD, Miller K, Robbins MC, Harrison PT, Waite SJ. The local lymph node assay: Results of a final inter-laboratory validation under field conditions. *Journal of Applied Toxicology* 1992; 12: 217–222.

53. Kimber I, Hilton J, Botham PA. Identification of contact allergens using the murine local lymph node assay: Comparisons with the Buehler occluded patch test in guinea pigs. *Journal of Applied Toxicology* 1990; 10: 173–180.

54. KIMBER I, MITCHELL JA, GRIFFIN AC. Development of a murine local lymph node assay for the determination of sensitizing potential. *Food and Chemical Toxicology* 1986; 24: 585–586.

55. KIMBER I, WEISENBERGER C. A murine local lymph node assay for the identification of contact allergens. Assay development and results of an initial validation study. *Archives of Toxicology* 1989; 63: 274–282.

56. OLIVER GJ, BOTHAM PA, KIMBER I. Models for contact sensitization–novel approaches and future developments. *The British Journal of Dermatology* 1986; 115(Suppl 31): 53–62.

57. KIMBER I, WEISENBERGER C. Anamnestic responses to contact allergens: Application in the murine local lymph node assay. *Journal of Applied Toxicology* 1991; 11: 129–133.

58. GERBERICK GF, RYAN CA, KERN PS, SCHLATTER H, DEARMAN RJ, KIMBER I, PATLEWICZ GY, BASKETTER DA. Compilation of historical local lymph node data for evaluation of skin sensitization alternative methods. *Dermatitis* 2005; 16: 157–202.

59. KIMBER I, DEARMAN RJ, BASKETTER DA, RYAN CA, GERBERICK GF. The local lymph node assay: Past, present and future. *Contact Dermatitis* 2002; 47: 315–328.

60. DIVKOVIC M, PEASE CK, GERBERICK GF, BASKETTER DA. Hapten-protein binding: From theory to practical application in the *in vitro* prediction of skin sensitization. *Contact Dermatitis* 2005; 53: 189–200.

61. MAISEY J, MILLER K. Assessment of the ability of mice fed on vitamin A supplemented diet to respond to a variety of potential contact sensitizers. *Contact Dermatitis* 1986; 15: 17–23.

62. MALKINSON FD. Studies on the percutaneous absorption of C14 labeled steroids by use of the gas-flow cell. *The Journal of Investigative Dermatology* 1958; 31: 19–28.

63. MALKOVSKÝ M, DORÉ C, HUNT R, PALMER L, CHANDLER P, MEDAWAR PB. Enhancement of specific antitumor immunity in mice fed a diet enriched in vitamin A acetate. *Proceedings of the National Academy of Sciences of the United States of America* 1983; 80: 6322–6326.

64. MALKOVSKÝ M, EDWARDS AJ, HUNT R, PALMER L, MEDAWAR PB. T-cell-mediated enhancement of host-versus-graft reactivity in mice fed a diet enriched in vitamin A acetate. *Nature* 1983; 302: 338–340.

65. MILLER K, MAISEY J, MALKOVSKÝ M. Enhancement of contact sensitization in mice fed a diet enriched in vitamin A acetate. *International Archives of Allergy and Applied Immunology* 1984; 75: 120–125.

66. KAMINSKY M, SZIVOS MM, BROWN KR. Application of the hill top patch test chamber to dermal irritancy testing in the albino rabbit. *Journal of Toxicology. Cutaneous and Ocular Toxicology* 1986; 5: 81–87.

67. FROSCH PJ, KLIGMAN AM. The Duhring chamber. An improved technique for epicutaneous testing of irritant and allergic reactions. *Contact Dermatitis* 1979; 5: 73–81.

68. HENDERSON CR, RILEY EC. Certain statistical considerations in patch testing. *The Journal of Investigative Dermatology* 1945; 6: 227–230.

69. CDRH. *Guidance for Industry and FDA Reviewers/Staff: Premarket Notification [510(k)] Submissions for Testing for Skin Sensitization to Chemicals in Natural Rubber Products*. Center for Devices and Radiological Health, U.S. Department of Health and Human Services, Washington, D.C., 1999.

70. SCHWARTZ L. The skin testing of new cosmetics. *Journal of the Society of Cosmetic Chemists* 1951; 2: 321–324.

71. SCHWARTZ L. Twenty two years' experience in the performance of 200,000 prophetic patch test. *The Southern Medical Journal* 1960; 53: 478–484.

72. BRUNNER MJ, SMILJANIC A. Procedure for evaluating skin-sensitizing power of new materials. *A. M. A. Archives of Dermatology and Syphilology* 1952; 66: 703–705.

73. TRAUB EF, TUSING TW, SPOOR HJ. Evaluation of dermal sensitivity; animal and human tests compared. *A. M. A. Archives of Dermatology and Syphilology* 1954; 69: 399–409.

74. SHELANSKI HA. Experience with and considerations of the human patch test method. *Journal of the Society of Cosmetic Chemists* 1951; 2: 324–331.

75. SHELANSKI HA, SHELANSKI MV. New technique of patch tests. *Drug and Cosmetic Industry* 1953; 73: 186.

76. GRIFFITH JF. Predictive and Diagnostic test for contact sensitization. *Toxicology and Applied Pharmacology* 1969; 3: 90–102.

77. GRIFFITH JF, BUEHLER E. Prediction of skin irritancy and sensitization potential by testing with animals and man. In: Drill VA, Lazar P, eds. *Cutaneous Toxicity*. Academic Press, New York, 1976; 155–173.

78. LACHAPELLE JM, MAIBACH HI. *Patch Testing and Prick Testing: A Practical Guide Official Publication of the ICDRG*. Springer-Verlag, New York, 2003.

79. KLIGMAN AM. The identification of contact allergens by human assay. I. A critique of standard methods. *The Journal of Investigative Dermatology* 1966; 47: 369–374.

80. KLIGMAN AM. Quantitative testing of chemical irritants. In: Steinberg TH, Newcomer VC, eds. *Evaluation of Therapeutic Agents and Cosmetics*. McGraw Hill, New York, 1964; 186–192.

81. KLIGMAN AM, EPSTEIN W. Some factors affecting contact sensitization in man. In: Shaffer JH, LoGrippo GA, Chase MW, eds. *Mechanisms of Hypersensitivity*. Little Brown, Boston, 1959; 713–722.

82. MARZULLI FN, MAIBACH HI. Antimicrobials: Experimental contact sensitisation in man. *Journal of the Society of Cosmetic Chemists* 1973; 24: 399–421.

83. GEORGE M, VAUGHAN JH. *In vitro* cell migration as a model for delayed hypersensitivity. *Proceedings of the Society for Experimental Biology and Medicine* 1962; 111: 514–521.

84. DAVID JR, REMOLD HG. Macrophage activation by lymphocyte mediators and studies on the activation of macrophage inhibitory factor (MIF) and its target cell. In: Nelson DS, ed. *Immunology of the Macrophage*. Academic Press, New York, 1976; 401–427.

85. ROCKLIN RE, MACDERMOTT RP, CHESS L, SCHLOSSMAN SF, DAVID JR. Studies on mediator production by highly purified human T and B lymphocytes. *The Journal of Experimental Medicine* 1974; 140: 1303–1316.

86. MOOREHEAD JW, MURPHY JW, HARVEY RP, HAYES RL, FETTERHOFF TJ. Soluble factors in tolerance and contact sensitivity to 2,4-dinitrofluorobenzene in mice, IV. Characterization of migration inhibition factor-producing lymphocytes and genetic requirements for activation. *European Journal of Immunology* 1982; 12: 431–436.

87. PEARMAIN GE, LYCETTE RR, FITZGERALD PH. Tuberculin-induced mitosis in peripheral blood lymphocytes. *Lancet* 1963; 1: 637–638.

88. ASPEGREN N, RORSMAN H. Short-term culture of leucocytes in nickel hypersensitivity. *Acta Dermato-Venereologica* 1962; 42: 412–417.

89. PAPPAS A, ORFANOS CE, BERTRAM R. Non-specific lymphocyte transformation *in vitro* by nickel acetate. A possible source of errors in lymphocyte transformation test (LLT). *The Journal of Investigative Dermatology* 1970; 55: 198–200.

90. EKWALL B. Screening of toxic compounds in mammalian cell cultures. *Annals of the New York Academy of Sciences* 1983; 407: 64–77.

91. MACLEOD TM, HUTCHINSON F, RAFFLE EJ. The uptake of labelled thymidine by leucocytes of nickel sensitive patients. *The British Journal of Dermatology* 1970; 82: 487–492.

92. GECZY AF, BAUMGARTEN A. Lymphocyte transformation in contact sensitivity. *Immunology* 1970; 19: 189–203.

93. MILLER AE JR, LEVIS WR. Studies on the contact sensitization of man with simple chemicals. I. Specific lymphocyte transformation in response to dinitrochlorobenzene sensitization. *The Journal of Investigative Dermatology* 1973; 61: 261–269.

94. DELESCLUSE J, TURK JL. Lymphocyte cytotoxicity: A possible in-vitro test for contact dermatitis. *Lancet* 1970; 11: 75–77.

95. BLOOMBERG BME, BRUYNZEEL DP, SCHEPER RJ. Advances in mechanisms of allergic contact dermatitis *in vitro* and *in vivo* research. In: Marzulli FN, Maibach HI, eds. *Dermatotoxicity*, 4th ed. Hemisphere, New York, 1991; 255–362.

96. GERBERICK GF, VASSALLO JD, BAILEY RE, CHANEY JG, MORRALL SW, LEPOITTEVIN JP. Development of a peptide reactivity assay for screening contact allergens. *Toxicological Sciences* 2004; 81: 332–343.

97. CHEW AL, MAIBACH HI. *Irritant Dermatitis*. Springer-Verlag, New York, 2006.

98. PROTTEY C. The molecular basis of skin irritation. In: Breuer MM, ed. *Cosmetics*, Vol. 1. Academic Press, London, 1978; 275–349.

99. PAGE AR, GOOD RA. A clinical and experimental study of the function of neutrophils in the inflammatory response. *The American Journal of Pathology* 1958; 34: 645–669.

100. PATRICK E, BURKHALTER A, MAIBACH HI. Recent investigations of mechanisms of chemically induced skin irritation in laboratory mice. *The Journal of Investigative Dermatology* 1987; 88: 24s–31s.

101. PATRICK E, MAIBACH HI. Comparison of the time course, dose response and mediators of chemically induced skin irritation in three species. In: Frosch P, Lachapelle JM, Rycroft R, Scheper RJ, eds. *Current Topics in Contact Dermatitis*. Springer-Verlag, Berlin, 1989; 399–404.

102. LAMMINTAUSTA K, MAIBACH HI. Exogenous and endogenous factors in skin irritation. *International Journal of Dermatology* 1988; 27: 213–222.

103. MATHIAS CG, MAIBACH HI. Dermatotoxicology monographs I. Cutaneous irritation: Factors influencing the response to irritants. *Clinical Toxicology* 1978; 13: 333–346.

104. WILHELM KP, MAIBACH HI. Factors predisposing to cutaneous irritation. *Dermatologic Clinics* 1990; 8: 17–22.

105. WOODING WH, OPDYKE DL. A statistical approach to the evaluation of cutaneous responses to irritants. *Journal of the Society of Cosmetic Chemists* 1967; 16: 809–829.

106. OFFICE OF THE FEDERAL REGISTRAR, NAOR. *Code of Federal Regulations*, Title 16, Commercial Practices, Chapter II, Consumer product safety commission, C: Federal Hazardous substances act regulations, Hazardous substances & articles; administration and enforcement regulations. 1985: 1500.1–1500.272.

107. PATIL S, PATRICK E, MAIBACH HI. Animal, human and *in vitro* test methods for predicting skin irritation. In: Marzulli F, Maibach HI, eds. *Dermatotoxicology Methods: The Laboratory Worker's Vade Mecum*. Taylor & Francis, Washington, D.C., 1998; 89.

108. JUSTICE J, TRAVERS J, VINSON L. The correlation between animal tests and human tests in assessing product mildness. *Proceedings of the Scientific Section Toilet Goods Association* 1961; 35: 12.

109. FROSCH PJ, SCHULZE-DIRKS A, HOFFMANN M, AXTHELM I, KURTE A. Efficacy of skin barrier creams (I). The repetitive irritation test (RIT) in the guinea pig. *Contact Dermatitis* 1993; 28: 94–100.

110. FROSCH PJ, SCHULZE-DIRKS A, HOFFMANN M, AXTHELM I. Efficacy of skin barrier creams (II). Ineffectiveness of a popular "skin protector" against various irritants in the repetitive irritation test in the guinea pig. *Contact Dermatitis* 1993; 29: 74–77.

111. PHILLIPS L II, STEINBERG M, MAIBACH HI, AKERS WA. A comparison of rabbit and human skin response to certain irritants. *Toxicology and Applied Pharmacology* 1972; 21: 369–382.

112. WAHLBERG JE. Measurement of skin-fold thickness in the guinea pig. Assessment of edema-inducing capacity of cutting fluids, acids, alkalis, formalin and dimethyl sulfoxide. *Contact Dermatitis* 1993; 28: 141–145.

113. MARZULLI FN, MAIBACH HI. The rabbit as a model for evaluating skin irritants: A comparison of results obtained on animals and man using repeated skin exposures. *Food and Cosmetics Toxicology* 1975; 13: 533–540.

114. ANDERSON C, SUNDBERG K, GROTH O. Animal model for assessment of skin irritancy. *Contact Dermatitis* 1986; 15: 143–151.

115. OPDYKE D, BURNETT C. Practical problems in the evaluation of the safety of cosmetics. *Proceedings of the Scientific Section Toilet Goods Association* 1965; 44: 3.

116. CALANDRA J. Comments on the Guinea pig immersion test. *CFTA Cosmetic Journal* 1971; 3: 47.

117. OPDYKE D. The guinea pig immersion test—A 20 year appraisal. *CFTA Cosmetic Journal* 1971; 3: 46.

118. MACMILLAN F, RAM R. Elvers WA comparison of the skin irritation produced by cosmetic ingredients and formulations in the rabbit, guinea pig, beagle dog to that observed in the human. In: Maibach HI, ed. *Animal Models in Dermatology*. Churchill Livingstone, Edinburgh, UK, 1975; 12.

119. GUPTA BN, MATHUR AK, SRIVASTAVA AK, SINGH S, SINGH A, CHANDRA SV. Dermal exposure to detergents. *Veterinary and Human Toxicology* 1992; 34: 405–407.

120. UTTLEY M, VAN ABBE NJ. Primary irritation of the skin: Mouse ear test and human patch test procedures. *Journal of the Society of Cosmetic Chemists* 1973; 24: 217–227.

121. PATRICK E, MAIBACH HI. A novel predictive assay in mice. *Toxicologist* 1987; 7: 84.

122. INOUE H, ASAKA T, NAGATA N, KOSHIHARA Y. Mechanism of mustard oil-induced skin inflammation in mice. *European Journal of Pharmacology* 1997; 333: 231–240.

123. HUMPHREY DM. Measurement of cutaneous microvascular exudates using Evans blue. *Biotechnic & Histochemistry* 1993; 68: 342–349.

124. TRUSH MA, EGNER PA, KENSLER TW. Myeloperoxidase as a biomarker of skin irritation and inflammation. *Food and Chemical Toxicology* 1994; 32: 143–147.

125. KLIGMAN AM, WOODING WM. A method for the measurement and evaluation of irritants on human skin. *The Journal of Investigative Dermatology* 1967; 49: 78–94.

126. MCFADDEN JP, WAKELIN SH, BASKETTER DA. Acute irritation thresholds in subjects with type I–type VI skin. *Contact Dermatitis* 1998; 38: 147–149.

127. LANMAN B, ELVERS WB, HOWARD CS. The role of human patch testing in a product development program. In: Proceedings of the Joint Conference of Cosmetic Sciences. The Toilet Goods Association, Washington, D.C., 1968; 135–145.

128. BATTISTA C, RIEGER M. Some problems of predictive testing. *Journal of the Society of Cosmetic Chemists* 1971; 22: 349–359.

129. WIGGER-ALBERTI W, HINNEN U, ELSNER P. Predictive testing of metalworking fluids: A comparison of 2 cumulative human irritation models and correlation with epidemiological data. *Contact Dermatitis* 1997; 36: 14–20.

130. FROSCH PJ, KLIGMAN AM. The chamber-scarification test for testing the irritancy of topically applied substances. In: Drill VA, Lazar P, eds. *Cutaneous Toxicity*. Academic Press, New York, 1977; 150.

131. FROSCH PJ, KLIGMAN AM. The chamber-scarification test for irritancy. *Contact Dermatitis* 1976; 2: 314–324.

132. KOOYMAN D, SNYDERM F. The test for mildness of soaps. *A. M. A. Archives of Dermatology and Syphilology* 1942; 46: 846–855.

133. CLARYS P, MANOU I, BAREL AO. Influence of temperature on irritation in the hand/forearm immersion test. *Contact Dermatitis* 1997; 36: 240–243.

134. ALLENBY CF, BASKETTER DA, DICKENS A, BARNES EG, BROUGH HC. An arm immersion model of compromised skin (I). Influence on irritation reactions. *Contact Dermatitis* 1993; 28: 84–88.

135. ALLENBY CF, BASKETTER DA. An arm immersion model of compromised skin (II). Influence on minimal eliciting patch test concentrations of nickel. *Contact Dermatitis* 1993; 28: 129–133.

136. ANDERSEN PH, MAIBACH HI. Skin irritation in man: A comparative bioengineering study using improved reflectance spectroscopy. *Contact Dermatitis* 1995; 33: 315–322.

137. BORENFREUND E, BABICH H, MARTIN-ALGUACIL N. Comparison of two in-vitro cytotoxicity assays: The neutral red (NR) and tetrazolium (MTT) tests. *Toxicology In Vitro* 1988; 2: 1–6.

138. BORENFREUND E, PUERNER JA. Toxicity determined *in vitro* by morphological alterations and neutral red absorption. *Toxicology Letters* 1985; 24: 119–124.

139. KNOX P, UPHILL PF, FRY JR, BENFORD J, BALLS M. The FRAME multicentre project on *in vitro* cytotoxicology. *Food and Chemical Toxicology* 1986; 24: 457–463.

140. MOSMANN T. Rapid colorimetric assay for cellular growth and survival: Application to proliferation and cytotoxicity assays. *Journal of Immunological Methods* 1983; 65: 55–63.

141. PARCE JW, OWICKI JC, KERCSO KM, SIGAL GB, WADA HG, MUIR VC, BOUSSE LJ, ROSS KL, SIKIC BI, MCCONNELL HM. Detection of cell-affecting agents with a silicon biosensor. *Science* 1989; 246: 243–247.

142. MOL MA, van de RUIT AM, KLUIVERS AW. NAD+ levels and glucose uptake of cultured human epidermal cells exposed to sulfur mustard. *Toxicology and Applied Pharmacology* 1989; 98: 159–165.

143. BLAKE-HASKINS JC, SCALA D, RHEIN LD, ROBBINS CR. Predicting surfactant irritation from the swelling response of a collagen film. *Journal of the Society of Cosmetic Chemists* 1986; 37: 199–210.

144. GORDON VC. An *in vitro* dermal safety test (SKINTEX dermal irritation assay). *Drug and Cosmetic Industry* 1990; 32.

145. GORDON VC, KELLY CP, BERGMAN HC. Skintex™, an *in vitro* method for determining dermal irritation. Fifth International Congress of Toxicology, Brighton, England, July 1989.

146. GORDON VC, KELLY CD, BERGMAN HC. Evaluation of Skintex™: An *in vitro* method for determining dermal irritation. *Toxicologist* 1990; 10: 75.

147. GRIFFITH JF, WEAVER JE, WHITEHOUSE HS, POOLE RL, NEWMANN EA, NIXON GA. Safety evaluation of enzyme detergents. Oral and cutaneous toxicity, irritancy and skin sensitization studies. *Food and Cosmetics Toxicology* 1969; 7: 581–593.

148. BULICH AA, GREENE MW, ISENBERG DL. Reliability of the bacterial luminescence assay for determination of the toxicity of pure compounds and complex effluents. In: Branson DR, Dickson KL, eds. *Aquatic Toxicology and Hazard Assessment: 4th Conference*. American Society for Testing and Materials (ASTM), Washington, D.C., 1981; 338–347.

149. SOCIETY OF TOXICOLOGY POSITION PAPER. Comments on the LD$_{50}$ and acute eye and skin irritation tests. *Fundamental and Applied Toxicology* 1989; 134: 621–623.

150. FLEISCHMAJER R, CONTARD P, SCHWARTZ E, MACDONALD ED II, JACOBS L II, SAKAI LY. Elastin-associated microfibrils (10 nm) in a three-dimensional fibroblast culture. *The Journal of Investigative Dermatology* 1991; 97: 638–643.

151. TRIGLIA D, BRAA SS, DONNELLY T, KIDD I, NAUGHTON GK. A three dimensional human dermal model substrate for *in vitro* toxicological studies. In: Goldberg AM, ed. *In Vitro Toxicology: Mechanisms and New Technology*. Mary Ann Liebert, New York, 1991; 351–362.

152. TRIGLIA D, BRAA SS, YONAN C, NAUGHTON GK. *In vitro* toxicity of various classes of test agents using the neutral red assay on a human three-dimensional physiologic skin model. *In Vitro Cellular & Developmental Biology* 1991; 27A: 239–244.

153. CANNON CL, NEAL PJ, KUBILUS J, KLAUSNER M, SWARTZENDRUBER DC, SQUIER CA, WERTZ PW. Lipid ultrastructure and barrier function characterization of a new *in vitro* epidermal model. *The Journal of Investigative Dermatology* 1994; 102: 600.

154. PERKINS MA, OSBORNE R, JOHNSON GR. Development of an *in vitro* method for skin corrosion testing. *Fundamental and Applied Toxicology* 1996; 31: 9–18.

155. FORBES PD, SAMBUCO CP, DEARLOVE GE, PARKER RM, KIORPES AL, WEDIG JH. Sample protocols for carcinogenesis and photocarcinogenesis. In: Marzulli FN, Maibach HI, eds. *Dermatotoxicology Methods: The Laboratory Worker's Vade Mecum*. Taylor and Francis, New York, 1997; 281–302.

156. FRANZ TJ. Percutaneous absorption on the relevance of *in vitro* data. *The Journal of Investigative Dermatology* 1975; 64: 190–195.

157. FRITSCH WC, STOUGHTON RB. The effect of temperature and humidity on the penetration of C14 acetylsalicylic acid in excised human skin. *The Journal of Investigative Dermatology* 1963; 41: 307–311.

158. ICCVAM (INTERAGENCY COORDINATING COMMITTEE ON THE VALIDATION OF ALTERNATIVE METHODS) AND NTP (NATIONAL TOXICOLOGY PROGRAM). *CorrositexR: An In Vitro Test Method for Assessing Dermal Corrosivity Potential of Chemicals*. National Institutes of Health, National Institute of Environmental Health Sciences, 1999; NIH Publication No. 99-4495. Available at: http://iccvam.niehs.nih.gov/docs/reports/corprrep.pdf.

159. BASKETTER DA, WHITTLE E, CHAMBERLAIN M. Identification of irritation and corrosion hazards to skin: An alternative strategy to animal testing. *Food and Chemical Toxicology* 1994; 32: 539–542.

160. OLIVER GJA, PEMBERTON MA, RHODES C. An *in vitro* skin corrosivity test—modifications and validation. *Food and Chemical Toxicology* 1986; 24: 507–512.

161. OLIVER GJA, PEMBERTON MA, RHODES C. The identification of corrosive agents for human skin *in vitro*. *Food and Chemical Toxicology* 1986; 24: 513–515.

162. WALKER AP, BASKETTER DA, BAVEREL M, DIEMBECK W, MATTHIES W, MOUGIN D, PAYE M, RÖTHLISBERGER R, DUPUIS J. Test guidelines for assessment of skin compatibility of cosmetic finished products in man. Task Force of COLIPA. *Food and Chemical Toxicology* 1996; 34: 651–660.

163. WHITTLE E, BASKETTER DA. The in-vitro skin corrosivity test: Development of a method using human skin. *Toxicology In Vitro* 1993; 7: 265–268.

Chapter 17

New Product Development for Transdermal Drug Delivery: Understanding the Market Opportunity

Hugh Alsop

INTRODUCTION

This chapter examines the new product development process and what factors are important in identifying a market opportunity and what needs to be considered when designing a product to capitalize on that opportunity. The focus of this chapter will be on drug delivery technologies for known molecules as opposed to new chemical entity (NCE) developments, and in particular will examine transdermal drug delivery technologies and their development path to market using a few examples.

TECHNOLOGY: PUSH OR PULL?

The global pharmaceutical industry of today faces many challenges: global pressure on health-care budgets and drug spending, rapidly expiring patent life of the major blockbuster drugs, and a declining output from innovative pharmaceutical research and development, which is constantly increasing in cost, complexity, and risk. Pharmaceutical companies are under pressure to maintain revenue growth and profitability, while producing products with real patient benefits and addressing the needs of health-care systems under increasing financial strain. Herein lies the opportunity for the drug delivery industry.

The premise of a drug delivery technology is to provide a way of delivering a therapeutic compound to the site of action where it can carry out its intended

Transdermal and Topical Drug Delivery: Principles and Practice, First Edition. Edited by Heather A.E. Benson, Adam C. Watkinson.
© 2012 John Wiley & Sons, Inc. Published 2012 by John Wiley & Sons, Inc.

purpose. Options include oral, buccal, intranasal, intravenous (IV), intramuscular, or transdermal delivery. The objective is to achieve either a particular blood concentration of the therapeutic compound or targeted delivery at a particular organ. Optimally delivering existing molecules to improve patient treatment is the fundamental premise of the drug delivery industry. Drug delivery products are able to improve therapeutic outcomes, compliance, and reduce the overall cost of treatment, and thus have historically had and will continue to have a positive commercial impact within the pharmaceutical industry.

By far the biggest area of drug delivery is now applying innovative technologies to improve existing drugs. This involves the development of new or improved ways of delivering drugs in order to solve a problem relating to bioavailability, efficacy, pharmacokinetics, dose, compliance, or side effects. Companies working in this space aim to develop systems that will not only increase the therapeutic value of a drug, but also its commercial value by providing a means of patent extension, point of differentiation, accelerated development, or new indications for an existing product. In many cases, NCE or innovative products are developed with suboptimal drug delivery. There may be a number of reasons for this, which could encompass a whole chapter in itself! For example, a number of new drugs reach approval with either a suboptimal dosing regimen (e.g., three times a day dosing), side effects caused by the mode of delivery (e.g., food effects or gastric problems), or an undesirable plasma profile (e.g., immediate release instead of sustained release [SR]). Most likely the originator has focused all their efforts on efficacy, safety, or toxicology, and therefore left optimizing the drug delivery lower down on their priorities list. However, this is where the opportunities present for drug delivery technologies, and transdermal technologies have been applied very effectively in the past to address and solve many of these issues.

According to a review by Bossart et al. in May 2010,* in the last 10 years, 213 drug delivery products were launched. In 2009 alone, 20 drug delivery products were approved, compared to nine biologicals.† The majority of the drug delivery approvals have employed the 505(b)(2) regulatory approval process with the U.S. Food and Drug Administration (FDA). The 505(b)(2) process has been in existence for 25 years and is intended for new applications of existing drugs that are of proven clinical efficacy and safety because they are already on the market. The process involves fewer and smaller clinical trials than an NCE, and thus the process is faster and cheaper than a new compound. It has been reported that in 2006, approximately 20% of new drugs were approved through the 505(b)(2) process. This increased to 43% in 2007 and more than half in 2008.

The advantages of transdermal drug delivery are that it provides a route of delivery that is noninvasive, provides steadier and sometimes more sustained pharmacokinetic delivery, that it allows for longer payout times, eliminates the first-pass

---

* Bossart J, Seto K, Kararli T. Delivery Report—Drug Delivery Products and Technologies—A Decade in Review: Approved Products 2000–2009. *Drug Delivery Technology*, May 2010, Vol. 10, No. 4.

† http://www.accessdata.fda.gov/scripts/cder/drugsatfda/index.cfm.

metabolism in the liver, and reduces side effects when compared to the more conventional methods of drug delivery. These benefits have been recognized widely and have led to the successful development and commercialization of a number of products such as Duragesic™, Vivelle-Dot®, and Androgel®.

However, transdermal drug delivery is not without its limitations. As discussed elsewhere in this book, this mode of delivery is generally more suited to small, lipophilic molecules that can cross the stratum corneum easily. It is also more suited to delivering a sustained, elevated pharmacokinetic profile, typical of most drugs used to treat chronic conditions requiring months if not years of treatment, such as hormone replacement therapy, chronic cancer pain, or Parkinson's disease. The skin is an effective barrier to many compounds, and these properties mean that no transdermal products have been developed to treat acute medical conditions that require rapid treatment with short duration of action.

So how does one identify the right opportunity or drug candidate suited for a particular transdermal drug delivery technology? Simplistically, the very first choice is between an NCE and an existing, approved compound.

History has shown that NCE development programs favor more traditional drug delivery modes such as the oral or injectable route. Indeed, over the last 5 years, approximately 100 new molecular entity New Drug Applications (NDAs)/Biologic License Applications (BLAs) have been approved by the FDA. Of these approvals, only one has been for a product employing a transdermal drug delivery system (Neupro™, by Schwarz Pharma, 2007). This product was developed by Schwarz but employs technology developed by a third party, LTS Lohmann Therapie-Systeme AG, who are also the manufacturers of the product. There are other examples of collaborations between "Big Pharma" and transdermal companies, but usually very little is disclosed about these collaborations and certainly none of these have resulted in approved products or even late-stage clinical development.

Transdermal drug delivery programs have therefore traditionally focused on existing molecules, either soon to be, or already off, patent. Their aim is to provide a means of developing an improved and differentiated product that has a shorter and lower cost development program due to its exploitation of a known molecule. So how does one identify the opportunity within these parameters? Does one go searching for a drug best suited to the technical properties of the technology? Or does one search for the unmet need and the real commercial opportunity? Theory says the unmet need should drive the search for the technology—however, in practice the technology platform often already exists, and companies go in search of suitable applications for this technology.

The particular application of the technology has to be determined through a thorough and objective evaluation. Four fundamental questions need to be explored:

1. What advantage over the current treatments does the technology represent?
2. Is the advantage incremental or revolutionary?
3. Is the advantage easily secured and protected through solid intellectual property (IP)?

4. Are the advantages easily identifiable to the key decision makers (physicians, specialists, pharmacists)?

Companies are best to avoid selecting a molecule solely because it is technically the best fit with the technology. Many drug delivery companies have often spent countless hours and dollars researching and developing their technology and the temptation is very strong to pursue a particular opportunity because it works exceptionally well with their technology. They will try to make the commercial justification fit, rather than objectively explore the opportunity and determine whether they are addressing a real problem for which no solution exists, or that for which the available solutions are suboptimal in some way.

It might then be obvious that the fundamental premise of a drug delivery program is that it must provide a better/faster/safer/cheaper way of delivering the drug. The identification and communication of the benefits that any transdermal drug delivery technology provides over the current treatment forms is the most critical element of the entire program. This must be clearly understood before significant funds are committed to a project. Confidence that the solution is required and consumers will pay for the product is essential. Will the key decision makers recognize the value of the product? Will the physicians/doctors/specialists understand the benefits of the new delivery method and therefore prescribe the product? Will patients and patient groups endorse the product?

Early on in the development program, it may be sufficient to have qualitative answers to these questions, based on feedback from key opinion leaders, general company understanding, or experience. A business case for the project should be established, which should include a target product profile and development plan for the opportunity. These documents should detail the key attributes of the product, the targeted indication, intended pharmacokinetic profile, proposed delivery form, differences to the innovator product, regulatory strategy, clinical development strategy, manufacturing strategy, IP strategy, estimates of manufacturing cost and selling price, and finally an estimate of the overall development cost through to registration. Balancing the development plan and cost should be a thorough examination of the market potential for the product, by analyzing the therapeutic category growth rates, competitor products, and market share trends.

However, as development progresses through the various clinical phases and the investment increases significantly, there will come a time that further, external validation of the fundamental benefits of the product is required. When significant investment is committed, it is no longer appropriate to rely on a broad, qualitative, experience-based assessment of the opportunity. Targeted qualitative and quantitative market research of both physicians and patients in the target market will be required. This will provide alignment between the opportunity and the solution, essential validation of the idea so that investment can proceed, and provide a rigor to the investment proposition. This process will also provide feedback on the solution to the development team, and therefore an opportunity to refine, reshape, and optimize the solution to better meet the customer's needs. The collation of this information is also very important for potential investors of the company, as it provides them with an objective, external validation of the opportunity and thus a level of confidence in their investment in the company.

Incremental versus Revolutionary Change?

A drug delivery product can lie anywhere on a spectrum from an incremental advance through to a revolutionary change. Historically, transdermal products have been incremental improvements on existing products, providing either a different dosing regimen or an improved safety profile. There have, however, been cases with other drug delivery technologies where the product development can be considered a revolutionary change. For example, the combination of a stimulant/appetite suppressant (phentermine) with an anticonvulsant (topiramate) that has weight loss properties to form the product Qnexa™, developed by Vivus. This is an example of taking two well-known compounds using a patented oral drug delivery technology and developing them for treatment of obesity, a condition for which there are no currently indicated pharmaceutical products. This is a high-risk, long-term revolutionary example utilizing a drug delivery technology.

An example of a low-risk, incremental improvement from the transdermal field is of the methylphenidate patch Daytrana®. The compound was better known for many years (since its introduction in the 1960s) by the trade name of Ritalin. More recently, it has been improved with an oral SR version approved in 1982 and then with a long-acting version in 2002. In 2006, the first transdermal methylphenidate product was approved in Daytrana. This product can be considered an incremental development in that it provides an alternate delivery method to oral, and provides a more sustained delivery profile of the drug over the day. The indication is the same, the patient population is the same, and the product doesn't really solve any real problem—it simply provides an alternative to the current dosage forms on the market.

Identifying Market Opportunity and Designing a Product to Fit

Market opportunities can present in many forms, and the identification of these opportunities should underpin and justify a drug development program. A problem must first exist for which a solution can be found. Without a real problem existing, any additional product offering provides the consumer just another choice with no discernible benefit. How would one market a "me-too" product? Price? Service? Quality? Brand? A combination of these attributes may be successful, but to be sure of success a product needs a unique selling proposition. In the drug delivery world, this proposition involves an improvement over an existing therapy in some way or providing a solution to a problem that exists with an existing drug.

An example of this is probably best explained by examining the development of the transdermal patch product Sancuso™. The selective 5-HT₃ receptor antagonist granisetron was developed as an antiemetic to treat nausea and vomiting following chemotherapy, and was first approved in the mid-1990s under the brand Kytril™. It is now a generic and available in either oral or injectable dosage forms. However, with these delivery modes originally developed for the product, a number of issues emerged after being on the market for some time. Chemotherapy is usually delivered through IV infusion, conducted either in a hospital bed or day procedure clinic. In many cases, it is administered over consecutive days and an antiemetic will be administered (either through oral or injectable dosing) in conjunction with the anticancer agents to control the inevitable emesis that will occur. However, with oral dosing, when a patient is being violently sick, the effective delivery of the antiemetic is compromised and thus a significant amount of the dose may not actually be absorbed.

Thus, the problem is immediately obvious: with oral dosing, how does one maintain adequate systemic availability of the antiemetic medication, when a patient is constantly being sick? With oral delivery being compromised by the fact the patient is constantly vomiting, a doctor may choose additional injections of the antiemetic. However these can be inconvenient, especially if a patient goes home between treatment regimens, and there is of course the aversion of many patients to yet more injections. Therefore, there had to be a more effective way of maintaining systemic levels of the antiemetic to prevent nausea and vomiting during the chemotherapy administration regimen.

This problem was identified by employees at ProStrakan, a Scottish pharmaceutical company, in about 2002. They reasoned that if a 5-HT_3 receptor antagonist was delivered through the skin over a period of time, they could maintain a therapeutic level in the blood that wouldn't be affected by how many times a person was sick. They examined the physicochemical properties of the 5-HT_3 receptor antagonists available at the time and concluded that granisetron may make a reasonable transdermal candidate. This led to ProStrakan initiating a pharmaceutical development program that eventually became Sancuso. Approved by the FDA in 2008, Sancuso is indicated for the prevention of nausea and vomiting in patients receiving moderately and/or highly emetogenic chemotherapy for up to 5 consecutive days. This is a classic example of how transdermal drug delivery technology has been employed to solve a problem with an existing drug, resulting in a new product with a patented, highly differentiated and unique selling proposition. The benefits to the patient are clear and thus a better treatment outcome results.

The Importance of Getting It Right

The importance of properly identifying the problem and then being confident your solution will be adopted by customers is critical. Ensuring the final product that is developed solves the problem in a way that is actually desired by the customer is even more important. The pharmaceutical development landscape is littered with failures, of which there are numerous drug delivery examples, transdermal included. However, perhaps the best example of getting this process wrong is exemplified by an example that it is not from the transdermal field. The product is the inhaled insulin product Exubera™, invented by Nektar, and approved by the FDA in January 2006 and then launched by Pfizer. While not a transdermal technology, it was a drug delivery technology applied to an existing molecule intended to provide a differentiated product, and so is very useful to examine how such a costly failure can occur and the resulting consequences, even when the marketing company is the largest pharmaceutical corporation in the world.

Forecasted to be a $2-billion blockbuster product for the drug giant, Exubera achieved only $9 million in sales in the first 9 months and was withdrawn from the market after barely 18 months following its approval. The original premise behind Exubera was that inhaled insulin would be an attractive alternative to patients who disliked injections. In theory, this made a lot of sense, as daily injections are supposed to be painful and inconvenient.

However, the solution that was developed was never accepted due to a number of practical drawbacks that Pfizer failed to consider, recognize, or address during the development of the product. First, the product was cumbersome and not easily used in public. The dosage was difficult to adjust, almost impossible to correlate with their existing injectable dose, and patients had to endure additional lung function tests while using the medication. It was never shown to be more effective than injectable insulin, and was at least 30% more expensive; thus, most managed care companies slotted the product into their most expensive drug tiers. It also didn't help that the modern insulin pens have advanced so much that they are far more convenient and less painful than they have historically been.

So while the original idea behind the product was sound, what was eventually developed and approved was so unpopular it died a very quick and expensive death. In the end, patients actually preferred the injections! Pfizer incurred a staggering $2.8-billion charge against the product—an enormous penalty for misreading the market so badly, even though the original idea was sound.

LINE EXTENSION FOR "BIG PHARMA"

As discussed elsewhere in this book, there are a number of companies working on a variety of transdermal drug delivery technologies. They range from passive drug delivery methods such as topical gels, creams, and patches to active methods such as electroporation and microneedles. The business model for many of these companies is very similar: develop products utilizing their own technology and advance them through the clinic as far as their financial resources allow, and then partner them for further development and/or sales and marketing. A few brave companies take on the challenge of selling the product they developed, but as a general statement products will be licensed to marketing partners for commercialization.

There are cases where drug delivery technologies are employed by "Big Pharma" to develop line extensions for their existing innovative medicines. Extended release (XR) and SR are common examples in the oral drug delivery world, and these have been employed successfully for many major products by "Big Pharma" companies to extend the life of some of their key franchises. In the transdermal world, Exelon™

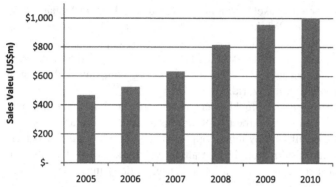

Figure 17.1   Exelon global sales, 2005–2010. Source: Novartis Annual Reports 2005, 2006, 2007, 2008, 2009 and 2010, www.sec.gov.

(rivastigmine) by Novartis is perhaps the most successful example of a transdermal technology being employed to extend the commercial life of a "Big Pharma" product. Exelon is indicated for the treatment of the symptoms of Alzheimer's disease, and was first launched by Novartis in June 2000 as a twice-daily capsule. The year 2008 saw the launch of generics from four different companies. In July 2007, the FDA approved a once-daily transdermal patch version of the product and this has proven popular with people with Alzheimer's disease and their caregivers due to the increased convenience of administration and its improved tolerability compared to oral rivastigmine. Transdermal administration reduces the incidence of gastrointestinal side effects, such as nausea and vomiting, by two-thirds. This clear differentiation from other marketed Alzheimer's disease drugs has allowed the patch to capture significant market share, and as can be seen in Figure 17.1, Exelon reached sales of US $1 billion in 2010, of which Novartis state the majority of sales are now coming from the patch.

Protection through Solid IP

Clearly a fundamental tenet of any drug delivery program is the strength of the IP protecting a product. Having sufficient protection from both an infringement and invalidity perspective underpins the commercial potential of any program. The Hatch–Waxman Act of 1984 (or more correctly, the amendment the Federal Food, Drug, and Cosmetic Act, Section 505(j) 21 U.S.C. 355(j)) describes the processes by which a generic manufacturer can file an Abbreviated New Drug Application (ANDA). Section 505(j)(2)(A)(vii)(IV), the so-called Paragraph IV, allows 180-day exclusivity to companies that are the "first to file" an ANDA against holders of patents for branded counterparts. Understanding how your product is protected from

* Datamonitor.

a Paragraph IV filing is critical, as the threshold for launching such challenges by the generic companies is getting lower and lower.

The transdermal world has seen two very public examples of such filings with both of the testosterone products Testim® and Androgel being hit with first-to-file challenges. Interestingly, both of these have patent challenges that have been closely followed by citizen's petitions to the FDA. An individual or a company can petition the FDA to "issue, amend, or revoke a regulation or order or take or refrain from taking any other form of administrative action."* It is certainly worth examining one of these cases to gain a more in-depth understanding of the processes involved from a specific example.

Testim was first approved in the United States on October 31, 2002. On October 24, 2008, Auxilium Pharmaceuticals, Inc. and CPEX Pharmaceuticals, Inc. announced that they received a notice from Upsher-Smith Laboratories, Inc. advising of the filing by Upsher-Smith of an ANDA containing a Paragraph IV certification against Testim. This Paragraph IV certification notice referred to CPEX's U.S. Patent No. 7,320,968 ("the '968 Patent"), which covers Testim. The Paragraph IV certification notice also stated that Upsher-Smith Laboratories, Inc. did not believe that the product for which it was seeking approval infringed the '968 Patent. The '968 Patent was listed in the Orange Book and will expire in January 2025.

On December 4, 2008, Auxilium and CPEX filed a lawsuit against Upsher-Smith Laboratories, Inc. for infringement of CPEX's U.S. Patent No. 7,320,968 ("the '968 Patent"), which covers Testim. The companies filed this lawsuit under the Hatch–Waxman Act in response to the notice from Upsher-Smith of its filing of an ANDA with the FDA containing a Paragraph IV certification. The Paragraph IV certification notice states that Upsher-Smith does not believe that the testosterone gel product for which it is seeking approval infringes the '968 Patent and that it would seek to market its product before the expiration of the '968 Patent.

Under the Hatch–Waxman Act, final FDA approval of Upsher-Smith's proposed product will be stayed until the earlier of 30 months or resolution of the patent infringement lawsuit. Should Upsher-Smith receive a tentative approval of its product from the FDA, it cannot lawfully launch its version of Testim in the United States before the earlier of the expiration of the currently pending 30-month stay or a district court decision in its favor. Upsher-Smith will also not be able to lawfully launch a version of Testim in the United States without the necessary final approval from the FDA. At the time of writing, this court case is ongoing and at this time the author is obviously unable to speculate on the outcome.

An additional defensive strategy against the Upsher-Smith product was adopted by Auxilium. On February 27, 2009, Auxilium Pharmaceuticals, Inc. submitted a citizen's petition to the FDA to request the Commissioner of Food and Drugs to take the actions set forth below with respect to the ANDA filed by Upsher-Smith Laboratories, Inc., ANDA No. 79-178, for testosterone transdermal gel 1%, citing

---

* Code of Federal Regulations, TITLE 21 (FOOD AND DRUGS), CHAPTER I, SUBCHAPTER A—GENERAL, PART 10—ADMINISTRATIVE PRACTICES AND PROCEDURES, Subpart B, Sec. 10.30 Citizen Petition.

Auxilium's product Testim as the reference listed drug (RLD). This citizen's petition is based on Upsher-Smith Laboratories Patent Certification Notice Letter.

The citizen's petition requested that the FDA require Upsher-Smith to demonstrate that the different inactive ingredients and formulation of the proposed product do not compromise its safety or efficacy by performing the following studies:

1. Transfer and hand-washing studies showing the proposed product does not have a greater potential for testosterone transfer than Testim despite its different formulation.

2. Showering studies showing that testosterone levels remain in the normal range and as high as they would be with Testim after showering or washing.

3. Studies showing the proposed product's different formulation does not result in increased risks, including skin irritation and sensitization studies.

4. Pharmacokinetic studies showing that the proposed product's different formulation does not affect bioavailability and bioequivalence.

Auxilium believed that these studies are required to ensure that the use of the proposed product is safe and effective. The FDA replied to Auxilium's petition on August 26, 2009. The key statement from the response document is as follows:

The practical effect of this determination is that any application for a testosterone gel product that has different penetration enhancers than the reference listed drug cannot be submitted as an ANDA and, instead, will have to be submitted as a NDA under section 505(b) of the Act.

The implications of this are important both for Auxilium and also for other developers of transdermal products. Upsher-Smith may be forced to refile the submission as an NDA under the 505(b)(2) rule and not as an ANDA. As an NDA, they will not be able to claim generic status against Testim and thus must generate prescriptions for their product by marketing it themselves. Additionally, they will have no patent protection themselves and therefore will be immediately open for people to file ANDAs against their product. Being forced to refile as an NDA means investment in money and time to generate the data the FDA require. The majority of this cost would be in a pivotal Phase III clinical trial. Upsher-Smith may not have the time or appetite for this investment, especially given the product will have no patent protection if it gains approval.

For developers of generic transdermal gel or cream products, this means the bar has been lifted significantly higher than the standard bioequivalence studies required, providing a further barrier for genericization of these products.

CONCLUSION

Drug delivery has historically delivered and promises to continue to deliver value-added products with a real ability to improve patient outcomes. Unfortunately, there is no exact formula for determining what will add value and how to improve patient outcomes. Whether the product represents a radical innovation or an incremental change, the attributes and benefits of the product must be clearly understood, accepted by both patients and prescribers, and be able to be strongly protected from the inevitable generic competition. Providing external validation of the benefits of a new product as early as possible in the development program will decrease the long-term risk of the project and increase the commercial viability.

Chapter 18

Transdermal and Topical Drug Delivery Today

Adam C. Watkinson

INTRODUCTION

This chapter examines the recent evolution of transdermal and topical drug delivery in man from a historical and commercial perspective. The focus is on the U.S. market, but where significant developments in technology or commercial success have occurred outside of the United States, these are included for completeness. Generally, products that have low commercial value and are also not of great technical interest are mentioned only briefly, if at all. Hence, this is not a comprehensive review of all commercially available topical and transdermal formulations (that would require more than this short chapter) but an examination of those that have contributed significantly to the evolution of the commercial landscape (by success or failure) associated with this mode of drug delivery.

TRANSDERMAL DRUG DELIVERY

Passive Transdermal Systemic Drug Delivery

At the time of writing, it is a little over 30 years since the launch of the first transdermal patch for passive systemic drug delivery in man. In the subsequent years, there have been approximately 20 drugs or drug combinations marketed in the United States and elsewhere as occlusive transdermal products for systemic delivery. The most significant of these products are listed in Table 18.1. Table 18.2 contains the pharmacokinetic and physicochemical properties of those drugs that have made it to the market in the United States. It is worth emphasizing that the values of the average molecular weight and LogP of these drugs is in line with those values commonly quoted as being ideal for transdermal delivery. Also of note is that the

Transdermal and Topical Drug Delivery: Principles and Practice, First Edition. Edited by Heather A.E. Benson, Adam C. Watkinson.
© 2012 John Wiley & Sons, Inc. Published 2012 by John Wiley & Sons, Inc.

Table 18.1   Passive Transdermal Drugs for Systemic Drug Delivery Launched in the United States and Europe

Drug	Indication	U.S. approval	Marketed in the EU
Scopolamine	Travel sickness	1979	Yes
Nitroglycerin	Angina	1982	Yes
Clonidine	Hypertension	1984	Yes
Estradiol	Female HRT	1986	Yes
Fentanyl	Chronic pain	1990	Yes
Testosterone	Hypogonadism	1995	Yes
Nicotine	Smoking cessation	1996	Yes
Estradiol and norethindrone acetate	Female HRT	1998	Yes
Ethinyl estradiol and norelgestromin	Female contraception	2001	Yes
Oxybutynin	Enuresis	2003	Yes
Methylphenidate	ADHD	2006	Yes
Selegiline	Depression	2006	Yes
Rivastigmine	Alzheimer's disease	2007	Yes
Rotigotine[a]	Parkinson's disease	2007	Yes
Granisetron	Chemotherapy-induced emesis	2008	–
Buprenorphine	Moderate to severe pain	2010	Yes

[a] Withdrawn from the United States in 2008.

systemic dose of all of these drugs is low and for many, very low indeed. These observations are worth emphasizing and clearly demonstrate the need for common sense and a practical attitude regarding what can be delivered through the skin from passive systems in man.

Of all these products, there is one that stands out as an obvious commercial success story. For many years Johnson & Johnson's (J&J) Duragesic™ fentanyl patch dominated the transdermal market and global sales peaked at in excess of $2 billion in 2004. By 2006, after patent expiration and the advent of generic competition, sales of Duragesic were still greater than $1.2 billion and by 2009 they were still approximately $900 million per annum. Despite the massive sales of Duragesic patches, it took some years after the expiration of the patents protecting the product for generic versions of these delivery systems to appear in the United States. This was in part due to J&J's vigorous protection of their market share and the submission of a citizen's petition to the U.S. Food and Drug Administration (FDA) aimed at blocking generic approvals. Despite these moves by J&J, Mylan Technologies gained approval for their fentanyl patch in January 2005, and Lavipharm™ followed with another in August 2006. Interestingly, in September 2005, Noven had a New Drug Application (NDA) for a generic fentanyl patch turned down by FDA on the

Table 18.2 Pharmacokinetic and Physicochemical Properties of Commercially Available Transdermally Delivered Drugs for Human Use

Drug	Relative molecular mass (Daltons)	Calculated LogP	Melting point (°C)	Maximum systemic daily dose (mg)
Ethinyl estradiol	296	4.5	141–142	0.02
Estradiol	272	4.1	173–179	0.1
Norelgestromin	327	4.4	112	0.15
Norethindrone acetate	341	4.0	161–162	0.25
Scopolamine	303	0.76	Liquid	0.3
Clonidine	230	1.4	130	0.3
Buprenorphine	468	3.4	209	1.7
Fentanyl	337	3.9	83–84	2.4
Granisetron	312	2.9		3.1
Oxybutynin	358	5.2	114	3.9
Rotigotine	316	5.0		6.0
Testosterone	288	3.5	155	10
Rivastigmine	250	2.1		9.5
Selegiline	187	3.0	Liquid	12
Nitroglycerin	227	2.3	Liquid	20
Nicotine	162	0.72	Liquid	21
Methylphenidate	233	2.6	Liquid	30
Mean	**296**	**3.2**	**–**	**3.1**

grounds of its high fentanyl content relative to Duragesic. However, there are now at least six generic fentanyl patches on the U.S. market (Mylan in 2005, Lavipharm in 2006, Actavis and Watson in 2007, Teva in 2008, and Noven in 2009). More recently, sales have declined slightly because of issues relating to product safety and further generic erosion, but to date, no other transdermal product has matched the commercial success of Duragesic.

Some of the reasons for the success of Duragesic hold valuable lessons for those attempting to emulate it with new approaches to transdermal drug delivery. The mantra of pharmaceutical companies often contains phraseology relating to the "meeting of unmet medical needs," and there is a strong case that Duragesic did this exceptionally well in an area of medicine (chronic pain) that has a lot of customers with the need met by the product. Therein probably resides the key to the future of transdermal drug delivery. There are certainly commercial returns to be made by incrementally improving currently available treatments, but the next "great leap forward" has to be based on an innovation that solves a problem that matters to a lot of people and that does so at a reasonable cost. The sales figures associated with transdermal fentanyl are unquestionably impressive and will ensure that the drug has a place in the pipeline of many drug delivery companies for years to come. Despite the dedication of much of the drug delivery world to reformulating a single opioid, there have been several other interesting and novel transdermal product launches over the last few years.

In relatively rapid succession, 2006 saw the approval of three new passive transdermal delivery systems. A rotigotine patch (Neupro™) for use in Parkinson's disease was launched in the EU by Schwarz Pharma (acquired by UCB in 2006) in early 2006 and subsequently approved by the FDA in May 2007 and launched in the United States in July of that year. Issues with crystallization of drug in the patches resulted in the product's withdrawal from the U.S. market in 2008. UCB, who currently market Neupro, initiated a cold chain (refrigerated supply chain) in Europe in 2008 that allowed existing patients to continue treatment with the product, and in June 2009 the European Medicines Agency (EMA) agreed to lift this supply restriction, making the product freely available in the EU again. However, despite suggesting to the FDA the implementation of a cold chain, UCB (who effectively bought Schwarz Pharma in 2006) was informed in April 2010 that reformulation of the product was required. This reformulation work is currently underway. Neupro is currently indicated in the EU for Parkinson's disease and restless leg syndrome and had netted nearly €59 million in 2010 by October.

The Emsam™ patch contains a monoamine oxidase inhibitor, selegiline, and is indicated for major depressive disorder. Emsam was approved by the FDA in February 2006 and launched in the US in 2007. Emsam represents the fruition of a joint venture, Somerset Pharmaceuticals, between Mylan Laboratories and Watson Pharmaceuticals. To date, however, Emsam sales in the United States have been disappointing and it is not yet registered in the EU.

After a great deal of work by Noven and Shire, April 2006 saw the FDA approval of Daytrana™, Noven's methylphenidate patch for ADHD (attention deficit hyperactivity disorder). This product was launched in the United States by Shire in June 2006 and attracted sales of $35 million in the first half of 2010. Interestingly, Noven recently (October 2010) reacquired the product from Shire and will sell it via their own sales force (Noven Therapeutics) in the United States.

Less recently, Oxytrol™ (oxybutynin for overactive bladder) was approved by the FDA in the first quarter (Q1) of 2003 and launched by Watson in the second quarter (Q2) of the same year. In its first 12 months of sales it realized about $30 million and has sold in the region of $30–40 million per annum since then. Exelon™, a rivastigmine trandermal patch, was approved in 2006 for mild to moderate dementia associated with Parkinson's disease, and in 2007 the rivastigmine transdermal patch became the first patch treatment for dementia (Alzheimer's disease).

Sancuso™ (developed and marketed by ProStrakan) was approved by the FDA in 2007 and launched in 2008. Sancuso delivers the 5-HT$_3$ antagonist granisetron for a 5-day period, over which it is used in the prevention of chemotherapy-induced nausea and vomiting. In 2009, U.S. sales of Sancuso were of the order of $11 million and it had registered higher sales levels into 2010 until a problem resulting from an FDA inspection at the product's manufacturer was revealed in August 2010. This has led to a supply shortage with more product not being available until 2011. The most recent U.S. proprietary transdermal approval was for Butrans (buprenorphine) from Purdue, which was approved by the FDA in June 2010 (note that a 7-day buprenorphine patch, Transtec, has been available in the EU since 2001). At the time of writing, the FDA has just accepted for review an NDA for a 7-day donepezil patch for the treatment of mild, moderate, and severe Alzheimer's disease. It is probably too early to pass judgment on how these more recent products will ultimately fare in the marketplace but it is unlikely that their sales will match those of fentanyl.

Older transdermal products that still yield significant sales exist in the form of a contraceptive patch (Ortho Evra™, launched in 2001), hormone replacement therapy (HRT) patches and gels (launched from the mid-1980s onwards), nicotine patches (launched from the early 1990s onwards), a clonidine patch (Catapres™, approved in the United States in 1990), and the testosterone gels discussed above (launched from 2000 onwards). Ortho Evra sales dipped (from a peak of over $400 million) because the greater dose of ethinyl estradiol delivered by the patch (than by oral contraceptives) was linked to an increased risk of thromboembolism. Despite these safety concerns and the inevitable associated litigation, the patch remains on the market in the United States and has sales of more than $200 million per annum.

HRT patch sales slowed for the same reason that all HRT therapies did after the first arm of the Women's Health Initiative (WHI) study was published in 2002.[1] This publication suggested that long-term combined (estrogen and progestogen) HRT increased the risk of breast cancer and thromboembolism. Two years later, the second arm of the WHI study suggested no increased risk for breast cancer for estrogen-only HRT[2] when commenced before the age of 60. It is now widely accepted that the data from these and more recent trials support the safe and beneficial use of HRT in the majority of women, who commence treatment near the menopause and before the age of 60. Furthermore, any risk of thromboembolism is small around the menopause and is not elevated with use of the transdermal route.[3,4] These more recent interpretations and understandings of the data seem set to reverse this trend and the decline in sales has now halted.

As well as the proprietary products outlined above, there are several generic versions of many of them available. These include patches containing fentanyl, estradiol, nicotine, clonidine, and nitroglycerin.

In addition to these occlusive systems, there are several nonocclusive passive transdermal formulations available that deliver drugs systemically. Despite the fact that there are at least nine individual formulations available that fall into this category, there are only four drugs delivered in this way. These are nitroglycerin (approved in 1988 and sold by Fougara), estradiol (Estrasorb™, approved in 2003; Estrogel™ in 2004; Elestrin™ in 2006; Divigel™ in 2007; and Evamist™ in 2007), testosterone (AndroGel™, approved in 2000; and Testim™, in 2002), and oxybutynin (Gelnique™, approved in 2009). From a sales perspective, the most notable of these nonocclusive products are those containing testosterone used for the treatment of hypogonadism in men. This market is currently (2010) worth in excess of $1 billion and, as with many pharmaceutical products, is predominantly (85%) in the United States. Although a proportion of testosterone product sales are injectables, oral, and implants, approximately 85% are transdermal, nonocclusive gels. Over the last 3 years, sales of such products (AndroGel in particular) have been experiencing between 15% and 20% growth year on year and, apart from the obvious exception of fentanyl, testosterone products represent one of the more lucrative areas of transdermal commercialization in recent years. An interesting addition to this market is likely to be Axiron™ (developed by Acrux and licensed to Eli Lilly in early 2010), a cutaneous solution that is applied into the axilla (armpit) with a no-touch applicator that was approved by the FDA in November 2010 and launched in the United States in April 2011.

Active Transdermal Systemic Drug Delivery

The Ionsys™ fentanyl iontophoretic device (J&J) was approved in the United States and Europe in 2006 and launched in Europe in early 2008. However, the product was suspended in Europe in November 2008 as a result of the corrosion of a component of the system in one batch of product. As this defect could potentially result in self-activation of the system, the risk of fentanyl overdose was deemed to outweigh the benefits. The EMEA thus recommended the suspension of the marketing authorization of Ionsys even though there have been no reports of serious adverse events associated with the malfunction of the device. The product is now currently unavailable in the United States also and listed by the FDA as discontinued. At the time of writing, the product is with Incline Therapeutics who have procured substantial ($43 million) Series A funding for the development of new patient safety features for the technology. Presumably these are to address the concerns of the EU and U.S. regulatory authorities outlined above.

In August 2011, NuPathe Inc. announced that it had received a Complete Response Letter (CRL) from the US FDA regarding their NDA for their sumatriptan iontophoresis patch (Zelrix) for migraine. The FDA acknowledged the efficacy of the patch but stated that some chemistry, manufacturing, and safety questions required further work. This means that NuPathe will not launch its migraine patch in the first half of 2012, as previously announced. Although this turn of events had a major impact on the company share price, NuPathe remain confident that they will achieve approval for the product.

TOPICAL DRUG DELIVERY

Passive Topical Local Drug Delivery

In contrast to the very few drugs (~20 worldwide) that are commercially available for systemic transdermal delivery, there are many that are applied to the skin and have a site of action either in or below the skin itself. A comprehensive review of these drugs and their various formulations is beyond the scope of this chapter but Table 18.3 contains a large number of examples simply to put the difference between systemic and local delivery into perspective. There are well in excess of 50 drugs delivered to and through the skin for local effect, more than twice the number deliv-

Table 18.3 Examples of Some Topical Drugs and Their Indications for Human Use

Drug	Indication/action	Drug	Indication/action
Aciclovir	Cold sores	Hydrocortisone	Pruritis, skin irritation, inflammatory dermatoses
Adapalene	Acne	Ibuprofen	Inflammation
Amorolfine	Onychomychoses	Isotretinoin	Acne
Azelaic acid	Acne	Ketoconazole	Antifungal
Benzalkonium chloride	Cuts, bites, grazes, and so on	Ketoprofen	Inflammation
Benzoyl benzoate	Scabies and pediculosis	Mometosome	Dermatoses
Benzyl peroxide	Acne	Methylprednisolone	Eczema, psoriasis
Benzydamine	Inflammation	Metronidazole	Rosacea
Betamethasone	Inflammatory dermatoses	Miconazole	Fungal infections
Bifonazole	Cutaneous infestations	Minoxidil	Hair loss
Bufexamac	Dermatitis, rashes	Mupirocin	Infected skin lesions
Camphor	Analgesic	Nicotinates	Rubecfacient/analgesic
Capsaicin	Arthritis pain, posthepatic neuralgia	Nystatin	Cutaneous candidiasis
Cetrimide	Skin cleanser	Permethrin	Scabies
Cicolopirox	Dermatitis	Phenoxyisopropanol	Pimples
Chlorhexidine	Infection	Piroxicam	Inflammation
Clindamycin	Acne	Triamcinolone	Inflammatory dermatoses
Clobetasone	Mild eczema, dermatitis	Tretinoin	Acne
Clotrimazole	Cutaneous infestations	Salicylic acid	Dermatitis keratolytic scalp psoriasis
Desonide	Dermatoses	Tazarotene	Acne, psoriasis
Dexpanthenol	Nappy rash	Terbinafine	Fungal infections
Dithranol	Psoriasis	Terpentine oil	Analgesic
Diclofenac	Inflammation	Tolnaftate	Topical fungal infections
Econazole	Fungal infections	Tretinoin	Acne
Erythromycin	Acne	Trilosan	Acne/pimples
Framycetin	Infection	Urea	Dry skin, eczema

ered systemically. This is likely to be the simple result of the required dose delivered through the skin usually being greater in systemic therapy than in local therapy. The dilution of delivered drug that occurs when it is placed into the systemic compartment and has a site of action distant from the site of application can be high, while a drug acting locally to its site of application on the skin will require a much lower degree of penetration to elicit its pharmacological effect. Furthermore, many topical drugs are targeted at skin diseases or used on broken skin where the barrier function is often hugely compromised, and therefore access of the drug to its site of action is relatively straightforward. Having said this, despite the apparent ease with which a topically applied drug may reach its target once it passes through the stratum corneum, such drugs, when applied to intact skin, are often very poorly bioavailable (many such formulations have bioavailabilities of <1%). This is a function of their nonocclusive nature, the excellent barrier properties of intact stratum corneum, and also the relatively poor understanding we have of how to optimize such formulations for efficient topical drug delivery. It is true that there are occlusive transdermal systems with poor bioavailability but the problem is greater for nonocclusive systems. Increasing bioavailability in the nonocclusive setting not only has the potential to reduce costs (via lower drug utilization) but also to reduce the risk of transfer of drug to individuals who may come into contact with the patient. A clear indication of the regulatory concern about such issues is the FDA response to the inadvertent transfer of testosterone from patients using gel products to women and children. All such products currently carry a black box warning in their labeling about restricting interactions with third parties to such times at which the product has been safely washed from the skin of the patient. Although these testosterone gels are used for systemic administration, it is quite feasible that such concerns be applied to local delivery if the nature of the active demands it. The utilization of lower drug loads in formulations also has positive environmental impacts, and this aspect of drug development is increasingly scrutinized by regulators worldwide.

A second product that has performed very well in the local topical delivery arena is Lidoderm. Lidoderm is a large patch that can be cut to appropriate sizes and delivers lidocaine locally for the relief of pain associated with postherpetic neuralgia. The product was approved in the United States in 1999 and is currently selling in excess of $750 million per annum for Endo Pharmaceuticals. This makes it one of the most successful topical/transdermal products of all time.

Active Topical Local Drug Delivery

The recent history of active drug delivery through the skin is, unfortunately, littered with products that made it to the market but, for various reasons, are no longer commercially available. An examination of some of these casualties of the marketplace is very pertinent if we are to learn lessons that may help future products to be more successful.

In 1995, the FDA approved an iontophoretic delivery system containing lidocaine and epinephrine for the local anesthesia of the skin. This product (from Iomed) is now listed as discontinued by FDA; exactly why is unclear. A second lidocaine and epinephrine iontophoretic device (Lidosite™ from Vyteris) was approved by FDA in May 2004 and launched in the United States in August 2007. However, poor market uptake of the device led to its withdrawal and the product is now listed as discontinued by FDA. Lidocaine seems to be the molecule of choice for those involved in the active topical drug delivery area. This is probably because it is a well-known, safe molecule that has reasonably simple clinical trial requirements for testing efficacy and safety. This is reflected in further attempts to market lidocaine devices for local anesthesia. In August 2004, FDA approved SonoPrep™ (from, at the time, Sontra), a device that enhanced the local delivery of lidocaine using ultrasound. Again, this product had poor market uptake and was eventually withdrawn in 2007. In August of the same year (2007) an intradermal lidocaine powder injector (Zingo™) was approved by the FDA and subsequently launched in the United States by Anesiva in June 2008. Less than 6 months later, in November 2008, the product was withdrawn from the market. The reasons appear to relate to limited market uptake and manufacturing challenges. The product was sold to another company in December of 2009 for $2.7 million and is still listed as discontinued by FDA (August 2011). There is certainly a clear pattern in these stories but thankfully, at the time of writing, there remains one active topical delivery device on the market. Synera™ (Zars Pharma) is a heat-activated topical lidocaine/tetracaine patch and was approved by the FDA in June 2005 and in the EU in April 2007. The product was launched in the United States in 2006 and in the EU in 2007 and, at the time of writing, is still available, although sales figures are not impressive. Zars Pharma was acquired by Nuvo Research Inc. in May 2011.

CONCLUSIONS

There will, no doubt, be further launches of passive transdermal products and most of these will sell reasonable numbers of units and return acceptable profits to their makers. One might even hope that some will follow the innovative approach used with rotigotine, a molecule selected with transdermal delivery in mind. The drug delivery problems associated with large molecules from the biotechnology sector are already prompting numerous potentially valuable solutions from within the transdermal sector. These solutions require more invasive delivery methods because of the physicochemical nature of the molecules involved, and these bring questions of their own relating to safety and therefore regulatory approval. Recent advances in microelectronics and miniaturization (nanotechnology) have the potential to allow the construction of portable powered devices at reasonable cost that may be used for controlling delivery in a bespoke way, possibly even to the point where feedback devices respond to biochemical changes in the body with appropriate delivery of drugs. Whatever technology is applied, it must be applied to the right problem at the right cost and in the right way for it to result in a product that will improve lives and meet those unmet needs that the pharmaceutical industry refers to almost incessantly. This is not a unique challenge in the industry, but it will require an intelligent and pragmatic blend of commercial and scientific knowledge and expertise to achieve.

REFERENCES

1. Writing Group for the Women's Health Initiative Investigators. Risks and benefits of estrogen plus progestin in healthy postmenopausal women: Principal results from the Women's Health Initiative Randomized Controlled Trial. *JAMA* 2002; 288(3): 321–333.
2. The Women's Health Initiative Steering Committee. Effects of conjugated equine estrogen in postmenopausal women with hysterectomy. *JAMA* 2004; 291(14): 1701–1712.
3. CANONICO M, OGER E, PLU-BUREAU G, CONARD J, MEYER G, LEVESQUE H, TRILLOT N, BARRELLIER MT, WAHL D, EMMERICH J, SCARABIN PY. Hormone therapy and venous thromboembolism among postmenopausal women: Impact of the route of estrogen administration and progestogens: The ESTHER study. *Circulation* 2007; 115(7): 840–845.
4. MACLENNAN AH. Evidence-based review of therapies at the menopause. *Int J Evid Based Healthcare* 2009; 7(2): 112–123.

Chapter 19

Current and Future Trends: Skin Diseases and Treatment

Simon G. Danby, Gordon W. Duff, and Michael J. Cork

INTRODUCTION

The skin serves as an important barrier that keeps moisture in the body and prevents the incursion of harmful exogenous agents, such as irritants and allergens, and resists the invasion of pathogens. A growing body of evidence suggests a primary role for the "skin barrier" in the pathogenesis of a broad range of inflammatory skin disorders, including contact dermatitis, ichthyosis, psoriasis, rosacea, and atopic dermatitis (AD).[1–3] Repeated barrier disruption, for instance, induces epidermal hyperplasia and inflammation.[4,5] Current medicine is based on the reactive treatment of these downstream consequences of skin barrier dysfunction, and includes the use of both anti-inflammatory and antiproliferative compounds (Fig. 19.1).[6–9] A greater understanding of the underlying skin barrier defect promises to first, identify susceptible individuals early on, and second, to deliver novel therapeutic options for targeted skin barrier repair with the potential to prevent the development of clinical disease.

This chapter focuses on the etiology of AD and current and future trends in its treatment. An appreciation of the role of the skin barrier in the development of AD (reviewed in Reference 2) is transforming the way in which the condition is treated. Current therapy involves treating clinical symptoms such as inflammation and pruritus, and managing provocation factors while artificially restoring barrier function in order to permit and encourage normal repair.[7] Future therapeutics being developed aim to actively repair the skin barrier defect and thereby avert the presentation of clinical symptoms. That early emollients with skin barrier repair properties improve the course of AD and are topical corticosteroid (TCS) sparing is a testament to this future promise.[10–12] AD is the first step in the atopic march, followed by food allergy, asthma, and allergic rhinitis.[13] Changing the way we treat a baby's skin from birth,

Transdermal and Topical Drug Delivery: Principles and Practice, First Edition. Edited by Heather A.E. Benson, Adam C. Watkinson.

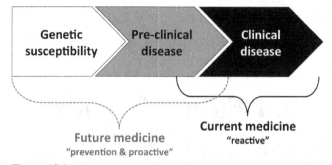

Figure 19.1   The future of medicine. There are three fundamental aspects/stages of disease: genetic susceptibility, pre-clinical disease, and clinical disease. Current medicine is mainly *reactive* and targets clinical disease. Future—*proactive* and *preventative*—medicine promises to delay or prevent the onset or development of clinical disease.

including wash products, topical oils, and emollients, may prevent some babies from developing AD and other conditions further along the atopic march.

THE SKIN BARRIER

Structure of the Skin Barrier

The "skin barrier" is a physical permeability barrier that prevents undue transepidermal water loss (TEWL) and protects the body from the external environment. The primary skin barrier is formed by the stratum corneum (SC), the uppermost layer of the epidermis. This layer is composed of terminally differentiated, anuclear keratinocytes referred to as corneocytes. Corneocytes have a flattened disc-like geometrical morphology, with a large surface area that increases twofold during maturation.[14] The SC is on average 20 corneocytes deep, spanning between 10 and 20 μm, depending on the body site (where the number of cell layers can range between 4 and 122).[15] The structure of the SC is often compared to a brick wall, where the bricks represent corneocytes.[16] Similar to motor, a complex mixture of lipids between the corneocytes, referred to as lipid lamellae, bonds the bricks together, creating a "weatherproof" barrier.

The plasma membrane of the corneocytes is fortified with insoluble proteins, including loricrin, involucrin, filaggrin, and small, proline-rich proteins.[17] The resulting water-impermeable "casing" is referred to as the cornified envelope (CE). Contained within the corneocytes is a range of humectants including lactic acid, sodium pyrrolidone carboxylic acid, urocanic acid, and urea, collectively known as the natural moisturizing factor (NMF).[18] The constituents of NMF are derived from the catabolism of the structural protein filaggrin during maturation of the corneocytes. NMF is essential for the retention of water within corneocytes and results in their optimal hydration and swelling, preventing the development of gaps between them.

Around the corneocytes, equimolar concentrations of cholesterol, phospholipids, and ceramides, arranged in multilamellar membrane sheets, make up the lipid lamellae.[19] The components of lipid lamellae are extruded into the extracellular space between the corneocytes from secretory lamellar bodies (LB).[20,21] In addition to preventing water loss, the lipid lamellae restricts the penetration of water-soluble materials between the corneocytes. Key ceramide species within the lamellar membranes interact with involucrin incorporated within the CE,[22–24] thereby binding the corneocytes within the lamellar mesh, to create a single coherent barrier.

Linking the corneocytes together are reinforced intercellular desmosomal junctions referred to as corneodesmosomes.[25] In the brick wall analogy, these can be visualized as iron rods running down through the bricks, providing additional strength to the wall. The incorporation of corneodesmosin marks the transition from desmosome to corneodesmosome.[26] Corneodesmosin is a 52-kDa protein, packaged in LB and secreted into the extracellular space at the transition between the nucleated layers of the epidermis and the SC.[27] LB also deliver a cocktail of proteases which progressively break down the corneodesmosomal junctions as the corneocytes mature. This results in the disassociation of mature corneocytes (or squames) in the uppermost layers of the SC. The process of corneocyte shedding, known as desquamation, counterbalances the generation of new keratinocytes in the basal layer so that the whole epidermis is continually renewed.[28]

The degradation of the corneodesmosomal junctions is largely attributed to the kallikrein-related peptidases (KLK), a family of serine proteases possessing either trypsin-like or chymotrypsin-like activity.[28] Eight trypsin-like KLK—KLK5 (previously *stratum corneum tryptic enzyme* [SCTE]), KLK6, KLK8, KLK10, KLK11, KLK13, and KLK14—and one chymotrypsin-like KLK—KLK7 (previously *stratum corneum chymotryptic enzyme*, SCCE)—have been specifically identified in the SC.[29] At least a further three, including KLK1, KLK3, and KLK9, have been found in total skin extracts. Other enzymes found in the SC and capable of degrading corneodesmosomal adhesion proteins include the cysteine proteases cathepsin L2 (*stratum corneum thiol protease*) and SC L-like enzyme,[30] and the aspartate protease cathepsin D.[31]

Under normal conditions the rate of desquamation is tightly controlled by a number of protease inhibitors delivered by LB ahead of the degradatory proteases, including Lymphoepithelial kazal-type 5 serine protease inhibitor (LEKTI).[32] LEKTI is composed of 15 potential serine proteinase inhibitory domains, at least four of which have confirmed activity against members of the kallikrein family, including KLK5, KLK6, KLK7, and KLK14. LEKTI, encoded by the *SPINK5* gene, is a member of a group of serine protease inhibitors of the Kazal type (SPINK), of which a second member has recently been identified in human skin.[31] Encoded by the *SPINK9* gene, LEKTI-2 was found to inhibit KLK5, but not KLK7 and KLK14 proteolytic activity. Human epidermis also expresses serine leukoprotease inhibitor (SLPI), elafin (*skin-derived antileukoprotease*), and alpha-2 macroglobulin-like 1 (α2ML1), which inhibit KLK7, and the cystatin protease inhibitors A, C, and M/E, which are specific for cysteine proteases.[31,33]

The primary barrier to the penetration of irritants and allergens through the skin is located in the lower part of the SC. This is the point at which the integrity of the barrier is greatest, where cornification (transition of keratinocytes into corneocytes) culminates prior to the natural breakdown of the SC. The thickness of the SC (the number of corneocyte layers and level of hydration)[34-37] and the maturity of the surface corneocytes (corneocyte surface area)[38] are important structural parameters that determine the effectiveness of this barrier at preventing the entry of irritants and allergens. These parameters vary at different sites of the body.[38-43] Sites with the thinnest SC and smallest (immature) corneocytes can be described as having low *skin barrier reserve*, and are at greatest risk to external insults, including irritant and allergen penetration[44-47] (Fig. 19.2).

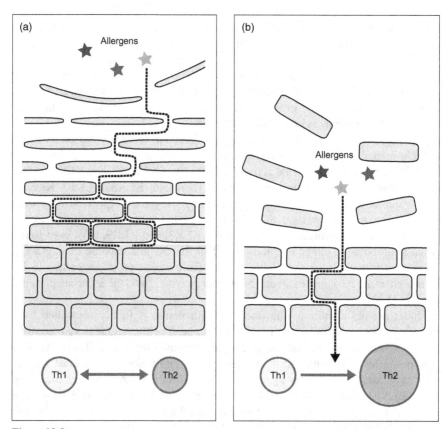

Figure19.2   There is a wide difference in the thickness of the SC at different body sites. The skin sites that are not predisposed to AD have a much thicker SC where the uppermost corneocytes have been permitted to mature (a), and as a result have higher skin barrier reserve (indicated by shading) to protect against irritant and allergen penetration. In contrast, the sites of predisposition to AD, such as the face and flexures, have the thinnest SC (b) and can be visualized as having a very low skin barrier reserve.

Skin Barrier Homeostasis

The structure of the skin barrier is regulated by its function as a permeability barrier. Poor permeability barrier function, defined by a decreased ability to retain water (increased permeability), is accompanied by increased ion flux with consequent perturbation of epidermal ion gradients.[48] A distinct gradient of calcium ions (Ca^{2+}) normally exists across the epidermis, starting with low levels in the basal layer(s) and progressively increasing toward the upper stratum granulosum (SG), where it peaks, before sharply declining across the SC.[48,49] Ca^{2+} regulates the expression of differentiation-dependent genes in keratinocytes, such as those encoding proteins of the CE.[50] As such, the Ca^{2+} gradient plays a key role in maintaining the different stages of differentiation. Other ions, including potassium, also exhibit specific gradients across the epidermis, which play important roles in regulating barrier homeostasis.[51] The maintenance of these ion gradients across the epidermis is interdependent on the ability of the epidermis, specifically the SC, to act as a permeability barrier.[48]

Acute barrier damage, by tape stripping, for example, causes rapid extracellular ion flux, resulting in the loss of Ca^{2+} in the SG.[52,53] This disruption of the Ca^{2+} gradient triggers rapid secretion of LB contents in the upper SG and restoration of permeability barrier function.[54] The altered distribution of Ca^{2+} in the nucleated layers of the epidermis inhibits differentiation and promotes proliferation to compensate for the loss of functional corneocytes as a result of barrier disruption.[50] If the permeability barrier is artificially restored using a vapor-permeable membrane, barrier repair does not take place, however the Ca^{2+} gradient is rapidly restored.[48] Similarly, if exogenous Ca^{2+} is applied to the skin, the repair process is inhibited.[51]

Barrier disruption also results in elevation of pH within the uppermost layers of the epidermis, and the subsequent elevation of serine protease activity.[55] Under normal circumstances, there is a pH gradient across the SC, starting with a pH close to 7 at the SG–SC interface and changing to an acidic pH, of around 5, in the superficial layers of the SC.[56–58] Localized pH within the SC regulates the activity of desquamatory proteases, protease inhibitors, and lipid synthesis enzymes, and therefore plays an important role in balancing formation and degradation of the skin barrier. For instance, a change in pH from 5.5 to 7.5 increases KLK7 activity by 50%.[28,59] On the other hand, the generation of lamellar components relies on the conversion of glycosylceramides and sphingomyelin into ceramides by *β-glucocerebrosidase* (β-GlucCer'ase) and *acid sphingomyelinase*, both of which have an acid optimum pH.[60–62] When the pH of the SC is increased, by the application of neutral/alkaline buffers, or by blocking the metabolic pathways involved in SC acidification, broad barrier abnormalities are observed.[63–66] This included rapid activation of serine proteases, with consequent breakdown of corneodesmosomes and degradation of lipid synthesis enzymes, and decreased β-GlucCer'ase activity, resulting in incompletely processed lipid lamellae membranes.

In addition to the role of pH in modulating skin barrier structure, it is an important element of the antimicrobial barrier. The acidic surface of the SC restricts colonization by pathogenic microorganisms and encourages persistence of normal microbial flora.[62] Furthermore, serine proteases, involved in desquamation, directly activate and further process antimicrobial peptides.[67] As such, the activity of these proteases is an important determinant in the antimicrobial properties of the skin. KLK7 is also capable of activating the proinflammatory cytokine interleukin (IL)-1.[68] Cytokines, including IL-1, IL-6, and tumor necrosis factor (TNF)-α, are released following skin barrier disruption and facilitate normal skin barrier repair.[5,69–73]

Alterations in trypsin-like serine protease activities, including KLK5 and KLK14, also play a key role in skin barrier homeostasis through their ability to activate the protease-activated receptor 2 (PAR2) signaling cascade by direct cleavage of PAR2.[55,74] PAR2 is a member of the PAR family of G-coupled receptors, involved in skin barrier homeostasis, inflammation, and pruritus.[75,76] Activation of PAR2 results in the inhibition of LB secretion and promotion of cornification (terminal differentiation), albeit with a delay of about 30 minutes.[77] This delay permits the secretion of the preformed pool of LB, triggered by extracellular Ca^{2+} flux. After this initial release of lamellar lipids, PAR2 activation prevents further LB secretion and promotes rapid cornification of the uppermost granular cells. This enhancement of cornification is thought to arise due to the PAR2-triggered increase in intracellular calcium, derived from internal stores, which occurs independently of extracellular Ca^{2+} levels.[78] A high intracellular concentration of calcium is required for profilaggrin processing and the aggregation and subsequent cross-linking of CE proteins.[17]

The opposing effects caused by disruption of the Ca^{2+} gradient and activation of the serine protease–PAR2 pathway following acute barrier disruption are thought to result in the regeneration of the skin barrier by the coordinated and rapid transition of granular cells into corneocytes encased in a preformed lamellar mesh.[77] The redefinition of the distinct layers of the epidermis in order to regenerate the damaged SC and restore permeability barrier function is undoubtedly a complex process involving both positive and negative signals that need to be targeted at specific regions of the epidermis.[79] Notably, inhibition of the serine protease–PAR2 pathway following skin barrier disruption, using serine protease inhibitors, was found to improve recovery of the permeability barrier.[55,80] Similarly, acute acidification of the SC was found to improve skin barrier structure and function owing to a reduced activity of serine proteases and enhanced activity of lipid synthesis enzymes.[81]

Variations in skin surface pH and serine protease activity at different body sites appear to correlate with the regional variation in skin barrier structure and function.[2] Together this suggests that differential regulation of the serine protease–PAR2 axis may, at least in part, determine regional skin barrier performance, including the extent of the skin barrier reserve, and subsequently regional variation in the susceptibility to the penetration of harmful exogenous agents and topically applied drugs. The serine protease–PAR2 axis (Fig. 19.3) is therefore an important target for improving and repairing the structure and function of the skin barrier. Notably, this axis plays an important role in the pathogenesis of a number of inflammatory skin disorders, including contact dermatitis, rosacea, ichthyosis, and AD.[31]

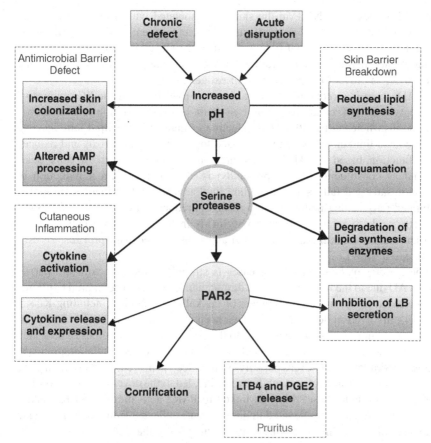

Figure 19.3   The serine protease–PAR2 axis. Acute and chronic disruption of the skin barrier leads to an elevation of SC pH, with consequent enhancement of serine protease activity. Serine proteases with trypsin-like activity have been shown to activate the PAR2 receptor on keratinocytes involved in epidermal homeostasis and inflammation. Activation of the serine protease–PAR2 axis following barrier disruption leads to: an antimicrobial barrier defect, cutaneous inflammation, skin barrier breakdown, and pruritus.

ATOPIC DERMATITIS

The skin of patients with AD is characterized by a thinner epidermis,[41,82] less mature surface corneocytes,[40,83] poor hydration, and an increased TEWL.[84–86] The reduced permeability barrier function of the SC broadly results from abnormal keratinocyte differentiation, defective lipid lamellae, and altered homeostasis. The expression of differentiation-dependent genes, including those encoding components of the CE, is broadly affected and compromises skin barrier structure.[87–89] The expression of filaggrin in particular is reduced and results in a structural defect and reduced levels of

374 Chapter 19 Current and Future Trends: Skin Diseases and Treatment

NMF.[18,90] Low levels of NMF in the skin are associated with dryness and scaling and correlate with the clinical severity and barrier impairment in AD.[18,91–93] Recently it was found that a deficiency of filaggrin leads to a reduced inflammatory threshold to irritants and allergens, demonstrating the importance of this protein to the ability of the barrier to prevent the permeation of exogenous agents.[94]

In AD, there is a reduction in the amount of total lipids in the SC owing to a significant deficit of ceramides found in both lesional and nonlesional skin.[95] Ceramide insufficiency results in the defective formation of the lipid lamellae and the corneocyte lipid envelope, and was found to correlate with xerosis and reduced barrier function based on TEWL measurements.[96,97] The pattern of fatty acids (free and as constituents of phospholipids) is also altered, with a reduction of omega-6 unsaturated fatty acids (including linoleic acid) and an increase in mono-unsaturated fatty acids (including oleic acid).[98] A reduced ratio of omega-6 unsaturated fatty acids to monounsaturated fatty acids in the skin of AD patients is an important marker of skin barrier function and is associated with pruritus, xerosis, and increased TEWL.

The activity of degradatory proteases is strongly associated with the barrier defect in AD due to the increased rate of desquamation observed compared to normal skin. Increased levels of seven members of the kallikrein family (including KLK5, 7, and 14), involved in desquamation, have been associated with AD.[85,99] The overexpression of human KLK in mice leads to the development of changes in their skin similar to those seen in chronic AD, such as a skin barrier defect, inflammation, and pruritus.[100] Similarly, KLK5 hyperactivity in mice, achieved by abrogating the expression of the serine protease inhibitor LEKTI, led to the development of AD-like lesions.[101] In the latter case, this was linked to PAR2 activation by KLK5. PAR2 expression was found to be elevated in human tissue collected from the lesional skin of patients with AD compared with controls, suggesting that both the direct action of serine proteases on the structure of the skin barrier and their role in activating PAR2 plays a role in the development of AD.[74]

Furthermore, skin surface pH of patients with AD is elevated at lesional and nonlesional sites.[62] Increased skin surface pH, associated with both elevated activity of serine proteases and the inhibition of enzymes involved in processing lamellar lipids,[65,102] leads to reduced SC integrity/cohesion and defective lipid lamellae with consequent reduction in skin barrier performance.[102] Through its modulation of serine protease activity, SC pH is also linked with the activation of PAR2 and subsequent inhibition of skin barrier repair and inflammation.[74] The finding that maintenance of an acidic pH can prevent the development of murine hapten-induced AD raises the importance of pH, and excessive protease activity, in the pathology of AD.[103]

Genetic Susceptibility to a Defective Skin Barrier

Changes in three groups of genes, encoding structural proteins, proteases, and protease inhibitors, predispose to a defective skin barrier in AD. The most important

genetic changes associated with AD identified to date are the loss-of-function mutations within the *FLG* gene, encoding the S100 fused-type protein (SFTP) profilaggrin, and the proform of filaggrin.[104–119] These mutations account for the reduced
expression of filaggrin and its breakdown products (NMF) in patients with AD.[18,90,120]
Mutations of the *FLG* gene were primarily identified as the underlying cause of
ichthyosis vulgaris (IV), which often occurs concomitantly with AD.[113] Approximately
15% of all AD patients carry an *FLG* loss-of-function mutation, which increases to
50% of severe cases.[121] Furthermore, a higher proportion of carriers develop AD at
an early age and display elevated levels of serum Immunoglobulin E (IgE) compared
to noncarriers.[122] *FLG* loss-of-function mutations have been associated with profound effects on the skin, including decreased SC hydration, elevated TEWL when
linked to disease severity, and elevated SC pH.[92,93,123] The elevation of SC pH is
thought to arise as a result of the reduction in acidic NMF components,[124,125] and
links *FLG* loss-of-function mutations to inhibition of lipid synthesis and activation
of the serine protease–PAR2 axis (Fig. 19.3). Carriers of *FLG* mutations possess a
defective skin barrier, the extent of which appears to be dependent on the degree of
filaggrin abrogation, and exhibit an increased susceptibility to irritant and allergen
penetration.[94,123,126,127] The contribution of elevated SC pH to the barrier abnormality
associated with *FLG* loss-of-function mutations requires further investigation.

The *FLG* gene is located within the epidermal differentiation complex (EDC,
chromosomal location 1q21), a cluster of genes encoding a range of proteins involved
in epidermal differentiation, many of which are incorporated in the CE such as
involucrin and loricrin.[128] Since the identification of the first *FLG* mutation, additional mutations associated with AD have been found in neighboring genes within
the EDC, including the gene encoding the SFTPs cornulin[129] and hornerin[130];
however, their significance in AD remains to be confirmed.

A reduced expression of protease inhibitors is also associated with AD; for
instance, several studies have linked mutations within the *SPINK5* gene, encoding
the serine protease inhibitor LEKTI with AD when maternally inherited.[119,131–133]
Mutations of the *SPINK5* gene are the underlying cause of Netherton syndrome, a
severe autosomal recessive disorder of the skin with atopic manifestations.[134,135]
Individuals with this disorder display marked barrier dysfunction, involving altered
desquamation and impaired keratinization as a result of elevated KLK5 and KLK7
activity.[136,137] Decreased expression of the cystatin A protease inhibitor, with dual
roles in epidermal differentiation and desquamation, was also found to be decreased
in AD, and attributed to a genetic variant of the *CSTA* gene associated with the
development of AD.[138,139]

Vasilopoulos and colleagues reported a significant association between a genetic
variant of the *KLK7* gene, which could potentially result in elevated expression of
the serine protease KLK7, and non-AD.[140] Two subsequent studies, however, have
failed to confirm an association with AD.[107,119] Despite this, KLK7 expression does
appear to be elevated in the skin of patients with AD compared to control subjects.[85,99,141] It has been suggested that the level of protease activity at the SC is an
important indicator of milder forms of barrier disruption, including sensitive skin,
in addition to AD.[142] This may explain the poor association between *KLK7* and AD,

where the control populations will have comprised subjects with a wide range of skin conditions. In support of this, the level of proteases quantified in samples of human SC was found to correlate with biophysical measures of skin condition, including hydration and TEWL.[142] Trypsin-like (including KLK5 and KLK14), tryptase-like plasmin and urokinase activities, but not chymotrypsin-like activities, were positively correlated to TEWL and negatively correlated with hydration. Interestingly, the type of protease activity found to correlate with skin barrier integrity is consistent with the types of protease capable of activating PAR2.[74]

Subclinical Skin Barrier Defect

The genetic factors discussed above result in an underlying skin barrier defect that is thought to predispose to AD. This skin barrier defect is characterized by fluctuations in permeability barrier function, measured as TEWL, that follow the phase of the disease. In the presence of active AD, TEWL is elevated even at sites far from active lesions.[143] On the other hand, in the absence of clinical symptoms of AD (for more than 5 years), baseline TEWL appears normal.[144] This led to the suggestion that it is the presence of active inflammatory lesions that leads to barrier impairment.[143] Contrary to this, the skin of patients with a history of AD (no clinical symptoms in the last 3 months) displays a greater susceptibility to the penetration of irritants and allergens,[145] as does the uninvolved skin of AD patients.[146,147] It is clear, therefore, that a defect exists, and that there are limits to the sensitivity of baseline TEWL measurements for detecting the underline defect. One must also consider the role of the so-called skin barrier reserve (Fig. 19.2).[47] The concept of a skin barrier reserve derives from the observation that a significant and repeated experimentally induced physical disruption to the SC by tape stripping is needed before an elevation in TEWL is observed in healthy human subjects.[85,148,149] This suggests that there is a great deal of scope for the presence of a defect that would not necessarily be identifiable by measuring permeability barrier function.

Filaggrin and its breakdown products, as already discussed, are important in the structure and function of the skin barrier. *FLG* loss-of-function mutations are associated with increased risk of contact sensitization[127,150] and enhanced percutaneous allergen penetration.[126] Kezic and coworkers recently demonstrated that at sites with no visible signs of skin disruption, there were significant differences in the concentrations of the filaggrin breakdown products sodium pyrrolidone carboxylic acid and urocanic acid, components of NMF.[151] These differences accurately reported the presence or absence of *FLG* loss-of-function mutations, and importantly demonstrate a subclinical change in skin barrier structure and function. A reduction of filaggrin, and subsequently NMF, levels in the skin is associated with elevated TEWL and increased skin surface pH, both features of AD.[92,123] Notably, the elevated skin surface pH associated with AD is found at unaffected sites, and becomes more pronounced as clinical symptoms arise, suggesting an association with AD severity.[62]

The lipid defect associated with AD, including the reduction in ceramides and alteration of fatty acid profiles, is also observed at both lesional and unaffected sites, and the extent of the defect compared to healthy controls correlates with the extent of the permeability barrier defect, measured as TEWL, and the severity of AD.[95] The presence of these changes, and their correlation with permeability barrier function and disease severity, highlights the predisposition to a skin barrier defect resulting from the genetic changes associated with AD, and moreover the need for interaction with additional factors to advance the disease (trigger the development of a flare).

It is important to recognize that many of the structural changes discussed, such as NMF levels, lipid profiles including ceramide levels, pH, and protease activity, can occur in seemingly healthy individuals (no clinical signs or history of AD) and correlate with xerosis, the changing of the seasons, and age.[91,95,152–154] Indeed, 40% of *FLG* loss-of-function mutation carriers never develop AD.[112] A predisposition to a defective skin barrier does not therefore necessarily lead to AD. The extent of the exiting predisposition (gene–gene interaction) and the interaction with environmental factors determine progression to AD. For instance, the risk of developing AD is increased significantly if *FLG* loss-of-function mutation carriers are exposed to cat, but not dog, allergens or where there is concomitant food sensitization early on in life.[155,156] The contribution of environmental factors to the risk conferred by genetic changes is an important area where further research is needed.

The degree of skin colonization in AD patients with *Staphylococcus aureus* (*S. aureus*) was found to correlate with disease severity.[157–160] *S. aureus* colonization is a common complication in AD patients, affecting more than 90% of patients with a mean density of up to ~20 million organisms/cm^2 in acute lesions.[161] Susceptibility to *S. aureus* colonization arises due to the elevated skin surface pH and reduced level of antimicrobial skin lipids.[62,162,163] In turn, *S. aureus* secretes a range of enzymes that break down the skin barrier, including several serine proteases known as exfoliative toxins, and the more recently identified V8 protease, which break down the skin barrier via cleavage of corneodesmosomes to facilitate colonization.[164–167] Bacterially derived *ceramidase* is also thought to be a confounding factor leading to ceramide insufficiency in the defective skin barrier.[168] Mites, such as the house dust mite (*Dermatophagoides pteronyssinu*), and cockroach allergens with proteolytic activity may also play a role in skin barrier breakdown directly and indirectly, via PAR2 activation.[169] These proteolytic allergens were specifically shown to delay skin barrier recovery and LB secretion in murine skin. Molds, such as *Alternaria alternata* (*A. alternata*), were also found to release proteases capable of activating PAR2.[170] *A. alternata* is the most common airborne fungi in indoor and outdoor environments, and may be responsible for allergic reactions in sensitive individuals.[171] In one study, 32% of AD patients had specific IgE against *A. alternata*.[171] Scabies mite (*Sarcoptes scabiei*) was recently shown to ingest filaggrin, which is subsequently broken down by the action of the Sar s3 protease.[172] Exposure to these allergens is an important environmental risk factor in the development/exacerbation of AD.[173,174]

A *subclinical skin barrier defect* therefore results from the interaction of genetic factors (gene–gene interaction) with environmental factors. A common target for this

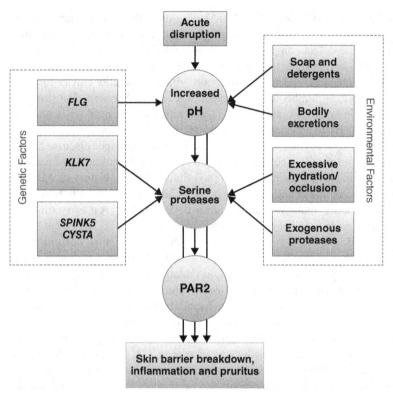

Figure 19.4   Interaction of genetic and environmental factors with the serine protease–PAR2 axis. Genetic factors, such as mutations in the *FLG*, *KLK7*, *SPINK5*, and *CYSTA* genes associated with the skin barrier defect in AD and environmental factors known to exacerbate AD drive activation of the serine protease–PAR2 pathway.

interaction is the serine protease–PAR2 axis, the activation of which helps explain their combined effect on skin barrier structure and function (Fig. 19.4). The normal skin barrier reserve provides a buffer to protect against natural variations in permeability barrier function and environmental conditions. Susceptibility to the development of AD appears to increase where this reserve is compromised at sites of natural predisposition where the reserve is small, during infancy where the barrier is not fully developed,[14,175] and when multiple negative gene–gene and gene–environment interactions combine.

Subclinical Inflammation

A consequence of acute or chronic skin barrier disruption is the release and activation of proinflammatory cytokines, including IL-1α, IL-1β, IL-18, TNF-α, and granulocyte–macrophage colony-stimulating factor (GM-CSF).[5,176,177] This event is an initial step in a cytokine cascade that leads to inflammation in AD. Serine proteases involved in desquamation, including KLK7 and KLK5, appear to play a key role in initiating this cascade. In response to skin barrier damage, SC pH rises, leading to increased activity of these proteases.[55] Subsequently, serine proteases, including KLK7, have been shown to activate IL-1α and IL-1β by direct cleavage of their 33-kDa proforms following release from the large cytoplasmic stores found within corneocytes.[68,178,179] Furthermore, activation of PAR2 on the surface of keratinocytes by proteases such as KLK5 and 14,[55,74] and also exogenous proteases derived from the house dust mite and *A. alternata*, for example,[170,180] triggers a signaling pathway resulting in the increased expression of TNF-α, IL-8, intercellular adhesion molecule 1, and thymic stromal lymphopoetin (TSLP).[101,170,181]

TSLP is an IL-7-like cytokine produced by epithelial cells in the lungs, gut, and the skin, in response to a range of stimuli, including protease activation of PAR2.[182] Elevated levels of TSLP are a feature of lesional skin in AD.[183] It is a potent activator of dendritic cells (DC), including Langerhans cells found within the basal and suprabasal layers of the epidermis.[183–185] The migration of activated DC to the draining lymph nodes triggers the proliferation of allergen-specific T lymphocyte cells and their differentiation into T helper (Th) type 2 (Th2) cells.[183] The activation of mast cells by TSLP also promotes Th2 polarization.[186] Th2 cells produce and release proallergic Th2 cytokines, including IL-4, IL-5, and IL-13 that trigger IgE production and eosinophilia characteristic of inflammation in AD.[187] Notably, the overproduction of IL-4 or IL-13 in the epidermis of transgenic mice results in the development of a pruritic inflammatory skin disease similar to AD.[188,189] DC recruit Th2 cells to the site of inflammation by the release of chemokines upon activation, including thymus and activation-regulated chemokine and macrophage-derived chemokine.[190] Furthermore, TSLP inhibits expression of the anti-inflammatory cytokine IL-10[191,192] and the Th1 cytokine IFNγ by DC, thereby favoring a Th2-dominant response.[183] IL-18, released by keratinocytes upon mechanical disruption of the skin barrier, has also been shown to promote the production of Th2 cytokines.[177]

A plethora of immune system defects are thought to combine in AD and promote progression to inflammation.[193] Whether these defects arise as a result of a skin barrier defect or inherent immune system defects is hotly debated. Genetic studies have revealed significant associations between mutations in candidate genes encoding proteins of both the skin barrier (such as the *FLG* gene encoding filaggrin) and the immune system and AD, suggesting that interaction between the two may be important in at least some cases.[121] In Netherton syndrome, skin barrier dysfunction was shown to be responsible for the development of AD-like inflammatory lesions.[101] In this case, unbridled KLK5 activity due to mutations within the *SPINK5* gene encoding the serine protease inhibitor LEKTI resulted in PAR2-dependent release of the proinflammatory mediator TSLP. In mice, inflammatory lesions develop as a result of the inducible expression of TSLP.[194] This suggests that the release of proinflammatory cytokines such as TSLP following skin barrier damage is sufficient, under certain circumstances, to trigger inflammation. Nevertheless, the association of mutations affecting the expression of immune system effectors with AD suggests an interaction, which may result in the reduction of inflammatory thresholds.

The uninvolved skin of patients with AD is characterized by *subclinical inflammation*.[187] This refers to the presence of a perivascular Th2 cell infiltrate, albeit at a low level, which is accompanied by increased levels of the Th2 cytokines IL-4 and IL-13. There are traces of hyperkeratosis, epidermal hyperplasia, and intercellular edema.[195] This clinically unaffected skin is prone to dryness and demonstrates an increased sensitivity to irritants.[196] The dry, xerotic skin of AD patients is characterized by decreased SC hydration, increased TEWL, elevated skin surface pH, an increased turnover rate of the SC, and smaller, less mature corneocytes.[197] Chemical irritation of this xerotic skin produces a much more severe, long-lasting, inflammatory response together with a delay in skin barrier repair. Persistent subclinical inflammation, concomitant with a skin barrier defect, therefore appears to lower the threshold for the development of inflammatory lesions.

Th2 cytokines have been shown to negatively affect the structure of the skin barrier. This includes the inhibition of ceramide synthesis[198,199] and the downregulation of key structural epidermal proteins, including filaggrin,[200] involucrin, loricrin,[201] and desmoglein 3, a component of desmosomal junctions.[202] Later, Howell and coworkers identified that IL-4 and IL-13 both inhibit profilaggrin and human β-defensin 3 expression indirectly by suppressing the expression of another protein encoded in the EDC, the S100 calcium binding protein 11 (S100/A11).[203] Notably, the selective abolition of IL-4 expression in mice results in improved skin barrier function.[204] This inflammation-induced suppression of skin barrier homeostasis is thought to compound the existing skin barrier defect present in patients with AD. Activated mast cells are expected to contribute to the amplification of both the skin barrier defect and the inflammatory reaction by releasing proteases such as *mast cell chymase* (MCC) and *β-tryptase*, respectively.[101,205] MCC is an important secondary protease that contributes to skin barrier breakdown during inflammation.[47] Mutations within the gene encoding this protease have been associated with AD.[206] β-Tryptase, on the other hand, could facilitate inflammation by activating PAR2 on mast cells, DC, and eosinophils.[207-210]

Clinical Disease

Accumulating evidence on the development of AD supports an event, normally early on in life, whereby skin barrier function is abrogated sufficiently to induce inflammation. The optimal combination of an existing genetically predetermined skin defect with the underdeveloped SC and adverse environmental conditions brings about this event, particularly at sites naturally low in skin barrier reserve. From this point, inflammation progresses in an escalating cycle, ultimately leading to the development of a flare. Clinically, AD is characterized by xerosis, pruritus, and erythematous lesions with increased TEWL.[2] Increased SC pH and protease activity are common consequences of skin barrier gene changes, and appear to play a central role in the development of the subclinical skin barrier defect and the perpetuation of the inflammatory cascade, ultimately leading to the development of a flare.

Historically, AD has been divided into two subtypes, "intrinsic" and "extrinsic," based on the presence of allergic sensitization.[187] Current opinion, however, favors a model whereby these subtypes represent different phases of the disease.[211] In this model, AD develops in early infancy as a nonatopic condition and later, in about 60%–80% of cases, progresses to "true" AD.[212] The penetration of allergens through the defective skin (permeability) barrier is a key event in the transition between the two stages.

Antigen-presenting cells (APC), including Langerhans cells and mast cells, capture antigens that penetrate through the weakened skin barrier. These cells express the high affinity IgE receptor, Fcε receptor I (FcεRI), and the low affinity IgE receptor, FcεRII, that bind to IgE. In AD, the expression of FcεRI and FcεRII is increased, along with elevated levels of serum IgE, and APC bearing IgE.[213] IgE+ Langerhans cells and mast cells activated by allergen binding strongly prime naïve T cells to produce Th2 cytokines, and thereby potentiate allergic inflammation. A predominance of Th2 cytokines is a feature of the acute phase of AD.[187] Recently, it was reported that FcεRI signaling induces elevated expression of TSLP receptor on the surface of DC in atopic subjects.[214] As a result, Th2 switching was selectively amplified when DC were coprimed with TSLP and cat allergen (variant of Fel d1). To this end, both allergen penetration through a damaged skin barrier and cytokine release (particularly TSLP) by keratinocytes in response to skin barrier damage play important, synergistic roles in the development of inflammatory lesions.

Cytokines released by Langerhans cells, mast cells, and keratinocytes during the acute phase of AD orchestrate the infiltration of inflammatory cells, including macrophages, eosinophils, and inflammatory dendritic epidermal cells (IDEC).[215] The ensuing infiltration of eosinophils and IDEC has been suggested to act as the switch from a Th2-type to a Th1-type response characteristic of the chronic phase of AD. The cytokine milieu in chronic AD comprises the Th1 cytokine IFN-γ, and elevated levels of IL-5 and GM-CSF, which enhance the survival of inflammatory cells and promote tissue remodeling.[187] Chronic inflamed skin is characterized by thickened plaques, lichenification, and dry fibrotic papules.

The course of disease does not end here. AD is often referred to as the first step along the *atopic march*.[13] This describes the observation that patients with AD often develop further atopic conditions such as food allergy, asthma, and allergic rhinitis. Recently the epidermal production of TSLP was identified as an important link between inflammation in AD and the development of asthma.[216]

TREATMENT OF AD

Reactive Inflammatory Treatment

Current treatment of AD is largely reactive (Fig. 19.5). When flares develop, short courses of anti-inflammatory compounds such as TCS are used to suppress inflammation.[7] The potency of TCS used depends on the severity of the disease and the site affected. Only mild TCS should be used at sites with a low skin barrier reserve

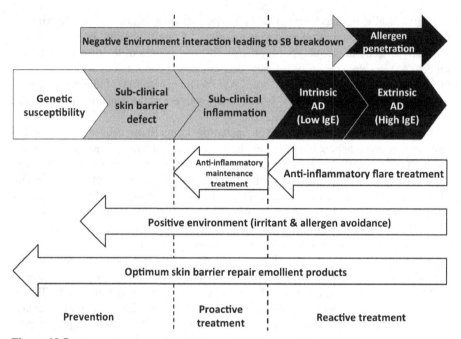

Figure 19.5   The progression and treatment of AD. The course of AD begins with a genetic susceptibility (white box) to a defective skin barrier, which alone does not lead to the development of disease. Negative environmental factors, discussed in the text, interact with genetic factors to determine the subclinical skin barrier defect (gray boxes). Theoretically this subclinical state is reversible by maintaining a positive environment. Environmental interaction (gray block arrow) with the skin barrier defect then drives disease progression through to the presentation of clinical disease (black boxes). A genetic predisposition to a reduced inflammatory threshold would also promote disease progression. Allergen penetration (black block arrow) through a defective skin barrier marks the progression from nonatopic disease, with low serum IgE (intrinsic AD), to atopic disease, with high serum IgE (extrinsic AD). White block arrows illustrate the effect of current and future treatment on the progression of AD.

due to their increased penetration through the skin and consequently the increased risk of adverse affects (reviewed in References 35 and 217). Most notably, TCS use is associated with skin atrophy. The short-term use of super-potent TCS and long-term use of mild–moderate TCS in humans is associated with reduced thickness of the SC, a reduced number of corneocytes layers in the SC, and elevated TEWL, indicative of reduced permeability barrier function.[148,149,218–222] Studies in mice demonstrated concomitant reductions in the number of LB, alteration of the structure of the lamellar matrices, and decreased persistence of corneodesmosomal junctions.[148,218] Together this evidence suggests a destructive effect of prolonged TCS use on the skin barrier. It is likely that the negative effect of TCS on the skin barrier accounts for, or at least contributes to, the rebound flare phenomenon.[223,224] Rebound flare occurs after topical steroids have been applied for several months.[225] This is due to a progressive thinning of the SC.[148,218,226]

Rebound flare, after the discontinuation of TCS, occurs both in the context of an underlying skin disease, such as AD, and also in normal skin after prolonged application of TCS.[223,224] Rebound flare is most common after the prolonged application of potent or moderately potent TCS to skin sites with a low skin barrier reserve (thin SC) such as the face.[218] The rebound flare following discontinuation of TCS has similarities to that observed following other forms of barrier disruption such as surfactants and tape stripping. An extreme form of rebound flare following the discontinuation of TCS is "the red burning skin syndrome."[225] In all the reported cases, patients had used TCS for prolonged periods on delicate skin sites such as the face and genitals. Patients initially developed pruritus followed by burning and erythema. Further application of TCS led to an exacerbation of the condition, described as corticosteroid addiction. The negative effects of prolonged TCS use on the skin barrier necessitate the use of only short reactive courses to treat flares, and demonstrate the need to assess the effect of treatments applied to the skin on the structure of the skin barrier.

Topical calcineurin inhibitors (TCI), such as tacrolimus and pimecrolimus, are an effective alternative anti-inflammatory treatment to mild–moderate potency TCS.[7] A number of large randomized clinical studies have demonstrated that topical treatment with tacrolimus or pimecrolimus can interrupt acute flares of AD, significantly reduce pruritus, and prevent exacerbation of AD after cessation of treatment.[227–230] Furthermore, the topical application of tacrolimus and pimecrolimus, unlike corticosteroids, has been associated with improvement in skin barrier function, measured as TEWL.[221,231,232] Whether these TCI simply permit normal barrier recovery or actively promote repair requires further investigation. The antipruritic action of TCI is also receiving much interest. Pruritus is an unpleasant and debilitating characteristic of AD, which also plays an important role in exacerbating the disorder by provoking the desire to scratch, leading to further skin barrier disruption and inflammation.[233] PAR2-induced release of leukotriene B4 and prostaglandin E2 has recently been shown to play a key role in the pathophysiology of itch.[234,235] This suggests that trypsin-like serine protease hyperactivity, associated with skin barrier dysfunction in AD, may be important in the etiology of pruritus, via activation of PAR2. Tacrolimus has been shown to inhibit PAR2-mediated pruritus in mice and reduce scratch behavior.[235] A greater understanding of the mechanisms of TCI action, specifically relating to an inhibitory action on PAR2 signaling, is essential in order to fully appreciate their ability to successfully treat AD. Whereas only the anti-inflammatory action of potent TCS are capable of suppressing severe inflammation in AD, combinations of both TCS and TCI appear to have greater efficacy than either of the two treatments when used as monotherapy.[236,237]

Proactive Inflammatory Treatment

AD has a chronic course of flares and remission.[238] Compromised skin barrier function,[227] the subclinical inflammatory cell infiltrate,[195] and increased expression of the high affinity IgE receptor (FcεRI)[239] lead to an increased propensity for the development of inflammatory flares. In acknowledgment of the contribution of subclinical inflammation to the development of further flares, long-term strategies employing the intermittent use of low doses of anti-inflammatory treatments are being adopted.[7] Following intensive treatment to clear flares, TCS and TCI have been successfully used to prevent the further development of flares and thereby prolong the period of remission.[238,240–244] TCI are particularly effective when used in this way because, in addition to suppressing subclinical inflammation, they support repair of skin barrier structure and function.[149,221,231] TCS, on the other hand, are associated with reduced skin barrier integrity, skin atrophy, and other diverse effects.[148,217,219,221,245]

The increased success in the management of AD by treating subclinical inflammation demonstrates its significance in the development of flares. The next step is to demonstrate whether treatment of the underlying skin barrier defect can prevent subclinical inflammation and thereby also improve remission.

Positive Environment

The relapsing course and severity of AD is associated with the interaction of environmental factors with an existing skin barrier defect.[238] The term "environmental factor" refers to anything from the environment that has a negative effect on the structure and function of the skin barrier and the development of inflammatory reactions.[47] As introduced earlier, this includes exogenous enzymes that break down the skin barrier, produced by colonizing bacteria and house dust mites, for example. Irritant chemicals and physical agents can also complicate the course of AD.[7] Patients with AD often develop sensitization to environmental allergens, including food allergens (cows milk, peanut, wheat, and/or soy protein), bacterial allergens (*S. aureus*), and aeroallergens (from the house dust mite and *A. alternata*, for example) associated with elevated serum IgE/transition to extrinsic AD.[171,246–248] Similarly, contact sensitization to chemical irritants such as nickel is frequently found in AD.[247] Sensitization to allergens and irritants is thought to occur as a result of a defective skin barrier, and subsequent exposure, through a defective barrier, triggers skin inflammation and exacerbates AD.[2,249] Avoidance of environmental triggers and factors that facilitate skin barrier breakdown is an important part of treatment both in terms of suppressing flares and extending periods of remission.[7,250,251] In the case of skin colonization with *S. aureus*, for example, a common complication in AD and a source of superantigens and degradatory enzymes (e.g., exfoliatoxins), antibacterial treatment has been shown to reduce the severity of disease in some circumstances[158,160]; however, a systematic review published in 2008 concluded that additional large studies with long-term outcomes are required before firm conclusions can be made.[252]

The role of the skin barrier defect in the persistence of dermatosis suggests that restoration of skin barrier function could prevent further relapses of AD by preventing the penetration of irritants and allergens.[253] The establishment of an artificial barrier over the skin using "barrier" creams/ointments to protect against contact irritants has shown some success in the treatment of contact dermatitis and supports the concept of skin barrier repair as a means of preventing relapses.[254] A systematic review of barrier creams for the treatment of occupational irritant hand dermatitis found a consistent trend for reduced numbers of new cases when a barrier cream intervention was made compared to no intervention; however, the human studies conducted to date are insufficiently powered to establish effectiveness.[255] In the case of napkin dermatitis, multiple environmental factors combine and contribute to its development.[256] The presence of urine under occlusion produces excessive skin hydration, leading to increased skin barrier permeability to potential irritants. Urine is also associated with the elevation of skin surface pH, which creates an optimum environment for the activity of fecal proteases and lipases. The prolonged exposure to these degradative enzymes under occlusion results in severe erythema and skin barrier disruption. Treatment of napkin dermatitis comprises effective cleansing of the napkin area to remove urine and fecal matter and the application of a barrier cream to protect against further skin contact with exogenous proteases and lipases.[257] Topical products that restore the skin pH to near normal (pH 4.5–5.5) are also important.

Washing the skin is an important environmental factor influencing the structure and function of the skin.[258] The way in which the skin is washed determines whether the effect is positive or negative. On one hand, effective cleansing is essential to remove contact irritants and other negative environmental agents such as saliva and food in perioral dermatitis and urine and feces in perianal dermatitis (napkin dermatitis).[259] Cleansing also reduces bacterial colonization of the skin, which is particularly important in AD due to high skin colonization with *S. aureus*.[161] The use of soap and harsh detergents (anionic surfactants) in wash products, however, is associated with skin dryness and irritation.[260,261] The negative effects of soap and some harsh detergents, such as the anionic surfactant sodium lauryl sulfate (SLS), is attributed in part to their ability to increase the surface pH of the skin, associated with degradation of the skin barrier and inhibition of repair.[2,261,262] The skin of patients with AD is characterized by an elevated surface pH that is directly related to disease severity,[62] which helps explain the increased susceptibility of these individuals to skin reactions following the use of soap and harsh detergents.

Washing the skin with soap and harsh detergents leads to increased TEWL concomitant with elevated skin surface pH.[261–263] The observed reduction in permeability barrier function is related to changes in the type and structure of SC lipids following surfactant application.[264,265] In addition to triggering inflammation itself, surfactants such as SLS have been shown to enhance the percutaneous penetration of other exogenous agents, including irritants and allergens.[266] Combined exposure to harsh surfactants and aeroallergens, for example, leads to an additive increase in skin irritation.[267] The effect of harsh surfactants, and the wash products containing them, vary greatly in their effect on the structure and function of the skin barrier.[268,269] Mild nonionic surfactants have been described with similar effects on the skin as using water alone and have been associated with beneficial effects.[258,261,270] Complexes of different mild surfactants, which together form large micelles, can produce less damaging effects on the skin barrier than water alone.[271] The use of alkaline soaps and harsh anionic surfactants is not recommended for patients with AD, and their avoidance is associated with improvement of the condition.[270,272]

Aside from the negative effects of harsh surfactants, water itself has been associated with mild skin irritation and dryness.[273-275] This irritation is largely observed under occlusive conditions and may be associated with the increased permeability of excessively hydrated skin and the concomitant elevation of protease activity under these conditions.[275] The loss of water-soluble skin actives, such as NMF, has been suggested as a mechanism by which soaking in water dries the skin.[276] Prolonged bathing in water may therefore damage the skin in AD rather than improve it. Water hardness has been linked to irritation of the skin.[275] Theoretically, the high levels of exogenous calcium are thought to inhibit the skin's natural repair mechanism.[51] In agreement with this, the hardness of wash water was shown to modulate the irritant effects of surfactants. In 1998, McNally and coworkers reported a significant association between the lifetime prevalence of AD and water hardness.[277] This association was also confirmed by a second study conducted in Japan.[278] In addition to the proposed direct effect of calcium on the skin barrier, hard water necessitates the use of increased amounts of soap or detergent to achieve a lather when washing. The optimal formulations of wash products contain ion chelators such as citric acid to reduce the level of free calcium and thereby improve lathering. This may be an unintended partial solution to the direct negative effects of hard water on the structure and function of the skin barrier. A multicenter, randomized controlled trial of ion exchange water softeners for the treatment of eczema in children is currently underway in the United Kingdom.[279] The role of water, water hardness, and ion chelators in the development/prevention and treatment of AD requires further investigation. Calcium ion chelators could be combined with the mildest surfactant complexes or polymeric surfactants to achieve optimal cleansing and positive effects on the skin barrier.

Skin Barrier Repair

The routine use of emollients is an important baseline treatment for AD.[7] Emollients are either small, very hygroscopic molecules (humectants) capable of penetrating the skin and binding water, or larger hydrocarbons that form an occlusive barrier able to retain moisture.[280] Traditional emollients are biologically inert, such as petrolatum, and as such artificially, and temporarily, restore permeability barrier function. This necessitates regular use, which is recommended to be approximately 150–200 g per week for children and 500 g per week for adults.[7] Complete emollient therapy describes the replacement of soap and detergent-based wash products with emollient-based alternatives.[251,281] Emollient use is associated with improvement in skin dryness, pruritus, and skin barrier function.[7] Their correct use was also shown to reduce the amount of corticosteroid used in a randomized controlled trial.[282] Despite this, there is limited evidence-based proof for the use of emollients owing to the limitation of clinical observations at assessing underlying changes in skin barrier function.[7] There is also a wide range of emollients with very different effects on the skin barrier. For example, aqueous cream is a particularly crude emollient that contains 1% SLS as an emulsifier.[283] When used as a leave-on emollient, aqueous cream enhances skin hydration yet causes significant skin barrier damage assessed by measuring TEWL.[284,285] An audit of adverse drug reactions to aqueous cream in children with AD reported immediate cutaneous reactions (burning, stinging, itching, and/or redness) in 56.3% of cases when used as a leave-on emollient.[286] This demonstrates the need to functionally test emollient-based products for their effect of the skin barrier to ensure that their overall effect is positive.

The growing recognition of the importance of the structure and function of the skin barrier has focused attention on the design of new emollients with biological activity, with the aim of repairing and maintaining its structure and function. Several strategies are being pursued, including the replacement of key structural components of the skin barrier, or their precursors, inhibition of protease activity/skin barrier breakdown, and maintenance of an acidic SC. New formulations containing native skin barrier constituents such as lamellar lipids and components of NMF are now appearing. The use of moisturizers containing urea (5%–10%), a component of NMF, resulted in a clinical improvement of AD.[10] Chamlin and colleagues demonstrated an improvement in childhood AD following the use of ceramide dominant SC lipids.[11] Vegetable oils are being investigated as a source of native skin lipids, and have revealed divergent biological effects. Olive oil, containing high levels of oleic acid, appears to damage the skin barrier, whereas sunflower oil, containing high levels of linoleic acid, promoted skin barrier repair.[287] In a randomized clinical study involving 68 patients with moderate AD, an emollient containing 2% sunflower oleodistillate was found to be corticosteroid sparing and improved lichenification, excoriation, and quality of life.[12,288] Whether this effect can be attributed to the presence of linoleic acid or another component of the distillate cannot be said and requires further investigation. For instance, the unsaponifiable fraction of canola oil was found to be the source of its anti-inflammatory properties.[289] Furthermore, it has been questioned whether patients with AD can metabolize linoleic acid following the finding that they have lower levels of linoleic acid metabolites in the skin.[257] These are just a few of the new advances being made, and each requires further investigation before we can be sure that particular active ingredients have a significant effect on treatment of AD above that of currently available emollient products.

ASSESSMENT OF SKIN BARRIER STRUCTURE AND FUNCTION

The development of new biologically active emollients intended to repair the skin barrier places greater emphasis on the need to analyze and quantify their effects *in vivo*. The presence of an underlying skin barrier defect only becomes evident clinically once the skin becomes inflamed. The clinical significance of anti-

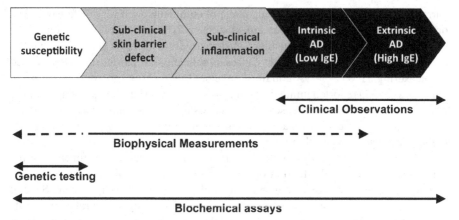

Figure 19.6   Skin assessment throughout the course of AD. The ability of different methodologies (detailed in Table 19.1) to assess the skin varies throughout the course of disease. Clinical assessments are informative only once the disease has presented, whereas biophysical and biochemical methods can be used to study the underlying skin barrier defect.

inflammatory treatments is based on their ability to visually reduce inflammation and reduce pruritus (itching). The clinical significance of skin barrier repair therapies will be the reduction in the number of flares (increased duration of remission), and/ or their ability to prevent the development of clinical disease. The first stage in the development of these new therapies must therefore be to demonstrate an ability to improve skin barrier structure and function and/or repair the underlying skin barrier defect. Clinical observations are only suitable during the late stages of disease, and are limited to the assessment of visual signs arising as a result of inflammation, such as skin irritation and xerosis and symptoms such as itching. To establish the effect of new and existing treatments for AD on the subclinical condition of the skin barrier, the use of more sensitive and informative biophysical and biochemical assays is essential (Fig. 19.6 and Table 19.1).

Appropriate biophysical tests and biochemical assays are required to demonstrate the positive effects of individual actives and determine the overall performance of a product. Emollients have traditionally been selected on their ability to hydrate the SC; however, as the case of aqueous cream exemplifies, the ability to hydrate the skin does not necessarily lead to improved skin barrier function. Optimum formulations will both provide hydration and decreased TEWL and percutaneous penetration of irritants and allergens. The skin barrier defect associated with AD is broad, and likely derives from multiple combinations of gene–gene and gene–environment interactions.[2] The ideal topical formulation will need to restore normal proliferation, differentiation, and desquamation across the epidermis, correct the lipid abnormality, and restore SC pH to normal. Demonstrating the ability of a complex formulation to address each of these factors will require a combination of *in vivo* methodologies in humans.

Table 19.1 Techniques for Noninvasive Assessment of Human Skin Barrier Structure and Function *In Vivo*

Method	Details	References
Biophysical measurements		
Basal TEWL	Measure of permeability function.	291–294
Skin barrier integrity	TEWL is measured during and after repeated tape stripping of the skin. The rate of increase in TEWL is dependent on the amount of damage caused by each tape strip, which is dependent on the structural integrity of the SC.	85, 148, 149, 284
SC cohesion	The amount of protein removed by each tape-strip required to reach a TEWL of 100 $g/m^2/h$ is assessed. This is a measure of intercorneocyte connectivity and is an indicator of the rate of desquamation.	85, 148
Hydration	Measure electrical capacitance, conductance, and impedance.	291, 292,295
Erythema	Colorimetric assessment of skin to quantify erythema/irritation.	296
Vasodilatation	Laser Doppler flowmetry is used to measure blood microcirculation, which is elevated during inflammation.	296, 297
Skin surface pH	A surface pH probe is used to estimate superficial SC pH. There is some question over the relevance of surface measurements to the actual pH of the SC; however, it remains a useful indicator.	62, 291
Epidermal thickness	Confocal microscopy used to measure epidermal thickness (<180 μm) and SC thickness. Ultrasound used to measure epidermal thickness (>50 μm) and dermal thickness. Raman can be used to determine SC thickness.	220, 292,298
Corneocyte morphology	Corneocyte surface area is related to their maturity and skin barrier thickness and is putatively a surrogate marker for proteolytic activity.	38, 40, 299
Molecular imaging of SC compounds	*In vivo* confocal Raman microspectroscopy for semiquantitative assessment of SC lipids, urea lactate, urocanic acid, and other components. Determination of SC water gradient.	175, 292, 300
Lipid structure	Attenuated total internal reflection Fourier-transform infrared spectroscopy used to determine lipid structure.	301
Biochemical assays		
Enzyme assays	Determination of the activity or quantity of SC proteases *ex vivo* in samples of SC collected on the back of adhesive discs.	153, 232,302

(Continued)

Table 19.1   *(Continued)*

Method	Details	References
Protein expression	Quantification of proteins, including structural proteins, proteases, or cytokines, collected on the back of adhesive tape.	303, 304
Chemical analysis	Quantification of NMF components, including sodium pyrrolidone carboxylic acid and urocanic acid, collected on the back of adhesive discs. Determination of sodium pyrrolidone carboxylic acid and urocanic acid predicts *FLG* genotype.	151, 305
Lipid analysis	Determination of the composition of the lipid lamellae, including ceramides, cholesterol, and free fatty acids.	154, 306
Genetic analysis		
Genotyping	Assessment of genetic predisposition to a defective skin barrier. Identification of changes/mutations in genes encoding key epidermal proteins including filaggrin, LEKTI, KLK7, and so on.	121, 307

The multifactorial nature of AD may mean that different groups of patients respond differently to different treatments based on their predisposition. This will inevitably make it harder to demonstrate a clinical effect, and may give cause to first establish the type of skin barrier defect a patient has. Subclinical assessment of skin barrier function, and the further development of novel technologies to do this, will pave the way to first identifying at-risk individuals early on in life (at birth) so that they can receive the necessary treatment to help prevent the development of clinical disease. This prevention of the development of AD may then in turn prevent the development of the other diseases in the atopic march, food allergy, asthma, and allergic rhinitis.[13] The observation that the route of sensitization to some foods, including peanuts, is through the skin and not by eating them[290] reinforces the importance of skin barrier breakdown as the first event in the development of the atopic march and not just AD.

CONCLUSION

The recognition that a defective skin barrier plays a primary role in the development of AD has led to a need to understand how every topical product affects the structure and function of the skin barrier. The aim now is to produce a combination of topical products with optimal "skin barrier-enhancing" properties to treat the underlying skin barrier defect. These products include optimal wash formulations, which should combine the mildest surfactants, specific ion chelating activity, and emollients. There is a wide spectrum of emollient formulations from aqueous cream containing 1% SLS, which has a very negative effect on the skin barrier, to sophisticated formulations, which have a positive effect. Vegetable-derived oils such as olive oil should be avoided because they contain high concentrations of oleic acid, which damages the skin barrier.[287] Some sunflower oils contain very low levels of oleic acid (mineral oils contain no oleic acid) and have a positive effect on the skin barrier.[12,287,288]

Treatment of the subclinical skin barrier defect promises to improve remission and even prevent the development of AD. The complex interaction of environmental agents and components of topical formulations with the skin barrier mean that comprehensive *in vivo* assessment of the effect of new, and existing, treatments needs to be made on human skin. There are now a host of sensitive biophysical and biochemical methods available, and under development, for the diagnosis of skin barrier structure and function. Using these techniques it is now possible to ensure that everything patients apply to their skin exerts only a positive effect on the skin barrier. In the future the ability to determine the structure and function of a neonate's skin barrier will permit the design of tailored skin care regimens aimed at preventing the emergence of AD and the atopic march.

REFERENCES

1. YAMASAKI K, DI NARDO A, BARDAN A, MURAKAMI M, OHTAKE T, CODA A, et al. Increased serine protease activity and cathelicidin promotes skin inflammation in rosacea. *Nature Medicine* 2007; 13(8): 975–980.
2. CORK MJ, DANBY SG, VASILOPOULOS Y, HADGRAFT J, LANE ME, MOUSTAFA M, et al. Epidermal barrier dysfunction in atopic dermatitis. *The Journal of Investigative Dermatology* 2009; 129(8): 1892–1908.
3. PROKSCH E, BRANDNER JM, JENSEN JM. The skin: An indispensable barrier. *Experimental Dermatology* 2008; 17(12): 1063–1072.
4. DENDA M, WOOD LC, EMAMI S, CALHOUN C, BROWN BE, ELIAS PM, et al. The epidermal hyperplasia associated with repeated barrier disruption by acetone treatment or tape stripping cannot be attributed to increased water loss. *Archives of Dermatological Research* 1996; 288(5–6): 230–238.
5. WOOD LC, JACKSON SM, ELIAS PM, GRUNFELD C, FEINGOLD KR. Cutaneous barrier perturbation stimulates cytokine production in the epidermis of mice. *The Journal of Clinical Investigation* 1992; 90(2): 482–487.
6. CLARK SC, ZIRWAS MJ. Management of occupational dermatitis. *Dermatologic Clinics* 2009; 27(3): 365–383, vii–viii.
7. DARSOW U, WOLLENBERG A, SIMON D, TAIEB A, WERFEL T, ORANJE A, et al. ETFAD/EADV eczema task force 2009 position paper on diagnosis and treatment of atopic dermatitis. *Journal of the European Academy of Dermatology and Venereology* 2009; 24: 317–328.
8. LAWS PM, YOUNG HS. Topical treatment of psoriasis. *Expert Opinion on Pharmacotherapy* 2010; 11(12): 1999–2009.
9. SCHEINFELD N, BERK T. A review of the diagnosis and treatment of rosacea. *Postgraduate Medicine* 2010; 122(1): 139–143.
10. BISSONNETTE R, MAARI C, PROVOST N, BOLDUC C, NIGEN S, ROUGIER A, et al. A double-blind study of tolerance and efficacy of a new urea-containing moisturizer in patients with atopic dermatitis. *Journal of Cosmetic Dermatology* 2010; 9(1): 16–21.

11. CHAMLIN SL, KAO J, FRIEDEN IJ, SHEU MY, FOWLER AJ, FLUHR JW, et al. Ceramide-dominant barrier repair lipids alleviate childhood atopic dermatitis: Changes in barrier function provide a sensitive indicator of disease activity. *Journal of the American Academy of Dermatology* 2002; 47(2): 198–208.

12. MSIKA P, DE BELILOVSKY C, PICCARDI N, CHEBASSIER N, BAUDOUIN C, CHADOUTAUD B. New emollient with topical corticosteroid-sparing effect in treatment of childhood atopic dermatitis: SCORAD and quality of life improvement. *Pediatric Dermatology* 2008; 25(6): 606–612.

13. SPERGEL JM, PALLER AS. Atopic dermatitis and the atopic march. *The Journal of Allergy and Clinical Immunology* 2003; 112(6 Suppl.): S118–S127.

14. STAMATAS GN, NIKOLOVSKI J, LUEDTKE MA, KOLLIAS N, WIEGAND BC. Infant skin microstructure assessed *in vivo* differs from adult skin in organization and at the cellular level. *Pediatric Dermatology* 2010; 27: 125–131.

15. YA-XIAN Z, SUETAKE T, TAGAMI H. Number of cell layers of the stratum corneum in normal skin—relationship to the anatomical location on the body, age, sex and physical parameters. *Archives of Dermatological Research* 1999; 291(10): 555–559.

16. ELIAS PM. Epidermal lipids, barrier function, and desquamation. *The Journal of Investigative Dermatology* 1983; 80(Suppl.): 44s–49s.

17. CANDI E, SCHMIDT R, MELINO G. The cornified envelope: A model of cell death in the skin. *Nature Reviews. Molecular Cell Biology* 2005; 6(4): 328–340.

18. HARDING C, RAWLINGS A. Natural moisturizing factor. In: Loden M, Maibach H, eds. *Dry Skin and Moisturizers*. CRC Press LLC, Boca Raton, FL, 2006; 187–209.

19. SCHURER NY, ELIAS PM. The biochemistry and function of stratum corneum lipids. *Advances in Lipid Research* 1991; 24: 27–56.

20. LAVKER RM. Membrane coating granules: The fate of the discharged lamellae. *Journal of Ultrastructure Research* 1976; 55(1): 79–86.

21. NORLEN L, AL-AMOUDI A, DUBOCHET J. A cryotransmission electron microscopy study of skin barrier formation. *The Journal of Investigative Dermatology* 2003; 120(4): 555–560.

22. MAREKOV LN, STEINERT PM. Ceramides are bound to structural proteins of the human foreskin epidermal cornified cell envelope. *The Journal of Biological Chemistry* 1998; 273(28): 17763–17770.

23. NEMES Z, MAREKOV LN, FESUS L, STEINERT PM. A novel function for transglutaminase 1: Attachment of long-chain omega-hydroxyceramides to involucrin by ester bond formation. *Proceedings of the National Academy of Sciences of the United States of America* 1999; 96(15): 8402–8407.

24. WERTZ PW, DOWNING DT. Covalent attachment of omega-hydroxyacid derivatives to epidermal macromolecules: A preliminary characterization. *Biochemical and Biophysical Research Communications* 1986; 137(3): 992–997.

25. LUNDSTROM A, SERRE G, HAFTEK M, EGELRUD T. Evidence for a role of corneodesmosin, a protein which may serve to modify desmosomes during cornification, in stratum corneum cell cohesion and desquamation. *Archives of Dermatological Research* 1994; 286(7): 369–375.

26. SERRE G, MILS V, HAFTEK M, VINCENT C, CROUTE F, REANO A, et al. Identification of late differentiation antigens of human cornified epithelia, expressed in re-organized desmosomes and bound to cross-linked envelope. *The Journal of Investigative Dermatology* 1991; 97(6): 1061–1072.

27. ISHIDA-YAMAMOTO A, SIMON M, KISHIBE M, MIYAUCHI Y, TAKAHASHI H, YOSHIDA S, et al. Epidermal lamellar granules transport different cargoes as distinct aggregates. *The Journal of Investigative Dermatology* 2004; 122(5): 1137–1144.

28. CAUBET C, JONCA N, BRATTSAND M, GUERRIN M, BERNARD D, SCHMIDT R, et al. Degradation of corneodesmosome proteins by two serine proteases of the kallikrein family, SCTE/KLK5/hK5 and SCCE/KLK7/hK7. *The Journal of Investigative Dermatology* 2004; 122(5): 1235–1244.

29. EISSA A, DIAMANDIS EP. Human tissue kallikreins as promiscuous modulators of homeostatic skin barrier functions. *Biological Chemistry* 2008; 389(6): 669–680.

30. BERNARD D, MEHUL B, THOMAS-COLLIGNON A, SIMONETTI L, REMY V, BERNARD MA, et al. Analysis of proteins with caseinolytic activity in a human stratum corneum extract revealed a yet

unidentified cysteine protease and identified the so-called "stratum corneum thiol protease" as cathepsin l2. *The Journal of Investigative Dermatology* 2003; 120(4): 592–600.

31. MEYER-HOFFERT U. Reddish, scaly, and itchy: How proteases and their inhibitors contribute to inflammatory skin diseases. *Archivum Immunologiae Et Therapiae Experimentalis* 2009; 57(5): 345–354.

32. DERAISON C, BONNART C, LOPEZ F, BESSON C, ROBINSON R, JAYAKUMAR A, et al. LEKTI fragments specifically inhibit KLK5, KLK7, and KLK14 and control desquamation through a pH-dependent interaction. *Molecular Biology of the Cell* 2007; 18(9): 3607–3619.

33. GALLIANO MF, TOULZA E, GALLINARO H, JONCA N, ISHIDA-YAMAMOTO A, SERRE G, et al. A novel protease inhibitor of the alpha2-macroglobulin family expressed in the human epidermis. *The Journal of Biological Chemistry* 2006; 281(9): 5780–5789.

34. CRONIN E, STOUGHTON RB. Percutaneous absorption of nicotinic acid and ethyl nicotinate in human skin. *Nature* 1962; 195: 1103–1104.

35. FELDMANN RJ, MAIBACH HI. Regional variation in percutaneous penetration of 14C cortisol in man. *The Journal of Investigative Dermatology* 1967; 48(2): 181–183.

36. MARZULLI FN. Barriers to skin penetration. *The Journal of Investigative Dermatology* 1962; 39: 387–393.

37. SCHAEFER KE, SCHEER K. Regional differences in CO2 elimination through the skin. *Experimental Medicine and Surgery* 1951; 9(2–4): 449–457.

38. ROUGIER A, LOTTE C, CORCUFF TP, MAIBACH H. Relationship between skin permeability and corneocyte size according to anatomic site, age and sex in a man. *Journal of the Society of Cosmetic Chemists* 1988; 39: 15–26.

39. BARKER DE. Skin thickness in the human. *Plastic and Reconstructive Surgery (1946)* 1951; 7(2): 115–116.

40. KASHIBUCHI N, HIRAI Y, O'GOSHI K, TAGAMI H. Three-dimensional analyses of individual corneocytes with atomic force microscope: Morphological changes related to age, location and to the pathologic skin conditions. *Skin Research and Technology* 2002; 8(4): 203–211.

41. LEE Y, HWANG K. Skin thickness of Korean adults. *Surgical and Radiologic Anatomy* 2002; 24(3–4): 183–189.

42. PLEWIG G, MARPLES RR. Regional differences of cell sizes in the human stratum corneum. I. *The Journal of Investigative Dermatology* 1970; 54(1): 13–18.

43. SOUTHWOOD WF. The thickness of the skin. *Plastic and Reconstructive Surgery (1946)* 1955; 15(5): 423–429.

44. DOTTERUD LK, KVAMMEN B, LUND E, FALK ES. Prevalence and some clinical aspects of atopic dermatitis in the community of Sor-Varanger. *Acta Dermato-Venereologica* 1995; 75(1): 50–53.

45. KUNZ B, RING J. Clinical features and diagnostic criteria of atopic dermatitis. In: Harper JI, Oranje A, Prose N, eds. *Textbook of Pediatric Dermatology.* Blackwell Science, Oxford, 2002; 199–214.

46. SCHUDEL P, WUTHRICH B. Clinical course of childhood atopic neurodermatitis. A catamnestic study of 121 cases. *Zeitschrift fur Hautkrankheiten* 1985; 60(6): 479–486.

47. CORK MJ, DANBY S, VASILOPOULOS Y, MOUSTAFA M, MACGOWAN A, VARGHESE J, et al. Gene-environment interactions in atopic dermatitis. *Drug Discovery Today: Disease Mechanisms* 2008; 5(1): e11–e31.

48. ELIAS P, AHN S, BROWN B, CRUMRINE D, FEINGOLD KR. Origin of the epidermal calcium gradient: Regulation by barrier status and role of active vs passive mechanisms. *The Journal of Investigative Dermatology* 2002; 119(6): 1269–1274.

49. FORSLIND B, WERNER-LINDE Y, LINDBERG M, PALLON J. Elemental analysis mirrors epidermal differentiation. *Acta Dermato-Venereologica* 1999; 79(1): 12–17.

50. ELIAS PM, AHN SK, DENDA M, BROWN BE, CRUMRINE D, KIMUTAI LK, et al. Modulations in epidermal calcium regulate the expression of differentiation-specific markers. *The Journal of Investigative Dermatology* 2002; 119(5): 1128–1136.

51. LEE SH, ELIAS PM, PROKSCH E, MENON GK, MAO-QUIANG M, FEINGOLD KR. Calcium and potassium are important regulators of barrier homeostasis in murine epidermis. *The Journal of Clinical Investigation* 1992; 89(2): 530–538.

52. MENON GK, ELIAS PM, LEE SH, FEINGOLD KR. Localization of calcium in murine epidermis following disruption and repair of the permeability barrier. *Cell and Tissue Research* 1992; 270(3): 503–512.

53. MAURO T, BENCH G, SIDDERAS-HADDAD E, FEINGOLD K, ELIAS P, CULLANDER C. Acute barrier perturbation abolishes the Ca²⁺ and K⁺ gradients in murine epidermis: Quantitative measurement using PIXE. *The Journal of Investigative Dermatology* 1998; 111(6): 1198–1201.

54. MENON GK, PRICE LF, BOMMANNAN B, ELIAS PM, FEINGOLD KR. Selective obliteration of the epidermal calcium gradient leads to enhanced lamellar body secretion. *The Journal of Investigative Dermatology* 1994; 102(5): 789–795.

55. HACHEM JP, HOUBEN E, CRUMRINE D, MAN MQ, SCHURER N, ROELANDT T, et al. Serine protease signaling of epidermal permeability barrier homeostasis. *The Journal of Investigative Dermatology* 2006; 126(9): 2074–2086.

56. OHMAN H, VAHLQUIST A. *In vivo* studies concerning a pH gradient in human stratum corneum and upper epidermis. *Acta Dermato-Venereologica* 1994; 74(5): 375–379.

57. SCHADE H, MARCHIONINI A. Der Säuremantel der Haut (Nach Gaskettenmessungen). *Journal of Molecular Medicine* 1928; 7(1): 1432–1440.

58. HANSON KM, BEHNE MJ, BARRY NP, MAURO TM, GRATTON E, CLEGG RM. Two-photon fluorescence lifetime imaging of the skin stratum corneum pH gradient. *Biophysical Journal* 2002; 83(3): 1682–1690.

59. EKHOLM IE, BRATTSAND M, EGELRUD T. Stratum corneum tryptic enzyme in normal epidermis: A missing link in the desquamation process? *The Journal of Investigative Dermatology* 2000; 114(1): 56–63.

60. HOLLERAN WM, TAKAGI Y, MENON GK, LEGLER G, FEINGOLD KR, ELIAS PM. Processing of epidermal glucosylceramides is required for optimal mammalian cutaneous permeability barrier function. *The Journal of Clinical Investigation* 1993; 91(4): 1656–1664.

61. SCHMUTH M, MAN MQ, WEBER F, GAO W, FEINGOLD KR, FRITSCH P, et al. Permeability barrier disorder in Niemann-Pick disease: Sphingomyelin-ceramide processing required for normal barrier homeostasis. *The Journal of Investigative Dermatology* 2000; 115(3): 459–466.

62. FLUHR J, BANKOVA LG. Skin surface pH: Mechanism, measurement, importance. In: Serup J, Jemec GB, Grove GL, eds. *Handbook of Non-Invasive Methods and the Skin*. CRC Press, Boca Raton, FL, 2006; 411–420.

63. BEHNE MJ, MEYER JW, HANSON KM, BARRY NP, MURATA S, CRUMRINE D, et al. NHE1 regulates the stratum corneum permeability barrier homeostasis. Microenvironment acidification assessed with fluorescence lifetime imaging. *The Journal of Biological Chemistry* 2002; 277(49): 47399–47406.

64. FLUHR JW, KAO J, JAIN M, AHN SK, FEINGOLD KR, ELIAS PM. Generation of free fatty acids from phospholipids regulates stratum corneum acidification and integrity. *The Journal of Investigative Dermatology* 2001; 117(1): 44–51.

65. HACHEM JP, MAN MQ, CRUMRINE D, UCHIDA Y, BROWN BE, ROGIERS V, et al. Sustained serine proteases activity by prolonged increase in pH leads to degradation of lipid processing enzymes and profound alterations of barrier function and stratum corneum integrity. *The Journal of Investigative Dermatology* 2005; 125(3): 510–520.

66. MAURO T, HOLLERAN WM, GRAYSON S, GAO WN, MAN MQ, KRIEHUBER E, et al. Barrier recovery is impeded at neutral pH, independent of ionic effects: Implications for extracellular lipid processing. *Archives of Dermatological Research* 1998; 290(4): 215–222.

67. YAMASAKI K, SCHAUBER J, CODA A, LIN H, DORSCHNER RA, SCHECHTER NM, et al. Kallikrein-mediated proteolysis regulates the antimicrobial effects of cathelicidins in skin. *The FASEB Journal* 2006; 20(12): 2068–2080.

68. NYLANDER-LUNDQVIST E, EGELRUD T. Formation of active IL-1 beta from pro-IL-1 beta catalyzed by stratum corneum chymotryptic enzyme *in vitro*. *Acta Dermato-Venereologica* 1997; 77(3): 203–206.

69. BARLAND CO, ZETTERSTEN E, BROWN BS, YE J, ELIAS PM, GHADIALLY R. Imiquimod-induced interleukin-1 alpha stimulation improves barrier homeostasis in aged murine epidermis. *The Journal of Investigative Dermatology* 2004; 122(2): 330–336.

70. JIANG YJ, LU B, CRUMRINE D, MAN MQ, ELIAS PM, FEINGOLD KR. IL-1alpha accelerates stratum corneum formation and improves permeability barrier homeostasis during murine fetal development. *Journal of Dermatological Science* 2009; 54(2): 88–98.

71. JENSEN JM, SCHUTZE S, FORL M, KRONKE M, PROKSCH E. Roles for tumor necrosis factor receptor p55 and sphingomyelinase in repairing the cutaneous permeability barrier. *The Journal of Clinical Investigation* 1999; 104(12): 1761–1770.

72. MAN MQ, WOOD L, ELIAS PM, FEINGOLD KR. Cutaneous barrier repair and pathophysiology following barrier disruption in IL-1 and TNF type I receptor deficient mice. *Experimental Dermatology* 1999; 8(4): 261–266.

73. WANG XP, SCHUNCK M, KALLEN KJ, NEUMANN C, TRAUTWEIN C, ROSE-JOHN S, et al. The interleukin-6 cytokine system regulates epidermal permeability barrier homeostasis. *The Journal of Investigative Dermatology* 2004; 123(1): 124–131.

74. STEFANSSON K, BRATTSAND M, ROOSTERMAN D, KEMPKES C, BOCHEVA G, STEINHOFF M, et al. Activation of proteinase-activated receptor-2 by human kallikrein-related peptidases. *The Journal of Investigative Dermatology* 2008; 128(1): 18–25.

75. RAMACHANDRAN R, HOLLENBERG MD. Proteinases and signalling: Pathophysiological and therapeutic implications via PARs and more. *British Journal of Pharmacology* 2008; 153(Suppl.): S263–S282.

76. STEINHOFF M, NEISIUS U, IKOMA A, FARTASCH M, HEYER G, SKOV PS, et al. Proteinase-activated receptor-2 mediates itch: A novel pathway for pruritus in human skin. *The Journal of Neuroscience* 2003; 23(15): 6176–6180.

77. DEMERJIAN M, HACHEM JP, TSCHACHLER E, DENECKER G, DECLERCQ W, VANDENABEELE P, et al. Acute modulations in permeability barrier function regulate epidermal cornification: Role of caspase-14 and the protease-activated receptor type 2. *The American Journal of Pathology* 2008; 172(1): 86–97.

78. MACFARLANE SR, SLOSS CM, CAMERON P, KANKE T, McKENZIE RC, PLEVIN R. The role of intracellular Ca^{2+} in the regulation of proteinase-activated receptor-2 mediated nuclear factor kappa B signalling in keratinocytes. *British Journal of Pharmacology* 2005; 145(4): 535–544.

79. FEINGOLD KR, SCHMUTH M, ELIAS PM. The regulation of permeability barrier homeostasis. *The Journal of Investigative Dermatology* 2007; 127(7): 1574–1576.

80. DENDA M, KITAMURA K, ELIAS PM, FEINGOLD KR. trans-4-(Aminomethyl)cyclohexane carboxylic acid (T-AMCHA), an anti-fibrinolytic agent, accelerates barrier recovery and prevents the epidermal hyperplasia induced by epidermal injury in hairless mice and humans. *The Journal of Investigative Dermatology* 1997; 109(1): 84–90.

81. HACHEM JP, ROELANDT T, SCHURER N, PU X, FLUHR J, GIDDELO C, et al. Acute acidification of stratum corneum membrane domains using polyhydroxyl acids improves lipid processing and inhibits degradation of corneodesmosomes. *The Journal of Investigative Dermatology* 2010; 130(2): 500–510.

82. WHITE MI, JENKINSON DM, LLOYD DH. The effect of washing on the thickness of the stratum corneum in normal and atopic individuals. *The British Journal of Dermatology* 1987; 116(4): 525–530.

83. HOLZLE E, PLEWIG G. Effects of dermatitis, stripping, and steroids on the morphology of corneocytes. A new bioassay. *The Journal of Investigative Dermatology* 1977; 68(6): 350–356.

84. HON KL, WONG KY, LEUNG TF, CHOW CM, NG PC. Comparison of skin hydration evaluation sites and correlations among skin hydration, transepidermal water loss, SCORAD index, Nottingham Eczema Severity Score, and quality of life in patients with atopic dermatitis. *American Journal of Clinical Dermatology* 2008; 9(1): 45–50.

85. VOEGELI R, RAWLINGS AV, BRETERNITZ M, DOPPLER S, SCHREIER T, FLUHR JW. Increased stratum corneum serine protease activity in acute eczematous atopic skin. *The British Journal of Dermatology* 2009; 161: 70–77.

86. SUGARMAN JL, FLUHR JW, FOWLER AJ, BRUCKNER T, DIEPGEN TL, WILLIAMS ML. The objective severity assessment of atopic dermatitis score: An objective measure using permeability barrier function and stratum corneum hydration with computer-assisted estimates for extent of disease. *Archives of Dermatology* 2003; 139(11): 1417–1422.

87. JENSEN JM, FOLSTER-HOLST R, BARANOWSKY A, SCHUNCK M, WINOTO-MORBACH S, NEUMANN C, et al. Impaired sphingomyelinase activity and epidermal differentiation in atopic dermatitis. *The Journal of Investigative Dermatology* 2004; 122(6): 1423–1431.

88. GUTTMAN-YASSKY E, SUAREZ-FARINAS M, CHIRICOZZI A, NOGRALES KE, SHEMER A, FUENTES-DUCULAN J, et al. Broad defects in epidermal cornification in atopic dermatitis identified through genomic analysis. *The Journal of Allergy and Clinical Immunology* 2009; 124(6): 1235–1244.

89. SUGIURA H, EBISE H, TAZAWA T, TANAKA K, SUGIURA Y, UEHARA M, et al. Large-scale DNA microarray analysis of atopic skin lesions shows overexpression of an epidermal differentiation gene cluster in the alternative pathway and lack of protective gene expression in the cornified envelope. *The British Journal of Dermatology* 2005; 152(1): 146–149.

90. SEGUCHI T, CUI CY, KUSUDA S, TAKAHASHI M, AISU K, TEZUKA T. Decreased expression of filaggrin in atopic skin. *Archives of Dermatological Research* 1996; 288(8): 442–446.

91. NAKAGAWA N, SAKAI S, MATSUMOTO M, YAMADA K, NAGANO M, YUKI T, et al. Relationship between NMF (lactate and potassium) content and the physical properties of the stratum corneum in healthy subjects. *The Journal of Investigative Dermatology* 2004; 122(3): 755–763.

92. NEMOTO-HASEBE I, AKIYAMA M, NOMURA T, SANDILANDS A, MCLEAN WH, SHIMIZU H. Clinical severity correlates with impaired barrier in filaggrin-related eczema. *The Journal of Investigative Dermatology* 2009; 129(3): 682–689.

93. SERGEANT A, CAMPBELL LE, HULL PR, PORTER M, PALMER CN, SMITH FJ, et al. Heterozygous null alleles in filaggrin contribute to clinical dry skin in young adults and the elderly. *The Journal of Investigative Dermatology* 2009; 129(4): 1042–1045.

94. SCHARSCHMIDT TC, MAN MQ, HATANO Y, CRUMRINE D, GUNATHILAKE R, SUNDBERG JP, et al. Filaggrin deficiency confers a paracellular barrier abnormality that reduces inflammatory thresholds to irritants and haptens. *The Journal of Allergy and Clinical Immunology* 2009; 124(3): 496–506.

95. PROKSCH E, JENSEN JM, ELIAS PM. Skin lipids and epidermal differentiation in atopic dermatitis. *Clinics in Dermatology* 2003; 21(2): 134–144.

96. DI NARDO A, WERTZ P, GIANNETTI A, SEIDENARI S. Ceramide and cholesterol composition of the skin of patients with atopic dermatitis. *Acta Dermato-Venereologica* 1998; 78(1): 27–30.

97. MEGURO S, ARAI Y, MASUKAWA Y, UIE K, TOKIMITSU I. Relationship between covalently bound ceramides and transepidermal water loss (TEWL). *Archives of Dermatological Research* 2000; 292(9): 463–468.

98. SCHAFER L, KRAGBALLE K. Abnormalities in epidermal lipid metabolism in patients with atopic dermatitis. *The Journal of Investigative Dermatology* 1991; 96(1): 10–15.

99. KOMATSU N, SAIJOH K, KUK C, LIU AC, KHAN S, SHIRASAKI F, et al. Human tissue kallikrein expression in the stratum corneum and serum of atopic dermatitis patients. *Experimental Dermatology* 2007; 16(6): 513–519.

100. HANSSON L, BACKMAN A, NY A, EDLUND M, EKHOLM E, EKSTRAND HAMMARSTROM B, et al. Epidermal overexpression of stratum corneum chymotryptic enzyme in mice: A model for chronic itchy dermatitis. *The Journal of Investigative Dermatology* 2002; 118(3): 444–449.

101. BRIOT A, DERAISON C, LACROIX M, BONNART C, ROBIN A, BESSON C, et al. Kallikrein 5 induces atopic dermatitis-like lesions through PAR2-mediated thymic stromal lymphopoietin expression in Netherton syndrome. *The Journal of Experimental Medicine* 2009; 206(5): 1135–1147.

102. HACHEM JP, CRUMRINE D, FLUHR J, BROWN BE, FEINGOLD KR, ELIAS PM. pH directly regulates epidermal permeability barrier homeostasis, and stratum corneum integrity/cohesion. *The Journal of Investigative Dermatology* 2003; 121(2): 345–353.

103. HATANO Y, MAN MQ, UCHIDA Y, CRUMRINE D, SCHARSCHMIDT TC, KIM EG, et al. Maintenance of an acidic stratum corneum prevents emergence of murine atopic dermatitis. *The Journal of Investigative Dermatology* 2009; 129(7): 1524–1535.

104. BARKER JN, PALMER CN, ZHAO Y, LIAO H, HULL PR, LEE SP, et al. Null mutations in the filaggrin gene (FLG) determine major susceptibility to early-onset atopic dermatitis that persists into adulthood. *The Journal of Investigative Dermatology* 2007; 127(3): 564–567.

105. BROWN SJ, RELTON CL, LIAO H, ZHAO Y, SANDILANDS A, WILSON IJ, et al. Filaggrin null mutations and childhood atopic eczema: A population-based case-control study. *The Journal of Allergy and Clinical Immunology* 2008; 121(4): 940–946 e3.

106. EKELUND E, LIEDEN A, LINK J, LEE SP, D'AMATO M, PALMER CN, et al. Loss-of-function variants of the filaggrin gene are associated with atopic eczema and associated phenotypes in Swedish families. *Acta Dermato-Venereologica* 2008; 88(1): 15–19.

107. HUBICHE T, GED C, BENARD A, LEAUTE-LABREZE C, MCELREAVEY K, de VERNEUIL H, et al. Analysis of SPINK 5, KLK 7 and FLG genotypes in a French atopic dermatitis cohort. *Acta Dermato-Venereologica* 2007; 87(6): 499–505.

108. MARENHOLZ I, NICKEL R, RUSCHENDORF F, SCHULZ F, ESPARZA-GORDILLO J, KERSCHER T, et al. Filaggrin loss-of-function mutations predispose to phenotypes involved in the atopic march. *The Journal of Allergy and Clinical Immunology* 2006; 118(4): 866–871.

109. MORAR N, COOKSON WO, HARPER JI, MOFFATT MF. Filaggrin mutations in children with severe atopic dermatitis. *The Journal of Investigative Dermatology* 2007; 127(7): 1667–1672.

110. NOMURA T, AKIYAMA M, SANDILANDS A, NEMOTO-HASEBE I, SAKAI K, NAGASAKI A, et al. Prevalent and rare mutations in the gene encoding filaggrin in japanese patients with ichthyosis vulgaris and atopic dermatitis. *The Journal of Investigative Dermatology* 2009; 129(5): 1302–1305.

111. NOMURA T, SANDILANDS A, AKIYAMA M, LIAO H, EVANS AT, SAKAI K, et al. Unique mutations in the filaggrin gene in Japanese patients with ichthyosis vulgaris and atopic dermatitis. *The Journal of Allergy and Clinical Immunology* 2007; 119(2): 434–440.

112. O'REGAN GM, SANDILANDS A, MCLEAN WH, IRVINE AD. Filaggrin in atopic dermatitis. *The Journal of Allergy and Clinical Immunology* 2008; 122(4): 689–693.

113. PALMER CN, IRVINE AD, TERRON-KWIATKOWSKI A, ZHAO Y, LIAO H, LEE SP, et al. Common loss-of-function variants of the epidermal barrier protein filaggrin are a major predisposing factor for atopic dermatitis. *Nature Genetics* 2006; 38(4): 441–446.

114. ROGERS AJ, CELEDON JC, LASKY-SU JA, WEISS ST, RABY BA. Filaggrin mutations confer susceptibility to atopic dermatitis but not to asthma. *The Journal of Allergy and Clinical Immunology* 2007; 120(6): 1332–1337.

115. RUETHER A, STOLL M, SCHWARZ T, SCHREIBER S, FOLSTER-HOLST R. Filaggrin loss-of-function variant contributes to atopic dermatitis risk in the population of Northern Germany. *The British Journal of Dermatology* 2006; 155(5): 1093–1094.

116. SANDILANDS A, O'REGAN GM, LIAO H, ZHAO Y, TERRON-KWIATKOWSKI A, WATSON RM, et al. Prevalent and rare mutations in the gene encoding filaggrin cause ichthyosis vulgaris and predispose individuals to atopic dermatitis. *The Journal of Investigative Dermatology* 2006; 126(8): 1770–1775.

117. SANDILANDS A, TERRON-KWIATKOWSKI A, HULL PR, O'REGAN GM, CLAYTON TH, WATSON RM, et al. Comprehensive analysis of the gene encoding filaggrin uncovers prevalent and rare mutations in ichthyosis vulgaris and atopic eczema. *Nature Genetics* 2007; 39(5): 650–654.

118. STEMMLER S, PARWEZ Q, PETRASCH-PARWEZ E, EPPLEN JT, HOFFJAN S. Two common loss-of-function mutations within the filaggrin gene predispose for early onset of atopic dermatitis. *The Journal of Investigative Dermatology* 2007; 127(3): 722–724.

119. WEIDINGER S, BAURECHT H, WAGENPFEIL S, HENDERSON J, NOVAK N, SANDILANDS A, et al. Analysis of the individual and aggregate genetic contributions of previously identified serine peptidase inhibitor Kazal type 5 (SPINK5), kallikrein-related peptidase 7 (KLK7), and filaggrin (FLG) polymorphisms to eczema risk. *The Journal of Allergy and Clinical Immunology* 2008; 122(3): 560–568 e4.

120. KEZIC S, KEMPERMAN PM, KOSTER ES, de JONGH CM, THIO HB, CAMPBELL LE, et al. Loss-of-function mutations in the filaggrin gene lead to reduced level of natural moisturizing factor in the stratum corneum. *The Journal of Investigative Dermatology* 2008; 128(8): 2117–2119.

121. BROWN SJ, MCLEAN WH. Eczema genetics: Current state of knowledge and future goals. *The Journal of Investigative Dermatology* 2009; 129(3): 543–552.

122. GREISENEGGER E, NOVAK N, MAINTZ L, BIEBER T, ZIMPRICH F, HAUBENBERGER D, et al. Analysis of four prevalent filaggrin mutations (R501X, 2282del4, R2447X and S3247X) in Austrian and

German patients with atopic dermatitis. *Journal of the European Academy of Dermatology and Venereology* 2010; 24(5): 607–610.

123. JUNGERSTED JM, SCHEER H, MEMPEL M, BAURECHT H, CIFUENTES L, HOGH JK, et al. Stratum corneum lipids, skin barrier function and filaggrin mutations in patients with atopic eczema. *Allergy* 2010; 65(7): 911–918.

124. KRIEN PM, KERMICI M. Evidence for the existence of a self-regulated enzymatic process within the human stratum corneum—An unexpected role for urocanic acid. *The Journal of Investigative Dermatology* 2000; 115(3): 414–420.

125. ELIAS PM. Barrier repair trumps immunology in the pathogenesis and therapy of atopic dermatitis. *Drug Discovery Today: Disease Mechanisms* 2008; 5(1): e33–e38.

126. FALLON PG, SASAKI T, SANDILANDS A, CAMPBELL LE, SAUNDERS SP, MANGAN NE, et al. A homozygous frameshift mutation in the mouse Flg gene facilitates enhanced percutaneous allergen priming. *Nature Genetics* 2009; 41(5): 602–608.

127. THYSSEN JP, JOHANSEN JD, LINNEBERG A, MENNE T, NIELSEN NH, MELDGAARD M, et al. The association between null mutations in the filaggrin gene and contact sensitization to nickel and other chemicals in the general population. *The British Journal of Dermatology* 2010; 162(6): 1278–1285.

128. MISCHKE D, KORGE BP, MARENHOLZ I, VOLZ A, ZIEGLER A. Genes encoding structural proteins of epidermal cornification and S100 calcium-binding proteins form a gene complex ("epidermal differentiation complex") on human chromosome 1q21. *The Journal of Investigative Dermatology* 1996; 106(5): 989–992.

129. LIEDEN A, EKELUND E, KUO IC, KOCKUM I, HUANG CH, MALLBRIS L, et al. Cornulin, a marker of late epidermal differentiation, is down-regulated in eczema. *Allergy* 2009; 64(2): 304–311.

130. ESPARZA-GORDILLO J, WEIDINGER S, FOLSTER-HOLST R, BAUERFEIND A, RUSCHENDORF F, PATONE G, et al. A common variant on chromosome 11q13 is associated with atopic dermatitis. *Nature Genetics* 2009; 41(5): 596–601.

131. KATO A, FUKAI K, OISO N, HOSOMI N, MURAKAMI T, ISHII M. Association of SPINK5 gene polymorphisms with atopic dermatitis in the Japanese population. *The British Journal of Dermatology* 2003; 148(4): 665–669.

132. NISHIO Y, NOGUCHI E, SHIBASAKI M, KAMIOKA M, ICHIKAWA E, ICHIKAWA K, et al. Association between polymorphisms in the SPINK5 gene and atopic dermatitis in the Japanese. *Genes and Immunity* 2003; 4(7): 515–517.

133. WALLEY AJ, CHAVANAS S, MOFFATT MF, ESNOUF RM, UBHI B, LAWRENCE R, et al. Gene polymorphism in Netherton and common atopic disease. *Nature Genetics* 2001; 29(2): 175–178.

134. KOMATSU N, TAKATA M, OTSUKI N, OHKA R, AMANO O, TAKEHARA K, et al. Elevated stratum corneum hydrolytic activity in Netherton syndrome suggests an inhibitory regulation of desquamation by SPINK5-derived peptides. *The Journal of Investigative Dermatology* 2002; 118(3): 436–443.

135. SPRECHER E, CHAVANAS S, DIGIOVANNA JJ, AMIN S, NIELSEN K, PRENDIVILLE JS, et al. The spectrum of pathogenic mutations in SPINK5 in 19 families with Netherton syndrome: Implications for mutation detection and first case of prenatal diagnosis. *The Journal of Investigative Dermatology* 2001; 117(2): 179–187.

136. COMEL M. Ichthyosis linearis circumflexa. *Dermatologica* 1949; 98(3): 133–136.

137. ROEDL D, TRAIDL-HOFFMANN C, RING J, BEHRENDT H, BRAUN-FALCO M. Serine protease inhibitor lymphoepithelial Kazal type-related inhibitor tends to be decreased in atopic dermatitis. *Journal of the European Academy of Dermatology and Venereology* 2009; 23(11): 1263–1266.

138. LEE YA, WAHN U, KEHRT R, TARANI L, BUSINCO L, GUSTAFSSON D, et al. A major susceptibility locus for atopic dermatitis maps to chromosome 3q21. *Nature Genetics* 2000; 26(4): 470–473.

139. VASILOPOULOS Y, CORK MJ, TEARE D, MARINOU I, WARD SJ, DUFF GW, et al. A nonsynonymous substitution of cystatin A, a cysteine protease inhibitor of house dust mite protease, leads to decreased mRNA stability and shows a significant association with atopic dermatitis. *Allergy* 2007; 62(5): 514–519.

140. VASILOPOULOS Y, CORK MJ, MURPHY R, WILLIAMS HC, ROBINSON DA, DUFF GW, et al. Genetic association between an AACC insertion in the 3'UTR of the stratum corneum chymotryptic enzyme gene and atopic dermatitis. *The Journal of Investigative Dermatology* 2004; 123(1): 62–66.

141. Saaf AM, Tengvall-Linder M, Chang HY, Adler AS, Wahlgren CF, Scheynius A, et al. Global expression profiling in atopic eczema reveals reciprocal expression of inflammatory and lipid genes. *PLoS ONE* 2008; 3(12): e4017.

142. Voegeli R, Rawlings AV, Doppler S, Schreier T. Increased basal transepidermal water loss leads to elevation of some but not all stratum corneum serine proteases. *International Journal of Cosmetic Science* 2008; 30(6): 435–442.

143. Seidenari S, Giusti G. Objective assessment of the skin of children affected by atopic dermatitis: A study of pH, capacitance and TEWL in eczematous and clinically uninvolved skin. *Acta Dermato-Venereologica* 1995; 75(6): 429–433.

144. Matsumoto M, Sugiura H, Uehara M. Skin barrier function in patients with completely healed atopic dermatitis. *Journal of Dermatological Science* 2000; 23(3): 178–182.

145. Jakasa I, Verberk MM, Esposito M, Bos JD, Kezic S. Altered penetration of polyethylene glycols into uninvolved skin of atopic dermatitis patients. *The Journal of Investigative Dermatology* 2007; 127(1): 129–134.

146. Yoshiike T, Aikawa Y, Sindhvananda J, Suto H, Nishimura K, Kawamoto T, et al. Skin barrier defect in atopic dermatitis: Increased permeability of the stratum corneum using dimethyl sulfoxide and theophylline. *Journal of Dermatological Science* 1993; 5(2): 92–96.

147. Jakasa I, de Jongh CM, Verberk MM, Bos JD, Kezic S. Percutaneous penetration of sodium lauryl sulphate is increased in uninvolved skin of patients with atopic dermatitis compared with control subjects. *The British Journal of Dermatology* 2006; 155(1): 104–109.

148. Kao JS, Fluhr JW, Man MQ, Fowler AJ, Hachem JP, Crumrine D, et al. Short-term glucocorticoid treatment compromises both permeability barrier homeostasis and stratum corneum integrity: Inhibition of epidermal lipid synthesis accounts for functional abnormalities. *The Journal of Investigative Dermatology* 2003; 120(3): 456–464.

149. Cork MJ, Varghese J, Sultan A, Guy RH, Lane ME, Al Enezi T (eds.). Therapeutic implications of the differential effects of topical corticosteroids and calcineurin inhibitors on the skin barrier. 5th George Rajka International Symposium on Atopic Dermatitis (ISAD), Kyoto, 2008.

150. Novak N, Baurecht H, Schafer T, Rodriguez E, Wagenpfeil S, Klopp N, et al. Loss-of-function mutations in the filaggrin gene and allergic contact sensitization to nickel. *The Journal of Investigative Dermatology* 2008; 128(6): 1430–1435.

151. Kezic S, Kammeyer A, Calkoen F, Fluhr JW, Bos JD. Natural moisturizing factor components in the stratum corneum as biomarkers of filaggrin genotype: Evaluation of minimally invasive methods. *The British Journal of Dermatology* 2009; 161(5): 1098–1104.

152. Conti A, Rogers J, Verdejo P, Harding CR, Rawlings AV. Seasonal influences on stratum corneum ceramide 1 fatty acids and the influence of topical essential fatty acids. *International Journal of Cosmetic Science* 1996; 18(1): 1–12.

153. Voegeli R, Rawlings AV, Doppler S, Heiland J, Schreier T. Profiling of serine protease activities in human stratum corneum and detection of a stratum corneum tryptase-like enzyme. *International Journal of Cosmetic Science* 2007; 29(3): 191–200.

154. Rogers J, Harding C, Mayo A, Banks J, Rawlings A. Stratum corneum lipids: The effect of ageing and the seasons. *Archives of Dermatological Research* 1996; 288(12): 765–770.

155. Marenholz I, Kerscher T, Bauerfeind A, Esparza-Gordillo J, Nickel R, Keil T, et al. An interaction between filaggrin mutations and early food sensitization improves the prediction of childhood asthma. *The Journal of Allergy and Clinical Immunology* 2009; 123(4): 911–916.

156. Bisgaard H, Simpson A, Palmer CN, Bonnelykke K, McLean I, Mukhopadhyay S, et al. Gene-environment interaction in the onset of eczema in infancy: Filaggrin loss-of-function mutations enhanced by neonatal cat exposure. *PLoS Medicine* 2008; 5(6): e131.

157. Bunikowski R, Mielke ME, Skarabis H, Worm M, Anagnostopoulos I, Kolde G, et al. Evidence for a disease-promoting effect of *Staphylococcus aureus*-derived exotoxins in atopic dermatitis. *The Journal of Allergy and Clinical Immunology* 2000; 105(4): 814–819.

158. Hauser C, Wuethrich B, Matter L, Wilhelm JA, Sonnabend W, Schopfer K. *Staphylococcus aureus* skin colonization in atopic dermatitis patients. *Dermatologica* 1985; 170(1): 35–39.

159. ZOLLNER TM, WICHELHAUS TA, HARTUNG A, VON MALLINCKRODT C, WAGNER TO, BRADE V, et al. Colonization with superantigen-producing *Staphylococcus aureus* is associated with increased severity of atopic dermatitis. *Clinical and Experimental Allergy* 2000; 30(7): 994–1000.

160. HUANG JT, ABRAMS M, TLOUGAN B, RADEMAKER A, PALLER AS. Treatment of *Staphylococcus aureus* colonization in atopic dermatitis decreases disease severity. *Pediatrics* 2009; 123(5): e808–e814.

161. LEYDEN JJ, MARPLES RR, KLIGMAN AM. *Staphylococcus aureus* in the lesions of atopic dermatitis. *The British Journal of Dermatology* 1974; 90(5): 525–530.

162. DRAKE DR, BROGDEN KA, DAWSON DV, WERTZ PW. Thematic review series: Skin lipids. Antimicrobial lipids at the skin surface. *Journal of Lipid Research* 2008; 49(1): 4–11.

163. MELNIK B. Disturbances of antimicrobial lipids in atopic dermatitis. *Journal der Deutschen Dermatologischen Gesellschaft* 2006; 4(2): 114–123.

164. HIRASAWA Y, TAKAI T, NAKAMURA T, MITSUISHI K, GUNAWAN H, SUTO H, et al. *Staphylococcus aureus* extracellular protease causes epidermal barrier dysfunction. *The Journal of Investigative Dermatology* 2010; 130(2): 614–617.

165. DUBIN G. Extracellular proteases of *Staphylococcus* spp. *Biological Chemistry* 2002; 383(7–8): 1075–1086.

166. AMAGAI M, YAMAGUCHI T, HANAKAWA Y, NISHIFUJI K, SUGAI M, STANLEY JR. Staphylococcal exfoliative toxin B specifically cleaves desmoglein 1. *The Journal of Investigative Dermatology* 2002; 118(5): 845–850.

167. NISHIFUJI K, SUGAI M, AMAGAI M. Staphylococcal exfoliative toxins: "Molecular scissors" of bacteria that attack the cutaneous defense barrier in mammals. *Journal of Dermatological Science* 2008; 49(1): 21–31.

168. OHNISHI Y, OKINO N, ITO M, IMAYAMA S. Ceramidase activity in bacterial skin flora as a possible cause of ceramide deficiency in atopic dermatitis. *Clinical and Diagnostic Laboratory Immunology* 1999; 6(1): 101–104.

169. JEONG SK, KIM HJ, YOUM JK, AHN SK, CHOI EH, SOHN MH, et al. Mite and cockroach allergens activate protease-activated receptor 2 and delay epidermal permeability barrier recovery. *The Journal of Investigative Dermatology* 2008; 128(8): 1930–1939.

170. KOUZAKI H, O'GRADY SM, LAWRENCE CB, KITA H. Proteases induce production of thymic stromal lymphopoietin by airway epithelial cells through protease-activated receptor-2. *Journal of Immunology* 2009; 183(2): 1427–1434.

171. HEDAYATI MT, ARABZADEHMOGHADAM A, HAJHEYDARI Z. Specific IgE against *Alternaria alternata* in atopic dermatitis and asthma patients. *European Review for Medical and Pharmacological Sciences* 2009; 13(3): 187–191.

172. BECKHAM SA, BOYD SE, REYNOLDS S, WILLIS C, JOHNSTONE M, MIKA A, et al. Characterization of a serine protease homologous to house dust mite group 3 allergens from the scabies mite *Sarcoptes scabiei. The Journal of Biological Chemistry* 2009; 284(49): 34413–34422.

173. DARSOW U, LAIFAOUI J, KERSCHENLOHR K, WOLLENBERG A, PRZYBILLA B, WUTHRICH B, et al. The prevalence of positive reactions in the atopy patch test with aeroallergens and food allergens in subjects with atopic eczema: A European multicenter study. *Allergy* 2004; 59(12): 1318–1325.

174. COLLOFF MJ. Exposure to house dust mites in homes of people with atopic dermatitis. *The British Journal of Dermatology* 1992; 127(4): 322–327.

175. NIKOLOVSKI J, STAMATAS GN, KOLLIAS N, WIEGAND BC. Barrier function and water-holding and transport properties of infant stratum corneum are different from adult and continue to develop through the first year of life. *The Journal of Investigative Dermatology* 2008; 128(7): 1728–1736.

176. NICKOLOFF BJ, NAIDU Y. Perturbation of epidermal barrier function correlates with initiation of cytokine cascade in human skin. *Journal of the American Academy of Dermatology* 1994; 30(4): 535–546.

177. OYOSHI MK, HE R, KUMAR L, YOON J, GEHA RS. Cellular and molecular mechanisms in atopic dermatitis. *Advances in Immunology* 2009; 102: 135–226.

178. NYLANDER-LUNDQVIST E, BACK O, EGELRUD T. IL-1 beta activation in human epidermis. *Journal of Immunology* 1996; 157(4): 1699–1704.

179. WOOD LC, ELIAS PM, CALHOUN C, TSAI JC, GRUNFELD C, FEINGOLD KR. Barrier disruption stimulates interleukin-1 alpha expression and release from a pre-formed pool in murine epidermis. *The Journal of Investigative Dermatology* 1996; 106(3): 397–403.

180. KATO T, TAKAI T, FUJIMURA T, MATSUOKA H, OGAWA T, MURAYAMA K, et al. Mite serine protease activates protease-activated receptor-2 and induces cytokine release in human keratinocytes. *Allergy* 2009; 64(9): 1366–1374.

181. BUDDENKOTTE J, STROH C, ENGELS IH, MOORMANN C, SHPACOVITCH VM, SEELIGER S, et al. Agonists of proteinase-activated receptor-2 stimulate upregulation of intercellular cell adhesion molecule-1 in primary human keratinocytes via activation of NF-kappa B. *The Journal of Investigative Dermatology* 2005; 124(1): 38–45.

182. HE R, GEHA RS. Thymic stromal lymphopoietin. *Annals of the New York Academy of Sciences* 2010; 1183: 13–24.

183. SOUMELIS V, RECHE PA, KANZLER H, YUAN W, EDWARD G, HOMEY B, et al. Human epithelial cells trigger dendritic cell mediated allergic inflammation by producing TSLP. *Nature Immunology* 2002; 3(7): 673–680.

184. EBNER S, NGUYEN VA, FORSTNER M, WANG YH, WOLFRAM D, LIU YJ, et al. Thymic stromal lymphopoietin converts human epidermal Langerhans cells into antigen-presenting cells that induce proallergic T cells. *The Journal of Allergy and Clinical Immunology* 2007; 119(4): 982–990.

185. RECHE PA, SOUMELIS V, GORMAN DM, CLIFFORD T, LIU M, TRAVIS M, et al. Human thymic stromal lymphopoietin preferentially stimulates myeloid cells. *Journal of Immunology* 2001; 167(1): 336–343.

186. ALLAKHVERDI Z, COMEAU MR, JESSUP HK, YOON BR, BREWER A, CHARTIER S, et al. Thymic stromal lymphopoietin is released by human epithelial cells in response to microbes, trauma, or inflammation and potently activates mast cells. *The Journal of Experimental Medicine* 2007; 204(2): 253–258.

187. LEUNG DY, BOGUNIEWICZ M, HOWELL MD, NOMURA I, HAMID QA. New insights into atopic dermatitis. *The Journal of Clinical Investigation* 2004; 113(5): 651–657.

188. CHAN LS, ROBINSON N, XU L. Expression of interleukin-4 in the epidermis of transgenic mice results in a pruritic inflammatory skin disease: An experimental animal model to study atopic dermatitis. *The Journal of Investigative Dermatology* 2001; 117(4): 977–983.

189. ZHENG T, OH MH, OH SY, SCHROEDER JT, GLICK AB, ZHU Z. Transgenic expression of interleukin-13 in the skin induces a pruritic dermatitis and skin remodeling. *The Journal of Investigative Dermatology* 2009; 129(3): 742–751.

190. KAKINUMA T, NAKAMURA K, WAKUGAWA M, MITSUI H, TADA Y, SAEKI H, et al. Thymus and activation-regulated chemokine in atopic dermatitis: Serum thymus and activation-regulated chemokine level is closely related with disease activity. *The Journal of Allergy and Clinical Immunology* 2001; 107(3): 535–541.

191. AKBARI O, DEKRUYFF RH, UMETSU DT. Pulmonary dendritic cells producing IL-10 mediate tolerance induced by respiratory exposure to antigen. *Nature Immunology* 2001; 2(8): 725–731.

192. ZUANY-AMORIM C, HAILE S, LEDUC D, DUMAREY C, HUERRE M, VARGAFTIG BB, et al. Interleukin-10 inhibits antigen-induced cellular recruitment into the airways of sensitized mice. *The Journal of Clinical Investigation* 1995; 95(6): 2644–2651.

193. BOGUNIEWICZ M, LEUNG DY. Recent insights into atopic dermatitis and implications for management of infectious complications. *The Journal of Allergy and Clinical Immunology* 2010; 125(1): 4–13. quiz 4–5.

194. YOO J, OMORI M, GYARMATI D, ZHOU B, AYE T, BREWER A, et al. Spontaneous atopic dermatitis in mice expressing an inducible thymic stromal lymphopoietin transgene specifically in the skin. *The Journal of Experimental Medicine* 2005; 202(4): 541–549.

195. MIHM MC, JR, SOTER NA, DVORAK HF, AUSTEN KF. The structure of normal skin and the morphology of atopic eczema. *The Journal of Investigative Dermatology* 1976; 67(3): 305–312.

196. UEHARA M, MIYAUCHI H. The morphologic characteristics of dry skin in atopic dermatitis. *Archives of Dermatology* 1984; 120(9): 1186–1190.

197. TAGAMI H, KOBAYASHI H, O'GOSHI K, KIKUCHI K. Atopic xerosis: Employment of noninvasive biophysical instrumentation for the functional analyses of the mildly abnormal stratum corneum

and for the efficacy assessment of skin care products. *Journal of Cosmetic Dermatology* 2006; 5(2): 140–149.

198. HATANO Y, KATAGIRI K, ARAKAWA S, FUJIWARA S. Interleukin-4 depresses levels of transcripts for acid-sphingomyelinase and glucocerebrosidase and the amount of ceramide in acetone-wounded epidermis, as demonstrated in a living skin equivalent. *Journal of Dermatological Science* 2007; 47(1): 45–47.

199. HATANO Y, TERASHI H, ARAKAWA S, KATAGIRI K. Interleukin-4 suppresses the enhancement of ceramide synthesis and cutaneous permeability barrier functions induced by tumor necrosis factor-alpha and interferon-gamma in human epidermis. *The Journal of Investigative Dermatology* 2005; 124(4): 786–792.

200. HOWELL MD, KIM BE, GAO P, GRANT AV, BOGUNIEWICZ M, DEBENEDETTO A, et al. Cytokine modulation of atopic dermatitis filaggrin skin expression. *The Journal of Allergy and Clinical Immunology* 2007; 120(1): 150–155.

201. KIM BE, LEUNG DY, BOGUNIEWICZ M, HOWELL MD. Loricrin and involucrin expression is down-regulated by Th2 cytokines through STAT-6. *Clinical Immunology* 2008; 126(3): 332–337.

202. KOBAYASHI J, INAI T, MORITA K, MOROI Y, URABE K, SHIBATA Y, et al. Reciprocal regulation of permeability through a cultured keratinocyte sheet by IFN-gamma and IL-4. *Cytokine* 2004; 28(4–5): 186–189.

203. HOWELL MD, FAIRCHILD HR, KIM BE, BIN L, BOGUNIEWICZ M, REDZIC JS, et al. Th2 cytokines act on S100/A11 to downregulate keratinocyte differentiation. *The Journal of Investigative Dermatology* 2008; 128(9): 2248–2258.

204. SEHRA S, YAO Y, HOWELL MD, NGUYEN ET, KANSAS GS, LEUNG DY, et al. IL-4 regulates skin homeostasis and the predisposition toward allergic skin inflammation. *Journal of Immunology* 2010; 184(6): 3186–3190.

205. BADERTSCHER K, BRONNIMANN M, KARLEN S, BRAATHEN LR, YAWALKAR N. Mast cell chymase is increased in chronic atopic dermatitis but not in psoriasis. *Archives of Dermatological Research* 2005; 296(10): 503–506.

206. MAO XQ, SHIRAKAWA T, ENOMOTO T, SHIMAZU S, DAKE Y, KITANO H, et al. Association between variants of mast cell chymase gene and serum IgE levels in eczema. *Human Heredity* 1998; 48(1): 38–41.

207. FIELDS RC, SCHOENECKER JG, HART JP, HOFFMAN MR, PIZZO SV, LAWSON JH. Protease-activated receptor-2 signaling triggers dendritic cell development. *The American Journal of Pathology* 2003; 162(6): 1817–1822.

208. MIIKE S, MCWILLIAM AS, KITA H. Trypsin induces activation and inflammatory mediator release from human eosinophils through protease-activated receptor-2. *Journal of Immunology* 2001; 167(11): 6615–6622.

209. MOORMANN C, ARTUC M, POHL E, VARGA G, BUDDENKOTTE J, VERGNOLLE N, et al. Functional characterization and expression analysis of the proteinase-activated receptor-2 in human cutaneous mast cells. *The Journal of Investigative Dermatology* 2006; 126(4): 746–755.

210. TEMKIN V, KANTOR B, WEG V, HARTMAN ML, LEVI-SCHAFFER F. Tryptase activates the mitogen-activated protein kinase/activator protein-1 pathway in human peripheral blood eosinophils, causing cytokine production and release. *Journal of Immunology* 2002; 169(5): 2662–2669.

211. BIEBER T. Atopic dermatitis. *The New England Journal of Medicine* 2008; 358(14): 1483–1494.

212. ILLI S, von MUTIUS E, LAU S, NICKEL R, GRUBER C, NIGGEMANN B, et al. The natural course of atopic dermatitis from birth to age 7 years and the association with asthma. *The Journal of Allergy and Clinical Immunology* 2004; 113(5): 925–931.

213. NOVAK N, KRAFT S, BIEBER T. Unraveling the mission of FcepsilonRI on antigen-presenting cells. *The Journal of Allergy and Clinical Immunology* 2003; 111(1): 38–44.

214. HULSE KE, REEFER AJ, ENGELHARD VH, PATRIE JT, ZIEGLER SF, CHAPMAN MD, et al. Targeting allergen to FcgammaRI reveals a novel T(H)2 regulatory pathway linked to thymic stromal lymphopoietin receptor. *The Journal of Allergy and Clinical Immunology* 2010; 125(1): 247–256. e1–8.

215. NOVAK N, BIEBER T, LEUNG DY. Immune mechanisms leading to atopic dermatitis. *The Journal of Allergy and Clinical Immunology* 2003; 112(6 Suppl.): S128–S139.

216. DEMEHRI S, MORIMOTO M, HOLTZMAN MJ, KOPAN R. Skin-derived TSLP triggers progression from epidermal-barrier defects to asthma. *PLoS Biology* 2009; 7(5): e1000067.
217. HENGGE UR, RUZICKA T, SCHWARTZ RA, CORK MJ. Adverse effects of topical glucocorticosteroids. *Journal of the American Academy of Dermatology* 2006; 54(1): 1–15, quiz 6–8.
218. SHEU HM, LEE JY, CHAI CY, KUO KW. Depletion of stratum corneum intercellular lipid lamellae and barrier function abnormalities after long-term topical corticosteroids. *The British Journal of Dermatology* 1997; 136(6): 884–890.
219. SHEU HM, TAI CL, KUO KW, YU HS, CHAI CY. Modulation of epidermal terminal differentiation in patients after long-term topical corticosteroids. *The Journal of Dermatology* 1991; 18(8): 454–464.
220. KOLBE L, KLIGMAN AM, SCHREINER V, STOUDEMAYER T. Corticosteroid-induced atrophy and barrier impairment measured by non-invasive methods in human skin. *Skin Research and Technology* 2001; 7(2): 73–77.
221. CORK MJ, ROBINSON DA, VASILOPOULOS Y, FERGUSON A. The effects of topical corticosteroids and pimecrolimus on skin barrier function, gene expression and topical drug penetration in atopic eczema and unaffected controls. *Journal of the American Academy of Dermatology* 2007; 56(Suppl. 2): AB69.
222. CORK MJ, VARGHESE J, HADGRAFT J, LANE ME, FERGUSON A, MOUSTAFA M. Differences in the effect of topical corticosteroids and calcineurin inhibitors on the skin barrier—implications for therapy. *The Journal of Investigative Dermatology* 2007; 127(S45): 545.
223. BJORNBERG A. Erythema craquele provoked by corticosteroids on normal skin. *Acta Dermato-Venereologica* 1982; 62(2): 147–151.
224. ZHENG PS, LAVKER RM, LEHMANN P, KLIGMAN AM. Morphologic investigations on the rebound phenomenon after corticosteroid-induced atrophy in human skin. *The Journal of Investigative Dermatology* 1984; 82(4): 345–352.
225. RAPAPORT MJ, LEBWOHL M. Corticosteroid addiction and withdrawal in the atopic: The red burning skin syndrome. *Clinics in Dermatology* 2003; 21(3): 201–214.
226. CORK MJ, ROBINSON DA, VASILOPOULOS Y, FERGUSON A, MOUSTAFA M, MACGOWAN A, et al. New perspectives on epidermal barrier dysfunction in atopic dermatitis: Gene-environment interactions. *The Journal of Allergy and Clinical Immunology* 2006; 118(1): 3–21. quiz 2–3.
227. ALOMAR A, BERTH-JONES J, BOS JD, GIANNETTI A, REITAMO S, RUZICKA T, et al. The role of topical calcineurin inhibitors in atopic dermatitis. *The British Journal of Dermatology* 2004; 151(Suppl. 70): 3–27.
228. ASHCROFT DM, DIMMOCK P, GARSIDE R, STEIN K, WILLIAMS HC. Efficacy and tolerability of topical pimecrolimus and tacrolimus in the treatment of atopic dermatitis: Meta-analysis of randomised controlled trials. *BMJ* 2005; 330(7490): 516.
229. NOVAK N, KWIEK B, BIEBER T. The mode of topical immunomodulators in the immunological network of atopic dermatitis. *Clinical and Experimental Dermatology* 2005; 30(2): 160–164.
230. RUER-MULARD M, ABERER W, GUNSTONE A, KEKKI OM, LOPEZ ESTEBARANZ JL, VERTRUYEN A, et al. Twice-daily versus once-daily applications of pimecrolimus cream 1% for the prevention of disease relapse in pediatric patients with atopic dermatitis. *Pediatric Dermatology* 2009; 26(5): 551–558.
231. ASCHOFF R, SCHWANEBECK U, BRAUTIGAM M, MEURER M. Skin physiological parameters confirm the therapeutic efficacy of pimecrolimus cream 1% in patients with mild-to-moderate atopic dermatitis. *Experimental Dermatology* 2009; 18(1): 24–29.
232. DANBY S, AL ENEZI T, SULTAN A, CHITTOCK J, CORK MJ (eds.). The effect of topical dermatological products on the epidermal barrier. Barrier Function of Mammalian Skin Gordon Research Conference 2009, Waterville Valley, 2009.
233. BUDDENKOTTE J, STEINHOFF M. Pathophysiology and therapy of pruritus in allergic and atopic diseases. *Allergy* 2010; 65(7): 805–821.
234. ZHU Y, PENG C, XU JG, LIU YX, ZHU QG, LIU JY, et al. Participation of proteinase-activated receptor-2 in passive cutaneous anaphylaxis-induced scratching behavior and the inhibitory effect of tacrolimus. *Biological & Pharmaceutical Bulletin* 2009; 32(7): 1173–1176.

235. ZHU Y, WANG XR, PENG C, XU JG, LIU YX, WU L, et al. Induction of leukotriene B(4) and prostaglandin E(2) release from keratinocytes by protease-activated receptor-2-activating peptide in ICR mice. *International Immunopharmacology* 2009; 9(11): 1332–1336.

236. NAKAHARA T, KOGA T, FUKAGAWA S, UCHI H, FURUE M. Intermittent topical corticosteroid/tacrolimus sequential therapy improves lichenification and chronic papules more efficiently than intermittent topical corticosteroid/emollient sequential therapy in patients with atopic dermatitis. *The Journal of Dermatology* 2004; 31(7): 524–528.

237. TOROK HM, MAAS-IRSLINGER R, SLAYTON RM. Clocortolone pivalate cream 0.1% used concomitantly with tacrolimus ointment 0.1% in atopic dermatitis. *Cutis* 2003; 72(2): 161–166.

238. THACI D, REITAMO S, GONZALEZ ENSENAT MA, MOSS C, BOCCALETTI V, CAINELLI T, et al. Proactive disease management with 0.03% tacrolimus ointment for children with atopic dermatitis: Results of a randomized, multicentre, comparative study. *The British Journal of Dermatology* 2008; 159(6): 1348–1356.

239. WOLLENBERG A, WEN S, BIEBER T. Phenotyping of epidermal dendritic cells: Clinical applications of a flow cytometric micromethod. *Cytometry* 1999; 37(2): 147–155.

240. BERTH-JONES J, DAMSTRA RJ, GOLSCH S, LIVDEN JK, VAN HOOTEGHEM O, ALLEGRA F, et al. Twice weekly fluticasone propionate added to emollient maintenance treatment to reduce risk of relapse in atopic dermatitis: Randomised, double blind, parallel group study. *BMJ* 2003; 326(7403): 1367.

241. BRENEMAN D, FLEISCHER AB, JR, ABRAMOVITS W, ZEICHNER J, GOLD MH, KIRSNER RS, et al. Intermittent therapy for flare prevention and long-term disease control in stabilized atopic dermatitis: A randomized comparison of 3-times-weekly applications of tacrolimus ointment versus vehicle. *Journal of the American Academy of Dermatology* 2008; 58(6): 990–999.

242. HANIFIN J, GUPTA AK, RAJAGOPALAN R. Intermittent dosing of fluticasone propionate cream for reducing the risk of relapse in atopic dermatitis patients. *The British Journal of Dermatology* 2002; 147(3): 528–537.

243. PESERICO A, STADTLER G, SEBASTIAN M, FERNANDEZ RS, VICK K, BIEBER T. Reduction of relapses of atopic dermatitis with methylprednisolone aceponate cream twice weekly in addition to maintenance treatment with emollient: A multicentre, randomized, double-blind, controlled study. *The British Journal of Dermatology* 2008; 158(4): 801–807.

244. WOLLENBERG A, REITAMO S, GIROLOMONI G, LAHFA M, RUZICKA T, HEALY E, et al. Proactive treatment of atopic dermatitis in adults with 0.1% tacrolimus ointment. *Allergy* 2008; 63(7): 742–750.

245. LUBACH D, BENSMANN A, BORNEMANN U. Steroid-induced dermal atrophy. Investigations on discontinuous application. *Dermatologica* 1989; 179(2): 67–72.

246. CAUBET JC, EIGENMANN PA. Allergic triggers in atopic dermatitis. *Immunology and Allergy Clinics of North America* 2010; 30(3): 289–307.

247. PONYAI G, HIDVEGI B, NEMETH I, SAS A, TEMESVARI E, KARPATI S. Contact and aeroallergens in adulthood atopic dermatitis. *Journal of the European Academy of Dermatology and Venereology* 2008; 22(11): 1346–1355.

248. de BENEDICTIS FM, FRANCESCHINI F, HILL D, NASPITZ C, SIMONS FE, WAHN U, et al. The allergic sensitization in infants with atopic eczema from different countries. *Allergy* 2009; 64(2): 295–303.

249. ELIAS PM, SCHMUTH M. Abnormal skin barrier in the etiopathogenesis of atopic dermatitis. *Current Opinion in Allergy and Clinical Immunology* 2009; 9(5): 437–446.

250. TAN BB, WEALD D, STRICKLAND I, FRIEDMANN PS. Double-blind controlled trial of effect of housedust-mite allergen avoidance on atopic dermatitis. *Lancet* 1996; 347(8993): 15–18.

251. LEWIS-JONES S, CORK MJ, CLARK C, COX H, GILMOUR E, LANCASTER W, et al. Atopic eczema in children—Guideline consultation: A systematic review of the treatments for atopic eczema and guideline for its management 2007. Available at: http://guidance.nice.org.uk/page.aspx?o=434713.

252. BIRNIE AJ, BATH-HEXTALL FJ, RAVENSCROFT JC, WILLIAMS HC. Interventions to reduce *Staphylococcus aureus* in the management of atopic eczema. *Cochrane Database of Systematic Reviews* 2008; (3): CD003871.

253. THYSSEN JP, CARLSEN BC, MENNE T, LINNEBERG A, NIELSEN NH, MELDGAARD M, et al. Filaggrin null-mutations increase the risk and persistence of hand eczema in subjects with atopic

dermatitis: Results from a general population study. *The British Journal of Dermatology* 2010; 163(1): 115–120.

254. SLADE HB, FOWLER J, DRAELOS ZD, REECE BT, CARGILL DI. Clinical efficacy evaluation of a novel barrier protection cream. *Cutis* 2008; 82(4 Suppl.): 21–28.

255. BAUER A, SCHMITT J, BENNETT C, COENRAADS PJ, ELSNER P, ENGLISH J, et al. Interventions for preventing occupational irritant hand dermatitis. *Cochrane Database of Systematic Reviews* 2010; (6): CD004414.

256. SHIN HT. Diaper dermatitis that does not quit. *Dermatologic Therapy* 2005; 18(2): 124–135.

257. YEN CH, DAI YS, YANG YH, WANG LC, LEE JH, CHIANG BL. Linoleic acid metabolite levels and transepidermal water loss in children with atopic dermatitis. *Annals of Allergy, Asthma & Immunology* 2008; 100(1): 66–73.

258. SUBRAMANYAN K. Role of mild cleansing in the management of patient skin. *Dermatologic Therapy* 2004; 17(Suppl. 1): 26–34.

259. HURWITZ S. *Clinical Pediatric Dermatology: A Textbook of Skin Disorders of Childhood and Adolescence*, 2nd ed. W.B. Saunders Company, Philadelphia, 1993.

260. IMOKAWA G. Comparative study on the mechanism of irritation by sulphate and phosphate type of anionic surfactants. *Journal of the Society of Cosmetic Chemists* 1980; 31: 45–66.

261. ANANTHAPADMANABHAN KP, MOORE DJ, SUBRAMANYAN K, MISRA M, MEYER F. Cleansing without compromise: The impact of cleansers on the skin barrier and the technology of mild cleansing. *Dermatologic Therapy* 2004; 17(Suppl. 1): 16–25.

262. KIM E, KIM S, NAM GW, LEE H, MOON S, CHANG I. The alkaline pH-adapted skin barrier is disrupted severely by SLS-induced irritation. *International Journal of Cosmetic Science* 2009; 31(4): 263–269.

263. PARK KB, EUN HC. A study of skin responses to follow-up, rechallenge and combined effects of irritants using non-invasive measurements. *Journal of Dermatological Science* 1995; 10(2): 159–165.

264. FULMER AW, KRAMER GJ. Stratum corneum lipid abnormalities in surfactant-induced dry scaly skin. *The Journal of Investigative Dermatology* 1986; 86(5): 598–602.

265. FROEBE CL, SIMION FA, RHEIN LD, CAGAN RH, KLIGMAN A. Stratum corneum lipid removal by surfactants: Relation to *in vivo* irritation. *Dermatologica* 1990; 181(4): 277–283.

266. FRANKILD S, ANDERSEN KE, NIELSEN GD. Effect of sodium lauryl sulfate (SLS) on *in vitro* percutaneous penetration of water, hydrocortisone and nickel. *Contact Dermatitis* 1995; 32(6): 338–345.

267. LOFFLER H, STEFFES A, HAPPLE R, EFFENDY I. Allergy and irritation: An adverse association in patients with atopic eczema. *Acta Dermato-Venereologica* 2003; 83(5): 328–331.

268. LODEN M, BURACZEWSKA I, EDLUND F. Irritation potential of bath and shower oils before and after use: A double-blind randomized study. *The British Journal of Dermatology* 2004; 150(6): 1142–1147.

269. LOFFLER H, HAPPLE R. Profile of irritant patch testing with detergents: Sodium lauryl sulfate, sodium laureth sulfate and alkyl polyglucoside. *Contact Dermatitis* 2003; 48(1): 26–32.

270. BLUME-PEYTAVI U, CORK MJ, FAERGEMANN J, SZCZAPA J, VANACLOCHA F, GELMETTI C. Bathing and cleansing in newborns from day 1 to first year of life: Recommendations from a European round table meeting. *Journal of the European Academy of Dermatology and Venereology* 2009; 23(7): 751–759.

271. WALTERS RM, FEVOLA MJ, LIBRIZZI JJ, MARTIN K. Designing cleansers for the unique needs of baby skin. *Cosmetics & Toiletries* 2008; December: 53–60.

272. BURKHART CG. Clinical assessment by atopic dermatitis patients of response to reduced soap bathing: Pilot study. *International Journal of Dermatology* 2008; 47(11): 1216–1217.

273. GALZOTE C, DIZON MZ, ESTANISLAO R, MATHEW N. Opportunities for mild and effective infant cleansing beyond water alone. *Journal of the American Academy of Dermatology* 2007; 56(Suppl. 2): AB158. [Abstract P2420].

274. HISCOCK H. The crying baby. *Australian Family Physician* 2006; 35(9): 680–684.

275. TSAI TF, MAIBACH HI. How irritant is water? An overview. *Contact Dermatitis* 1999; 41(6): 311–314.

276. ROBINSON M, VISSCHER M, LARUFFA A, WICKETT R. Natural moisturizing factors (NMF) in the stratum corneum (SC). II. Regeneration of NMF over time after soaking. *Journal of Cosmetic Science* 2010; 61(1): 23–29.

277. MCNALLY NJ, WILLIAMS HC, PHILLIPS DR, SMALLMAN-RAYNOR M, LEWIS S, VENN A, et al. Atopic eczema and domestic water hardness. *Lancet* 1998; 352(9127): 527–531.

278. MIYAKE Y, YOKOYAMA T, YURA A, IKI M, SHIMIZU T. Ecological association of water hardness with prevalence of childhood atopic dermatitis in a Japanese urban area. *Environmental Research* 2004; 94(1): 33–37.

279. THOMAS KS, SACH TH. A multicentre randomized controlled trial of ion-exchange water softeners for the treatment of eczema in children: Protocol for the Softened Water Eczema Trial (SWET) (ISRCTN: 71423189). *The British Journal of Dermatology* 2008; 159(3): 561–566.

280. WIECHERS JW, DEDEREN JC, RAWLINGS AV. Moisturization mechanisms: Internal occlusion by orthorhombic lipid phase stabilizers—a novel mechanism of action of skin moisturization. In: Rawlings AV, Leyden JJ, eds. *Skin Moisturization*, 2nd ed. Informa Healthcare, New York, 2009; 309–321.

281. CORK MJ. *Complete Emollient Therapy. The National Association of Fundholding Practices Official Yearbook*. BPC Waterlow, Dunstable, UK, 1998; 159–168.

282. GRIMALT R, MENGEAUD V, CAMBAZARD F. The steroid-sparing effect of an emollient therapy in infants with atopic dermatitis: A randomized controlled study. *Dermatology* 2007; 214(1): 61–67.

283. CAL K. Unwelcome skin penetration enhancers: A fly in the ointment. *Journal of Cosmetic Dermatology* 2009; 8(2): 144–145.

284. AL ENEZI T, SULTAN A, CHITTOCK J, MOUSTAFA M, DANBY S, CORK MJ (eds.). Breakdown of the Skin Barrier induced by aqueous cream: Implications for the management of atopic eczema. 89th Annual Meeting of the British Association of Dermatologists, Glasgow, 2009.

285. TSANG M, GUY RH. Effect of aqueous cream BP on human stratum corneum *in vivo*. *The British Journal of Dermatology* 2010; 163(5): 954–958.

286. CORK MJ, TIMMINS J, HOLDEN C, CARR J, BERRY V, WARD SJ, et al. An audit of adverse drug reactions to aqueous cream in children with atopic eczema. *Pharmaceutical Journal* 2003; 271: 746–747.

287. DARMSTADT GL, MAO-QIANG M, CHI E, SAHA SK, ZIBOH VA, BLACK RE, et al. Impact of topical oils on the skin barrier: Possible implications for neonatal health in developing countries. *Acta Paediatrica* 2002; 91(5): 546–554.

288. EICHENFIELD LF, MCCOLLUM A, MSIKA P. The benefits of sunflower oleodistillate (SOD) in pediatric dermatology. *Pediatric Dermatology* 2009; 26(6): 669–675.

289. LODEN M, ANDERSSON AC. Effect of topically applied lipids on surfactant-irritated skin. *The British Journal of Dermatology* 1996; 134(2): 215–220.

290. LACK G, FOX D, NORTHSTONE K, GOLDING J. Factors associated with the development of peanut allergy in childhood. *The New England Journal of Medicine* 2003; 348(11): 977–985.

291. AGERO AL, VERALLO-ROWELL VM. A randomized double-blind controlled trial comparing extra virgin coconut oil with mineral oil as a moisturizer for mild to moderate xerosis. *Dermatitis* 2004; 15(3): 109–116.

292. DARLENSKI R, SASSNING S, TSANKOV N, FLUHR JW. Non-invasive *in vivo* methods for investigation of the skin barrier physical properties. *European Journal of Pharmaceutics and Biopharmaceutics* 2009; 72(2): 295–303.

293. ELKEEB R, HUI X, CHAN H, TIAN L, MAIBACH HI. Correlation of transepidermal water loss with skin barrier properties *in vitro*: Comparison of three evaporimeters. *Skin Research and Technology* 2010; 16(1): 9–15.

294. FLUHR JW, FEINGOLD KR, ELIAS PM. Transepidermal water loss reflects permeability barrier status: Validation in human and rodent *in vivo* and ex vivo models. *Experimental Dermatology* 2006; 15(7): 483–492.

295. VERGNANINI AL, AOKI V, TAKAOKA R, MADI J. Comparative effects of pimecrolimus cream vehicle and three commercially available moisturizers on skin hydration and transepidermal water loss. *The Journal of Dermatological Treatment* 2010; 21(3): 126–129.

296. FLUHR JW, KUSS O, DIEPGEN T, LAZZERINI S, PELOSI A, GLOOR M, et al. Testing for irritation with a multifactorial approach: Comparison of eight non-invasive measuring techniques on five different irritation types. *The British Journal of Dermatology* 2001; 145(5): 696–703.

297. CAL K, ZAKOWIECKI D, STEFANOWSKA J. Advanced tools for *in vivo* skin analysis. *International Journal of Dermatology* 2010; 49(5): 492–499.

298. NOUVEAU-RICHARD S, MONOT M, BASTIEN P, de LACHARRIERE O. *In vivo* epidermal thickness measurement: Ultrasound vs. confocal imaging. *Skin Research and Technology* 2004; 10(2): 136–140.

299. LEE S, PARK YK, KIM YK, KANG JS. An experimental study on corneocytes of acutely and chronically irritated skin. *Archives of Dermatological Research* 1983; 275(1): 49–52.

300. O'REGAN GM, KEMPERMAN PM, SANDILANDS A, CHEN H, CAMPBELL LE, KROBOTH K, et al. Raman profiles of the stratum corneum define 3 filaggrin genotype-determined atopic dermatitis endophenotypes. *The Journal of Allergy and Clinical Immunology* 2010; 126(3): 574–580.

301. DAMIEN F, BONCHEVA M. The extent of orthorhombic lipid phases in the stratum corneum determines the barrier efficiency of human skin *in vivo*. *The Journal of Investigative Dermatology* 2010; 130(2): 611–614.

302. DANBY S, MOUSTAFA M, MACGOWAN A, WARD S, CORK MJ (eds.). Skin Protease Inhibitors: A new treatment for atopic dermatitis. 5th George Rajka International Symposium on Atopic Dermatitis, Kyoto, 2008.

303. de JONGH CM, VERBERK MM, SPIEKSTRA SW, GIBBS S, KEZIC S. Cytokines at different stratum corneum levels in normal and sodium lauryl sulphate-irritated skin. *Skin Research and Technology* 2007; 13(4): 390–398.

304. HENDRIX SW, MILLER KH, YOUKET TE, ADAM R, O'CONNOR RJ, MOREL JG, et al. Optimization of the skin multiple analyte profile bioanalytical method for determination of skin biomarkers from D-Squame tape samples. *Skin Research and Technology* 2007; 13(3): 330–342.

305. ROBINSON M, VISSCHER M, LARUFFA A, WICKETT R. Natural moisturizing factors (NMF) in the stratum corneum (SC). I. Effects of lipid extraction and soaking. *Journal of Cosmetic Science* 2010; 61(1): 13–22.

306. ISHIKAWA J, NARITA H, KONDO N, HOTTA M, TAKAGI Y, MASUKAWA Y, et al. Changes in the ceramide profile of atopic dermatitis patients. *The Journal of Investigative Dermatology* 2010; 130(10): 2511–2514.

307. BARNES KC. An update on the genetics of atopic dermatitis: Scratching the surface in 2009. *The Journal of Allergy and Clinical Immunology* 2010; 125(1): 16–29. e1–11; quiz 30–31.

Index

Transdermal and Topical Drug Delivery: Principles and Practice, First Edition. Edited by Heather A.E. Benson, Adam C. Watkinson.
© 2012 John Wiley & Sons, Inc. Published 2012 by John Wiley & Sons, Inc.

Printed in the United States
By Bookmasters